Policy and Health

This rich volume provides a comprehensive look at how policy leads to better health. Leading RAND thinkers, working in different disciplines, create an all-encompassing framework for students, scholars, and policymakers. Along the way, they tell us what is known and what still needs to be known about how policy and practice lead to better health outcomes in developing countries. Drawing on their broad experience in Asia, the authors begin by exploring the health effects of macroeconomic development, education, and technology. After making compelling arguments about the need for policymakers to use—and demand—evidence-based policy, they investigate the epidemiologic disease of persistent infectious diseases and the rapid ascendancy of chronic diseases in the elderly in the context of how effectively appropriate state-of-the-art clinical medicine addresses illness and promotes well-being. Peabody and his co-authors argue that while prioritization can be based on the effectiveness of the medical interventions, microeconomic principles must be invoked to influence behaviors and conserve public resources in order to improve health through pricing or funding strategies. Special emphasis is placed on examining equity-improving solutions to ascertain how and where they have helped the poor, women, and other vulnerable populations. And the authors cast a critical eye on the vexing problem of changing the health behaviors of both providers and consumers. The book concludes with a discussion of politics, priorities, the private sector, and what role Ministries or Departments of Health should play as they seek to translate policy objectives into better health for their population.

T0381531

RAND Studies in Policy Analysis

Editor: Charles Wolf, Jr., Senior Economic Advisor and
Corporate Fellow in International Economics

Policy analysis is the application of scientific methods to develop and test alternative ways of addressing social, economic, legal, international, national security, and other problems. The RAND Studies in Policy Analysis series aims to include several significant, timely, and innovative works each year in this broad field. Selection is guided by an editorial board consisting of Charles Wolf, Jr. (editor), and David S. C. Chu, Paul K. Davis, and Lynn Karoly (associate editors).

Other Titles in the Series:

David C. Gompert and F. Stephen Larrabee (editors), *America and Europe: A Partnership for a New Era*

Policy and Health
Implications for Development in Asia

John W. Peabody
M. Omar Rahman, Paul J. Gertler,
Joyce Mann, Donna O. Farley,
Jeff Luck, David Robalino, Grace M. Carter
RAND

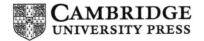
CAMBRIDGE
UNIVERSITY PRESS

PUBLISHED BY THE PRESS SYNDICATE OF THE UNIVERSITY OF CAMBRIDGE
The Pitt Building, Trumpington Street, Cambridge, United Kingdom

CAMBRIDGE UNIVERSITY PRESS
The Edinburgh Building, Cambridge CB2 2RU, UK
40 West 20th Street, New York NY 10011–4211, USA
477 Williamstown Road, Port Melbourne, VIC 3207, Australia
Ruiz de Alarcón 13, 28014 Madrid, Spain
Dock House, The Waterfront, Cape Town 8001, South Africa

http://www.cambridge.org

© RAND 1999

First published 1999
First paperback edition 2005

Typeset in Palatino 10/11 pt. in MS Word [TB]

A catalogue record for this book is available from the British Library

ISBN 0 521 66164 1 hardback
ISBN 0 521 61990 4 paperback

The findings, interpretations and conclusion expressed are entirely those of the authors
and should not be attributed to any individual we consulted, the Asian Development Bank
(ADB), the World Bank (WB), the World Health Organization (WHO), the United States
Agency for International Development (USAID), and ABT Associates, to their affiliated
organizations, or to members of their Boards of Executive Directors or the countries they
represent. These organizations do not guarantee the accuracy of the data included in this
book and accept no responsibility whatsoever for any consequence of their use. The
boundaries, colors, denominations and other information shown on any map or table do
not imply on the part of these organizations any judgement or the legal status of any
territory or the endorsement or acceptance of such boundaries.

Countries vary enormously in the health status of their populations—even after controlling for income and education levels. They vary in the amount of resources their health systems draw from the rest of the economy. And they vary in the extent to which their health financing mechanisms shield individuals from the risks of major health care expenditures. Governments' health policies vary as well: Some governments attempt to finance (or mandate the financing of) basic clinical services for all their populations, while others rely on out-of-pocket user fees or private voluntary insurance for much of the financing. Some focus public spending on public health and effective, targeted disease control, while others spend heavily on a few major tertiary facilities. Some governments provide the services they finance, while others use public resources to purchase services from private providers. It is the role of health policy analysis to assess whether these and other government choices affect performance in improving health, controlling costs, and spreading risk.

In this volume, John Peabody and an impressive team of coauthors assemble and interpret a broad range of material and provide a coherent overview of both current conditions and recent trends in health status, health expenditures, and health coverage in Asia—a region whose economic, social, and cultural diversity raises most of the policy issues facing health sectors in any country. The authors are careful not to be too prescriptive. That is not the role of this book. Important policy choices—such as R&D investment, level of public spending, or the long-term goal of social insurance—need to be made at the national level. That said, countries can learn a great deal from one another and from the experiences of their own past. The purpose of policy research—and one of the accomplishments of this lucid volume—is to place international experience at the disposal of national decisionmakers and those who advise them.

As a result, the book fills a major gap in the available literature on the key policy issues in health, regardless of the country or region being studied. As such, it will find a place on the desks of a broad range of analysts, development specialists, and health professionals worldwide. Indeed, this volume may well find its strongest niche in a teaching context for students and those who want a comprehensive, multidisciplinary approach to health in developing countries. And of course today's students become tomorrow's policy analysts and decisionmakers.

Policy and Health: Implications for Development in Asia provides a rich source of data and technical analysis, yet conveys its messages with clarity. It will be many years before it is replaced (although given the pace of change in Asia, a second edition may be needed sooner than the authors anticipated!). The authors have provided us with a resource of lasting value.

Dean T. Jamison
Professor of Education and School of Public Health,
University of California, Los Angeles
October, 1998

For almost two decades, the economy of Thailand grew at an average rate of 11.5 percent a year, but in July 1997 a simmering financial crisis resulted in the forced depreciation of the Thai baht. The crisis soon spread, and by the beginning of 1999, Indonesia, Korea, and Malaysia had experienced two consecutive years of negative economic growth for the first time in 30 years. Equity and real estate markets, which had boomed with the surfeit of domestic and foreign capital, suddenly collapsed under the weight of rising current account deficits and poorly regulated financial intermediaries. The financial contagion also spread to the Philippines, where the peso fell 39 percent, and to the more established economies of Hong Kong and Singapore. Other parts of the world, particularly Latin America and the transition economies of Eastern Europe, have also been severely affected by the crisis.

The crisis in Asia risks undermining one of the most remarkable economic and social achievements in modern history. Absolute poverty had been nearly eliminated in Korea, Malaysia, and Thailand. In 1975, six out of ten East Asians lived on less than a dollar a day; by 1995, this figure was down to roughly two out of ten. Although the precise figure is not known, tens of millions have been dragged back down into poverty by the crisis. For example, by the end of 1998, Thailand had 800,000 newly unemployed workers, and in Indonesia, the figure was a staggering 20 million people.

The health sector has been severely affected by the crisis, and this has had deleterious consequences on the health of the poor and other vulnerable populations. Rising unemployment, for example, has directly decreased spending on health. In Thailand, the poor spend 10 percent of their income on health compared to only 2 percent spent by the rich. Studies consistently show that utilization is very much influenced by income—regardless of the clinical conditions—and that decreases in utilization lead to higher death rates. There are many manifestations of the economic crisis on health and social welfare beyond direct decreases in the utilization of health services: Imported raw materials for generic drugs rose 70 percent in Indonesia; rising food prices have led to malnutrition in Viet Nam; girls have been forced to leave school early in China to look for work; and private clinics have closed in Korea.

Policymakers—particularly in times of crisis—are faced with a challenge and an opportunity. The challenge is to protect the poor and elderly, as well as women and children, from the consequences of poor health. But, the economic crisis also provides an opportunity to implement significant policy change that is sometimes politically infeasible in times of relative calm. It is an opportunity to strengthen and refocus activities directed toward the poor, to liberalize the regulations governing the private sector, to increase public support for prevention programs, and to improve the quality of clinical care through strategies that increase competition or link payment to clinical services.

Even without a crisis, the issues facing Asian policymakers are legion. Nearly two-thirds of the world's population lives in Asia, over 400 languages are spoken, and Asia's economies range from the richest in the world (Japan) to one of the fastest growing (China), to some of the poorest (Bangladesh and Nepal). In addition, Asia is experiencing the demographic transition to an older population as a result of a decline in female fertility and an increase in child survival, which has led to an epidemiologic shift toward chronic diseases such as coronary artery disease and cancer. Simultaneously, many Asian countries still face persistent problems with infectious diseases such as tuberculosis and malaria.

Clearly, Asia mirrors many of the most important health and policy development issues that face the global health sector today. Asia's struggles and successes thus provide lessons for policymakers everywhere—and reflect the massive policy challenge that all countries face.

The goal of this book is to help policymakers, researchers and students—in Asia and elsewhere—meet that challenge and understand the best policy options available to them in the next 5–10 years. But what does it mean to find the "best policy options"? Most would agree that the best policy options are those that are both effective and efficient—effective in that they have the most impact on the measure of most concern: improving the health outcomes and general welfare of the people treated; efficient in that they accomplish this with the most economical use of resources.

Thus, the real question is: "How do policymakers ensure they have the best chance of choosing effective *and* efficient policy options?" The answer, we argue, is that policy must be "evidence-based"—based on the best evidence available—evidence that will compel governments to pursue suitable interventions.

Of course, this is easier said than done. It is not just that the evidence needed is often missing or hard to come by if it does exist; it is that the kinds of evidence needed vary so much across the many areas of concern in the health sector. In this book, we examine five such areas of concern: (1) assessing the burden of disease; (2) allocating public (and private) health expenditures; (3) ensuring equity and access to health care; (4) improving health behaviors of individuals and providers; and (5) implementing health care policies.

To evaluate and summarize the evidence, we assembled a multidisciplinary team of researchers. For assessing the burden of disease, we brought to bear the disciplines of epidemiology and clinical medicine. Economics and health financing were the key disciplines used to examine the allocation of health expenditures; understanding what was needed to ensure a minimum level of care and access to services required the disciplines of ethics and systems analysis. To learn how to improve individual and provider behavior, we relied on the disciplines of social science and psychology. Finally, to understand how to get policies implemented, we drew on management science and organizational theory.

To derive our findings, we looked at an enormous amount of information—ultimately choosing over 900 sources, culling national data from every country, and reviewing the literature in all these disciplines. We feel so strongly that evidence-based policymaking is critical that we devote a full chapter to it. While the large tables in the chapter may seem more the province of an appendix (where such data are usually found), we use them for illustrative purposes to help readers understand the importance of data, the difficulty of getting them, and the data gaps that currently exist. We also use the tables to simplify data aggregations and make them accessible for the reader who is not quantitatively inclined.

In the evidence chapter and the five chapters that follow, we take a top-down, policy-oriented perspective. We have organized each chapter around what we consider to be the most important questions and answers in that area of concern. While such an approach has the downside of potentially excluding interesting material, we feel it has the much greater upside of providing focus and organization within very large research areas.

Each chapter therefore begins with a summary table detailing what we consider the fundamental questions in the area of concern, their bottom-line answers, and the most pertinent options for policymakers. Within a chapter, each section—designated by an offset heading—develops one question and explores the evidence underlying its answer. Policy options are discussed at the end of the chapter.

Within each chapter, we include a number of "boxes." These boxes, though not cited explicitly within the text, are directly related to the textual discussions around them and serve to further elucidate key concepts or present specific, concrete examples within Asia. We also elected to combine the references presented in the text with the bibliography, so that readers interested in exploring issues in more detail have a good starting point for investigating the relevant scientific literature.

Of course, a work of this size and scope would not have been possible without the contributions of a number of people. This book was prepared by a team led by John W. Peabody and comprising M. Omar Rahman, Paul J. Gertler, Joyce Mann, Donna O. Farley, Grace M. Carter, Jeff Luck, and David Robalino. The editor was Paul Steinberg and the manuscript was prepared by Joanna Nelsen. Research assistance was provided by Daochi Tong and Hongjun Kan, copyediting by Miriam Polon. The figures were prepared by the Publications Department at RAND. Research and extensive content were provided by Joseph Schmitt, Stephen Bickel, Keith Vom Eigen and Matthew Sanders. Boxes were also prepared by Dana Goldman, John W. Molyneaux, Steven Asch and Shan Cretin.

Earlier drafts of the book benefited greatly from data contributions of the World Health Organization (WHO), Western Pacific Regional Office, Manila, Philippines; the WHO South-East Regional Office, New Delhi, India; the WHO Eastern Mediterranean Office, Alexandria, Egypt; the World Bank, Washington, D.C.; the United States Agency for International Development, Washington, D.C.; and ABT Associates, Bethesda, Maryland. We also wish to acknowledge all the researchers and institutions whose work appears in this volume—in particular, Dean Jamison, who authored several of the key references and provided advice to us as we made revisions to the manuscript; James Socknat, who arranged for the collection of World Bank country-level health information and material; and B. P. Kean and Than Sein, who, along with Jens Jorgensen, provided or coordinated much of the country health statistics from WHO. The manuscript was reviewed by Albert Williams, RAND; Julia Walsh, University of California, Berkeley; James Lawson, University of New South Wales; John Caldwell, Australian National University, Canberra, and Jacques van der Gaag, World Bank and the University of Amsterdam. Their comments and suggestions were extremely valuable.

The early research and analysis for this book was carried out as part of a project sponsored by the Asian Development Bank (ADB). The project investigations prepared background material for a separate report, "Health Policy in Asia and the Pacific: Options for Developing Countries," which will be produced by the ADB as a Health Policy Document. Thus, the authors also wish to thank the ADB and, in particular, those connected with that project, who greatly assisted our efforts on this book. These include Dr. Benjamin Loevinsohn, Senior Health Specialist, who provided excellent technical comments and suggestions, and Mr. Edward Haugh, Manager, Education, Health and Population (West) Division, who provided valuable help coordinating the project. Important inputs were also provided during an ADB-sponsored consultative meeting, held July 3–5, 1996 in Manila, from Mario Taguiwalo and Orville Solon of the University of the Philippines; Andrew Creese, J.W. Lee, and (later) Ilona Kickbush of the World Health Organization; and Lenore Manderson, University of Queensland Medical School, Australia.

Finally, we are grateful to the many colleagues we consulted during this effort, in particular, Charles Wolf, RAND; Jia Wang, UCLA Center for Pacific Rim Studies; Nicholas Prescott, World Bank; Joanna Yu, National Health Insurance Task Force, Taipei; Rebecca Agoncillo, WHO; William Newbrander, Management Sciences for Health; and Meiwita Iskander, University of Indonesia. Many others contributed directly or indirectly to this volume and are too numerous to include. All errors, omissions, and opinions are those of the authors.

John W. Peabody, M.D., DTM&H, Ph.D.
West Los Angeles Veterans Affairs Medical Center
Senior Scientist, RAND
Assistant Professor of Medicine, UCLA

TABLE OF CONTENTS

FIGURES

BOXES

Box Tables

Box Figures

OVERVIEW: THE ROLE AND RESPONSIBILITY
OF GOVERNMENTS IN THE HEALTH SECTOR

As recently as 1960, a child born into poverty anywhere in the world had only a one-in-four chance of reaching his fifth birthday, while a person age 15 had a life expectancy of 67 years. Today, vaccines protect eight out of ten of the world's children, more than nine out of ten infants will enroll in school, and the average adult will live into his eighth decade. Around the world, the health gains made in the past two generations are arguably the greatest accomplishment of civilization. What makes these gains so remarkable is that they have been accomplished by people living on every continent on the globe—people representing a panoply of cultures, social structures, and values. Amid this diversity, there is a consistent belief that all societies, and the governments that represent them, are responsible for improving the well-being of the population.

In the health sector, this responsibility means understanding the many factors that go into improving people's health. Some of the most important factors—such as national economic development, education, particularly of women, and the creation of technologies that lead to more effective clinical care—lie outside of what is typically viewed as the health sector. Although these factors are not directly involved with the financing, organization, and delivery of health care, they are substantive sectoral inputs into any country's effort to create better health for its population, and, thus, need to be understood in any health policy context.

Other factors—such as optimally using limited resources or encouraging the use of the most effective medical treatments—are the obvious domain of health policymaking, and these also need to be understood from a dispassionate, empirical perspective. The implication, we will argue, means not being fettered by single-discipline paradigms when making health care policy; it also means not wasting economic or social opportunities; and it means using the best available data to derive and evaluate health-sector solutions.

Given the stakes—measured in terms of lives and resources—two basic questions need to be answered: What is the evidence supporting government policies? And what policies should governments pursue? Even when answers are proposed and policies enacted, it is not always clear how the interventions will turn out and whether the right policies were implemented. And so the same two questions need to be asked again in a process of continual iteration, so that better policies can be developed and better ideas put forward.

This book begins by trying to answer these broad questions, and so talks directly about how policymakers can make better decisions. The focus in the subsequent chapters ranges from clinical interventions to management strategies. The emphasis is on finding the best available evidence from global experiences that leads to improvement in health status. To do this, we critically evaluate data and underlying theories, identify gaps, and delineate policy implications.

Geographically, the book focuses on Asia and the Pacific—a region that dominates the world and that has nearly two-thirds of the global population. It is a region in the midst of enormous change and sometimes crisis, driven by economic, demographic, and epidemiologic forces that pose significant challenges to the health sector. With the enormous diversity of its geographies and societies, and of its politics and economies, it is also a region that captures many of the most important issues in health and development.

HEALTH-SECTOR REFORM IN ASIA

Health-sector reform has brought about sweeping transformations in health policy throughout Asia. In just 12 years, for example, the Republic of Korea completely changed its financing of health care by introducing a national system of insurance that now provides universal care for all citizens. In Papua New Guinea, macroeconomic crises and structural adjustment led to the reorganization of the political landscape, and in 1995, a new five-year National Health Plan used burden of disease, cost-effectiveness, and locally defined health priorities as the basis for policy. Political changes in Viet Nam over the past five years now permit entrepreneurial opportunities—today over 60 percent of health care is provided through the private sector. These examples reflect a pattern of accelerated health-sector reform by governments throughout Asia and around the world.

Policymakers in post–World War II Asia faced many serious health problems. Infectious and parasitic diseases such as malaria, tuberculosis, polio, measles, and tetanus were rampant. Widespread malnutrition associated with poverty weakened immune systems and thus worsened the seriousness of illnesses. High fertility rates and poor birth spacing threatened the health of both mother and child.

At the national government level, policymakers over the past four decades have responded by funding and sometimes implementing immunization drives, pest-control projects, and health education campaigns. Large hospitals and widespread systems of primary-care clinics were established to treat catastrophic and common illnesses. At the international level, additional intervention and support for family planning helped lower fertility rates and improve birth spacing. These efforts helped decrease infectious diseases, increase access to care, and reduce infant mortality, while improving maternal health.

Almost all the developing countries of Asia are involved in health-sector reform today. These efforts, according to one researcher, now include primary health care, sectoral finance, planning and development management and organizational review, rationalizing the role of the private sector and nongovernmental organizations (NGOs), improving gender staffing mechanisms and reducing gender disparities, health systems research, resource mobilization for health and the social sectors, and making better use of available resources. (See Asian Development Bank (ADB), 1994a; Ali, 1996.) And this is not all. Recent or current reforms include decentralization in the Philippines, efforts to create a private sector in the central Asian republics and in Mongolia, and the simultaneous introduction of universal health care and cost containment in Taiwan.

This interest in health-sector reform is motivated primarily by the belief that reforms will lead to better health by more efficiently using limited resources. Though health reforms are influenced by many factors, including each country's unique social, economic, medical, political, and cultural forces, change can be seen throughout Asia: In Indonesia, social disparities between urban and rural populations and economic development led to an overhaul in health care financing, which produced improved access to care through a redistribution of public resources. The explosive AIDS epidemic in Thailand spurred policy initiatives that now focus on changing personal behaviors to limit further spread of the disease. In Cambodia and Laos, as war yields to peace, political energies have turned to health and welfare, and the resources formerly used to wage war are now available to help the sick, the poor, and the disenfranchised. In Sri Lanka and South India, anthropologic research points to social and political influences on health. The combination of a cultural interest in diagnosing and treating diseases, a tradition of open politics and political consensus, and the marked degree of female autonomy associated with high levels of maternal education translate into early utilization, quick referral, and higher-quality medical care and better outcomes. (See Caldwell, 1993.)

The health sector reform we have witnessed in Asia has been impressive in scope and has involved a significant amount of policy innovation. However, a fundamental question remains: Have the reforms made a difference in improving the health status of the people of Asia? We answer this question below, first looking at health status gains over the past 35 years and then examining the most important factors behind those gains.

ASIA'S HEALTH STATUS: FROM 1960 TO THE PRESENT

Since 1960, health indicators across Asia have dramatically improved. Table 1.1 shows three common health status indicators in 19 countries—life expectancy at birth, deaths per 1,000 children age five and under, and deaths per 1,000 infants less than one year old (the infant mortality rate, or IMR)—and 35-year time trends for the first two of the indicators. The countries are sorted by gross national product (GNP) per capita, with the poorest at the top and the richest at the bottom.

The trends demonstrate that health status improved across the board in Asia and the Pacific as life expectancy rose and child mortality fell in all countries. Over a span of 35 years, the average under-five child mortality rates in Asia have been more than halved, from 220 per 1,000 live births in 1960 to 90 in 1994. (See Loevinsohn, 1996.)

The trend can be seen even more dramatically pictorially. Figure 1.1 shows a map of the region that represents the change in child mortality rates between 1960 and 1996.

Of course, this picture of improving health status is somewhat oversimplified. As we mentioned above, Asia is in the midst of a profound demographic and

Table 1.1

Health Status Indicators for Selected Asian Countries Sorted by GNP

Country	GNP Per Capita 1994 ($)	Life Expectancy at Birth			Child Mortality Rate (per 1,000 live births)			IMR (1994)
		1960	1994	% change	1960	1994	% change	
Nepal	200	44	53	20.5	290	118	−59.3	84
Viet Nam	200	44	65	47.7	232	46	−80.1	35
Bangladesh	220	46	55	19.6	247	117	−52.6	91
Mongolia	300	47	63	34.0	185	76	−58.9	58
Lao PDR	320	44	51	15.9	233	138	−40.8	94
India	320	47	60	27.7	236	119	−49.6	79
Bhutan	400	38	50	32.0	324	193	−40.0	125
Pakistan	430	49	61	24.5	221	137	−38.0	95
China	530	43	68	58.1	209	43	−79.4	35
Sri Lanka	640	58	72	24.1	130	19	−85.4	15
Indonesia	880	46	62	34.8	216	111	−48.6	71
Philippines	950	59	66	11.9	102	57	−44.1	44
Pap. New Guinea	1,240	47	56	19.1	248	95	−61.7	67
Fiji	2,250	63	71	13.2	97	27	−72.1	22
Malaysia	3,480	58	71	22.4	105	15	−85.7	12
Thailand	5,410	52	69	32.7	146	32	−78.1	27
Korea, Rep. of	8,260	53	71	34.0	124	9	−92.7	8
Singapore	22,500	65	75	15.4	40	6	−85.0	5
Japan	34,630	68	79	16.2	40	6	−85.0	4

SOURCE: United Nations International Children's Emergency Fund (UNICEF), 1996; World Health Organization (WHO),1996a; World Bank, 1996a.

epidemiologic shift that is having an impact on the improving health status we see. In demographic terms, nearly three out of every five inhabitants in the world live in the Asia and Pacific region. Many more of these people are moving to cities. Already, 9 of the world's 14 cities with over 10 million people are in Asia; by 2020, 55 percent of Asians will live in urban centers. The population growth rate (between 1985 and 1990), however, has already slowed to 1.85 percent. (See ADB, 1994b).

Such demographic changes are the results of changes both in fertility and in childhood and adult mortality. The decline in deaths is the result of an epidemiologic shift away from communicable diseases, particularly for the young, and toward more chronic and degenerative conditions that affect the elderly. Fertility declines further shift the age structure from the young to the old. The resulting demographic transition manifests itself in an "aging population," whereby diseases associated with insufficient nutrition and infection give way to diseases associated with degenerative conditions. As a result, the health status of Asian countries is changing dramatically and rapidly.

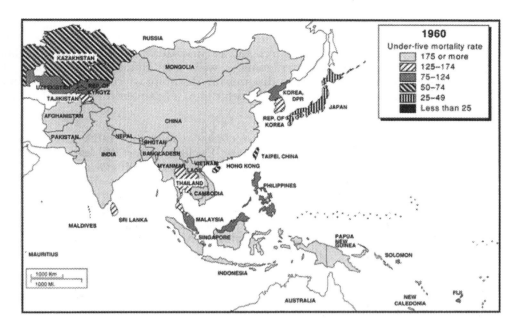

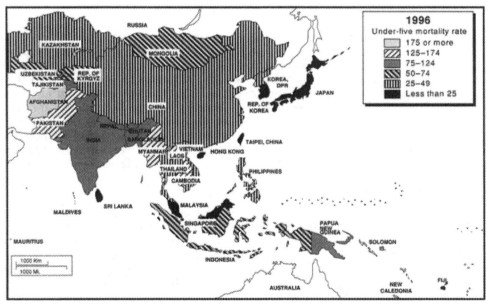

SOURCE: UNICEF, 1996.

Figure 1.1—Trends in Under-Five Mortality Rates in Asia (1960–1996)

These demographic results are further influenced by concurrent changes in behaviors associated with increased personal wealth. For example, dietary choices lead to an increased percentage of caloric intake from cholesterol and saturated fats that, in turn, lead to an increased incidence of cardiovascular or cerebrovascular disease and death. Similarly, smoking, ubiquitous throughout

Asia, and the chewing of tobacco in the betel quid, seen in South Asia and the Pacific, are two behaviors that lead to lung and oral cancers, respectively. World Bank projections show that, compared to industrialized countries where mortality from vascular disease and malignancy will not change significantly, the percentage of deaths from these diseases in developing countries will almost double over the next 30 years (from 26 percent to 49 percent). (See Bulatao et al., 1990.)

The gains in life expectancy and the declines in mortality rates that we see in Table 1.1 are one cause of population aging. Declines in fertility are another, often more important, cause. Commonly used indicators of health status, however, tend to focus only on diseases that affect younger populations; as these indicators of health status improve, they are not counterbalanced by reports and statistics of increasing adult mortality. In fact, if we look at health status indicators associated with more-chronic conditions—like cardiovascular diseases—we see increases for the wealthier and more-developed countries in the region. (See also Jamison et al., 1993.)

Still, despite this qualification, the improvement in health status in Asia is dramatic and provides grounds for optimism. The question is, what drives this dramatic improvement?

FACTORS DRIVING THE IMPROVEMENT IN HEALTH STATUS

Is this marked improvement in health (strictly speaking, the improvement in health status indicators) in Asia the product, at least in part, of health-sector reform and good policy? Four factors have improved the health status of Asians in important ways. For two of these factors—advances in economic development and education—the evidence is compelling. For the other two—improvements in medical technology and in the amount of public funding for health care service—the evidence is less direct but still persuasive. Putting these factors aside, however, how much can we expect health reform—and, therefore, better health policy—to further improve health status? Before trying to answer this fundamental question about policy, we discuss the four factors in more detail.

The Impact of Economic Development

In East Asia and the Pacific, the annual economic growth rate has been extraordinary by any historic measure: Between 1980 and 1994, the region's economy grew at 6.8 percent, which was, in turn, built on a 4.9 percent growth rate over the previous 15 years. Not surprisingly, health status today is substantially better in countries that, as a result of strong economic growth, are among the wealthiest. Recalling that the countries shown in Table 1.1 are listed by GNP, all three measures of health outcomes in the table improve as one moves down the rows. This is most evident in the child mortality statistics, where wealthy countries experienced more than a 50 percent larger decline in child mortality than did poorer countries. Almost all countries also experienced 15–30 percent increases in life expectancy.

Growth and development over time, as measured by variations in per capita income between countries, are very strongly associated with improved health status, as shown in Figure 1.2, which plots selected countries in Asia by their

---

Box 1.1: Economic Growth with Equity in East Asia: A Miracle or Just Good Policy?

In just thirty years' time, four Asian countries or areas—Singapore, South Korea, Taiwan, and Hong Kong—have set historical standards on what is possible in development. These four can already boast of per capita incomes of US $8,260 and first-world living standards for their populations. Now, three other Asian countries—Malaysia, Indonesia, and Thailand—have begun the steep, albeit uneven, ascent of rapid economic development.

These seven Asian countries—diverse in culture, population, and natural resources—are the only Asian economies that have sustained both increasing economic growth *and* better equity (where equity is defined as having access to health care, education, and other basic needs). The results of shared growth in the "East Asian Miracle" countries mean that the number of people living in absolute poverty—lacking such basic necessities as shelter and food—has dropped greatly. In Malaysia, for example, in 1970, 49 percent lacked basic necessities, but by 1990 this number had decreased to 10 percent. (See World Bank, 1993c.)

Why did equity improve with economic growth? This part of the miracle was not miraculous. Largely, it was a result of getting many elements of development policy right. For one thing, macroeconomic policy was sound: Private investment was encouraged, monetary policy promoted price stability, and prices were not allowed to become grossly distorted by excessive trade tariffs and quotas. Agricultural productivity also increased (although total agricultural production declined as a percentage of GDP), and rural economies were not taxed excessively in favor of urban development. Just as important, government policies focused on developing human capital: Universal education increased the skills of the labor force, particularly girls, eliminating the gender gap in education more rapidly than in other developing economies. Finally, technology was encouraged and introduced to match post-secondary education and technical training.

Analysts of the East Asian miracle and the recent economic crisis have tried to isolate the various factors that contribute to growth and sustainability, using cross-economy regressions. These show that government policy plays a key role. The most important of these policies is ensuring universal primary education. In the "East Asian Miracle" countries, this was by far the single largest contributor to economic growth. Government policy also encouraged growth in other ways. Economic targets were set and financial incentives were introduced to encourage technology. In Taiwan, for example, the government protected small technology firms from import competition (but only for a fixed period of time) and lowered interest rates for direct development of targeted industries. Empirical cross-national studies show the importance of blending the right amount of technology with human and financial capital. Under these conditions, economies can converge and the less developed countries can grow at a faster rate than the more developed economies. (See Barro, 1997.) These remarkable developments have recently been threatened by the 1997–1998 collapse of the financial and capital markets. The crisis, many believe, is the result of poor regulation of the financial markets and investor speculation in highly inflated or risky assets. Lack of financial transparency, insider relations, and undisciplined foreign lending are long-standing problems that, when combined with fixed exchange rates, exposed resource misallocation and produced a sudden collapse of confidence. (See Stiglitz, 1998.) These events highlight how uneven and precarious development can be. And while the expectation is that growth will return to East Asia, these events also show that it will depend on sound policy and a commitment to equity.

---

gross domestic product (GDP) per capita and by their levels of under-five child mortality. Increased income allows people to purchase more food, better housing, and higher-quality medical care, all of which are associated with a proportionate rise in regional health status.

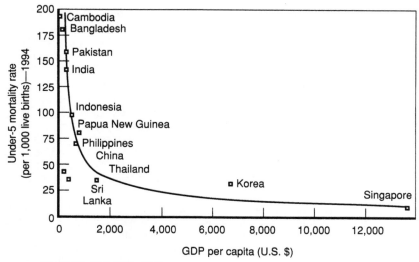

SOURCE: UNICEF, 1996.

**Figure 1.2—Association of Improved Under-Five Child Mortality
with Individual Economic Wealth in Asia**

Because countries vary in how they value goods and services, many experts argue that a better measure is to compare the same bundle of goods and services—a correction known as purchasing power parity adjustments. When these adjustments are done (as shown in Figure 1.3), we see that it tends to make the lower-income countries a little less poor (i.e., shifts the curve to the right) but

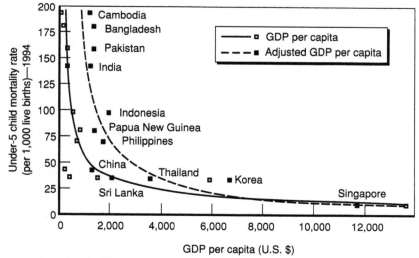

SOURCES: Adapted from UNICEF, 1996; Jamison et al., 1993.

**Figure 1.3—Association of Improved Under-Five Child Mortality with Individual
Economic Wealth Versus Purchasing Parity Adjustment in Asia**

it does not alter the strong relationship between income (or purchasing power) and health.

Interestingly enough, there is evidence that the converse is also true—i.e., that poor economic performance leads to *declining* health status. In a recent study, researchers performed a cross-national time-series analysis on health and income per capita in the developing world. They estimated that over a half-million child deaths in the developing world in 1990 can be attributed to poor economic performance in the 1980s.[1] (See Pritchett and Summers, 1996.)

The Impact of Education

Education, particularly of girls and women, plays a major role in improving health. In most societies, women are responsible for a broad range of household activities that are important for better health—they prepare food, care for a sick child, and allocate family resources. A number of investigations show that an educated mother is also more likely to work outside the home (and increase family income), more likely to ensure that children attend school, more likely to go to health facilities for prenatal care, and more likely to have a healthier child. (See Summers, 1994.) Educated women are more likely to postpone having children and to have fewer children, which contributes to increased maternal and child survival. For example, in Indonesia, Sri Lanka, and Thailand, when women had seven or more years of education, it reduced the odds of their having a child dying before age two by 41 percent. (See Hobcraft, 1993; Cleland and Ginneken, 1988.)

Education is interrelated with a host of social factors that, mediated by economic development, lead to better health. As Caldwell and other researchers argue, social, religious, and cultural values define women's opportunities for education, which, in turn, influence health decisions. Demographic Health Survey (DHS) data show that women who have been to school and are from higher social classes are more likely to use medical services and to have a supervised delivery. (See Elo, 1992.)

In a study that used a 1988 DHS survey in Thailand, researchers found that utilization rates of maternal and child health (MCH) services by women between the ages of 15 and 49 were significantly influenced by the individual woman's level of education. (See Raghupathy, 1996.) The most significant predictor of utilization was the completion of a secondary education.

In traditional Muslim countries—where the education of girls has been considered unnecessary and counter to the injunction for men to protect their women—cross-national studies suggest that the education gap between boys and girls and overall low education levels of both boys and girls are associated with worse health status. The data indicate that the impact of these disparities, namely higher child mortality, is manifest years later among their sons and daughters.

---

[1]The researchers used instrumental variables to isolate exogenous effects of income growth on health status from country-specific factors and time trends.

(See Caldwell, 1993.) Cultures that promote universal education produce citizens who are more aware of hygiene and who demand better health care facilities and higher-quality care. A discussion of the effects of education level on health outcomes is taken up in Chapter 5.

The Impact of Medical Technology Growth

Although it is very hard to compellingly demonstrate that the growth of medical technology improves the overall health status of a country, the role of medical technology in improving health outcomes of *individuals* is not hard to infer, particularly when talking about many communicable and even some noncommunicable diseases. Smallpox, for example, has been eradicated through immunization, and polio may soon follow. Since antibiotics became available in the 1940s, clinicians have had progressively more options to fight bacterial pathogens. Other developments for treating noncommunicable disease are nearly as remarkable. Anesthesia allows for dramatic surgical interventions, and the manipulation of genetic material has made it possible to produce vast quantities of insulin that is indistinguishable from naturally occurring, human-produced insulin.

The question of benefit in developing countries has another dimension: When were effective, inexpensive technologies made available for widespread use? For example, X-rays have long been used to decrease morbidity from fractures and accurately guide treatment, but only recently has relatively inexpensive roentgen technology been available to people living in rural areas of Asia.

The benefit of technology on overall health can be inferred by looking at health status over time. Figure 1.4 graphs the under-five mortality rate as a function of real GDP per capita (each point represents a country), for the years 1960, 1975, and 1990 (the GDP per capita curves from Figures 1.2 and 1.3). We have already shown that when GDP per capita increases, mortality rates are reduced. Here, we focus on the effect that "time" has on the under-five mortality rate. Indeed, the rate diminishes over time in all countries, regardless of the level of GDP per capita. Although many factors that affect the mortality rate, such as education and social change, are improving over time, the introduction of effective medical technology is certainly one of the most important. This figure shows the persistent and dramatic gains in health as income increases to about $3,000 per capita.

Despite gains from medical technologies, there is potential for much greater gains in developing countries. New medical technologies are needed that are appropriate to many of the poorer countries in Asia. In 1992, over $56 billion was spent on health research. But of this, only 3.6 percent was concerned with the health issues of developing countries—problems that account for the vast majority of disease and illness in 80 percent of the world's population. For example, research on diarrheal disease and pneumonia—two diseases that together account for 15 percent of the total burden of disease—accounted for just 0.2 percent of the total spent on health R&D (US $32 million and US $48–$68 million, respectively). The 1996 WHO Ad Hoc Committee on Health Research Relating to Future Intervention Options concluded that stark imbalances exist between the allocation of research funds and the most important diseases, particularly those of women and children.

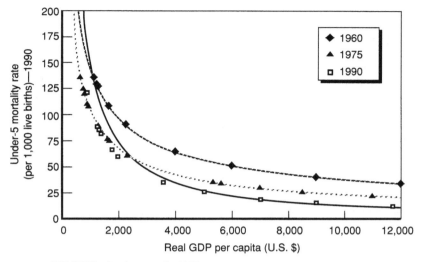

SOURCE: Jamison et al., 1996.

Figure 1.4—Reductions in Child Mortality in Asian Countries from 1960 to 1990

Future research and technology will deliver on the promise of a rotavirus vaccine which, when generally available, is projected to reduce diarrhea mortality by 13 percent every year. By contrast to preventive technology, recent advances in neuroscience suggest the possibility that spinal cord regeneration may eventually be available to treat traumatic quadriplegia. In the next generation, expected changes in demographics, the emergence of new and chronic diseases, and increased world travel will bring an obvious need for scientific advances to improve health.

Instead of concentrating on untreated conditions, research efforts have emphasized applications in tertiary health care that have only marginal benefits. This trend began shortly after World War II and continues today, as the largest investments are poured into the development of cardiovascular drugs, increasingly advanced diagnostic and monitoring equipment, and new tools for surgery. This is not surprising, since nearly all the research that underlies the development of new pharmaceuticals, medical devices, and other health-related technologies is carried out in the United States, Japan, Germany, and a handful of other industrialized countries. Logically, the fruits of these efforts are designed to fit the markets and patterns of use in these countries best.

The current failure of available technologies to satisfy the needs of the poor in developing countries has several origins, which include the lack of investment incentives for the private sector, the scarcity of scientists with intimate knowledge of local health care needs, and the multifaceted nature of the technical problems that underlie health care problems in underserved areas. (See WHO Ad Hoc Committee, 1996.) To make matters worse, engineers trying to garner acceptance as peers in the international scientific community do the overwhelming majority of their research on high technology and tertiary care. Meanwhile, the disproportionate expenditure of effort on inappropriate technologies consumes valuable resources.

Before we leave the medical technology discussion, it is important to point out that improvements in other technologies—specifically, information technologies (such as the increasing availability of telephones, facsimiles, and electronic mail)—can also have an impact on improving health status by enabling information—whether about optimal medical guidelines for a rural clinic or budget reconciliation for a district health office—to be collected, analyzed, and transmitted faster and at a lower cost than ever before in history. Enormous advances in computing capabilities using vastly improved software also make it possible to store and analyze large data sets and keep track of utilization, costs, and health outcomes in every Ministry of Health (MOH). These improvements increase awareness about health problems and decrease the time lag before useful medical technologies are implemented. A consortium of medical journals—led by the *Journal of the American Medical Association* and the *British Medical Journal*—and an NGO, Project HOPE, have recently teamed up to plan a global dissemination system of peer-reviewed biomedical and clinical information linking researchers and clinicians—a system that will cross national boundaries and obviate physical distances. (See WHO Ad Hoc Committee, 1996.)

The Impact of Public Spending on Health

In the past 35 years, Asian governments have made significant public investments in health care to ameliorate disparities and improve health status. Since 1960, there has been a four-fold increase in the amount of money that developing governments in Asia have spent on improving their people's health. (See Loevinsohn, 1996.) Among developing countries in Asia, spending now ranges from $5 per capita in Laos to $154 in Kazakhstan (1990 figures). As a percentage of GDP, government spending on health ranges from 1 percent in Laos and the Philippines to 2.8 percent in China and Papua New Guinea. (See World Bank, 1993a.) These health expenditures, in turn, have led to concurrent increases in income and labor productivity, which, in circular fashion, provide more individual and government income to spend on private and public health expenditures. Economic development and education, therefore, lead to increases in total spending on health (defined as both public and private). The total health expenditures as a percentage of GDP in Asia are 6.0 percent in India, approximately 4.5 percent in other Asian and Pacific countries, and 3.5 percent in China. (See World Bank, 1993a.)

Spending more on health, however, does not necessarily mean better health. There are several reasons for this, of which three are the most important. First, government spending may not be *allocated* productively. In more-developed countries, where health care is more likely to depend on public financing, much of the money spent is on the elderly in the last one or two years of life in expensive tertiary-level hospitals. This is unlikely to have an impact on longevity. Increasing life expectancy by increasing spending on health in affluent countries, therefore, is subject to diminishing returns when the common treatable causes of death have been eliminated or reduced.

Table 1.2 shows that, as in more-developed countries, Asian governments spend a large percentage of their health budgets on hospital care. Although we do not have the data, it is unlikely that the portion of those resources that is spent on the elderly will increase life expectancy.

Table 1.2

Relative Spending on Hospitals in Selected
Asian and Pacific Countries

Country	Health Expenditures as Percentage of Total Government Spending	Percentage of Health Budget Allocated to Hospitals
Bangladesh	3.9	56
China	4.2	67
India	6.7	71
Indonesia	3.8	59
Korea, Republic of	2.2	50
Malaysia	6.8	59
Myanmar	6.8	33
Nepal	4.3	50
Papua New Guinea	10.0	43
Philippines	3.3	58
Sri Lanka	4.5	70
Thailand	6.1	58
Mean	5.2	56

SOURCE: Griffin, 1992a.

Second, in all countries, public and private spending may not be *technically* optimal. More providers and more insurance lead to more physician visits and more hospitalizations, but this does not always lead to better health. (See Fuchs, 1994a.) Unproven technology, for example, is seductive, partly because it is offered to patients who are ill or who face a life-threatening problem and have little way of understanding medical diagnoses or the efficacy of treatments and partly because patients and doctors want to "do something" even if it may not work.

The Opportunity Costs and Benefits of Different Public Investment Strategies

We have argued that better health is a core policy objective of developing countries. It shows the success (or failure) of a nation's effort to care for its people. It is also an investment in human capital that will influence the supply and productivity of the labor force and is therefore a factor in future national development.

Although improving health status is clearly desirable, however, it is less clear how governments should invest their resources to actually improve health status. As we showed above, a number of elements contribute to improving health status—both indirectly and directly, and both in the long-term and the short-term. For example, as we saw in Figure 1.3, empirical evidence shows that health status, as measured by infant and adult mortality rates, is strongly correlated with per capita income and economic growth. Therefore, government policies that invest in producing higher national income—e.g., by eliminating currency restrictions, lowering trade barriers, or spending on infrastructure such as roads

---

Box 1.2: How Much Money Should Asian Governments Spend on Health?

Much of the world's health spending is in Organization for Economic Cooperation and Development (OECD) countries—countries that are among the world's most market-oriented. In 1995, the total global spending on health was US$ 2.46 trillion, equal to 9.1 percent of the world's GDP. What is dramatically shown in Table 1.2.1 is that Asia, which has 60 percent of the world's population, spends only 3.4 percent of global expenditures on health, while the OECD countries, with 15 percent of global population, spent 88 percent of global expenditures on health.

Table 1.2.1

Health Expenditures, Regions of the World, Using 1990–1995 Data

Region	Percent of World Pop.	Percent of Global Health Expend.	Percent of GDP Spent on Health	Percent of GDP Spent on Health Sector by Public Sector	Total Expend. on Health (billion US$)
OECD Nations	15.0	88.0	9.8	6.2	2159.6
South Asia, East Asia and Pacific	59.7	3.4	3.9	1.3	84.1
Eastern Europe and Central Asia	8.5	2.4	5.5	4.5	60.1
Latin America and Caribbean	8.3	4.6	7.2	3.0	114.0
Middle East and North Africa	2.1	0.9	4.4	2.7	21.4
Sub-Saharan Africa	6.5	0.7	5.6	2.8	16.2
Total	100.0*	100.0	9.1	5.5	2455.4

DATA SOURCES: World Bank. 1997. *Health, Nutrition, & Population.* Washington, DC: The World Bank; World Bank, 1997. *World Development Report,* Washington, D.C: The World Bank. *Numbers do not add to 100 due to rounding. OECD figures exclude the Republic of Korea, an OECD nation, which is listed with East Asia.

The table also shows that the high-income countries spend a much larger percentage of public money than the governments of middle- and low-income countries. Of the 9.1 percent of world GDP spent on health, 5.5 percent is financed from public funds and 3.6 percent is financed from private funds. Even in the United States, which is the only high-income OECD country that fails to finance or mandate universal access, the public sector spends 7.0 percent of its total GDP on health. (The private sector spends an additional 7.5 percent.) (1995 data, see World Bank, 1997a.) Other OECD countries all finance a basic benefits package and allow more-expensive levels of care to be privately financed. Overall, OECD government expenditures are high and range from 5.4 to 7.7 percent (1995 data). Total spending in these wealthier countries (with the notable exception of the U.S.), however, ranges only from 6.9 to 9.8 percent.

Gertham has shown that the greater the proportion of OECD public spending on health (as a proportion of both public and private total expenditures), the lower the total spending on health. (See Gertham et al., 1992.) In another cross-sectional study by Aiyer, Jamison, and Lodoño, increased spending by the public sector in Latin America was strongly associated with better health outcomes, while increased private spending was weakly and negatively associated with better outcomes. (See Aiyer et al., 1995.)

---

and telecommunications—may improve health by accelerating growth or facilitating access to care. However, improving health status by raising national income is both an indirect and long-term route to improving health status. Such would also be the case for improving health status by improving technology, one of the other contributing elements discussed above.

There are, however, more direct and shorter-term routes to improving health status. As discussed above, investing resources in health care services directed toward vulnerable populations is the most obvious way. However, compelling

(The dependent variable in these equations is life achievement—defined as a simple transformation of life expectancy to avoid the nonlinearity that results from the existence of biological limits to life.)* Oil-producing countries, however, run counter to this. Although they have often high levels of per capita income, their health indicators lag behind other countries of similar income and wealth.

What is the right level of public spending for developing countries? World Bank analysts argue that 1 percent of GDP is needed for public health expenditures and an additional 2–3 percent is needed to universally finance essential clinical and public health services. (See Sachs, 1996; Jamison, 1996.) Figure 1.2.1 shows health outcomes as a function of total spending (public and private) on health and government spending in Asia and other parts of the world. Outcomes are defined as life achievement,* and are a function of public and private spending holding national income and education constant. This figure, which uses cross-sectional data, suggests that optimal public spending may be as high as 2.3–2.9 percent of a country's GDP.

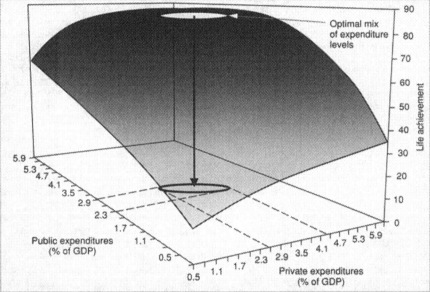

Figure 1.2.1—Effects of Public and Private Expenditures on Health Outcomes

* The equation for life achievement is as follows:

Life Achievement = 1/(Max Years – e(x)), where e(x) is life expectancy at birth (x = 0).

Max years can be chosen as the life expectancy of the country in the sample + 1 with the highest life expectancy. This way, the life achievement variable would be normalized to 1 [0,1].

evidence—shown above and in Chapter 5—also shows that spending in the education sector has a direct and immediate effect on improving health status, as does spending on water and sanitation projects.

Given the variety of shorter-term policy interventions that improve individual health status—spending on health, education, nutrition, water, or sanitation—the policy question is: Where should governments invest their scarce resources most efficiently to achieve the best health outcome for their population?

> **Box 1.3: Modeling Opportunity Costs: Investing in Health**
> **Versus Investing in Education**
>
> Evidence shows that education is effective in improving health, but can we conclude that education is a *better* investment than resources spent directly for health? Gertler et al. addressed this question by using a simple model of the health production function. (See Gertler et al., 1990.) Their dependent variables reflected health status (child mortality rate, crude death rate), while their independent policy variables included health care expenditures per capita, education (using literacy as a proxy), overall consumption levels, calorie intake, and general living condition. Overall living conditions—which can be assessed by examining access to public services, safe drinking water, and safe sewerage systems—were proxied by population density. Their resulting model was as follows:
>
> Health Status = f(Health Expenditure + Education + Overall Consumption
> + Food Consumption + Living Conditions)
>
> This estimation confirmed that education is an important factor in producing health. The results indicated that a 10 percent increase in literacy rate was associated with an increase of 1.91 years in life expectancy at birth, a 4 percent reduction in infant mortality rate, and a 7 percent reduction in child mortality rate. The results also showed that infant and child mortality rates fell when general living conditions improved.
>
> However, the most important result of the estimation was the weak correlation between health expenditure and health outcome. The estimation results indicated that a 10 percent increase in health care expenditures was associated with an increase of 0.4 years of life expectancy at birth, a 4.1 percent reduction in the infant mortality rate, and an 8.7 percent reduction in the child mortality rate. A 10 percent increase in expenditures corresponded to only $16.82 per capita on average in 1986.
>
> This model has several important limitations. It did not divide health expenditures into public versus out-of-pocket spending and did not directly compare the effects of spending on education with the effects of spending on health. We need to know, for example, how much it would cost to raise the literacy rate by 10 percent before we can answer the question of which investment is more efficient in improving the health status of a nation. Also, the model only indicated the average effect of improving education among all the countries; we would like to know the marginal impact. If, for example, a country raises its literacy rate from 20 to 30 percent, that increase would be 50 percent greater than an increase from 70 to 80 percent (only 14% greater). Another limitation is that the model was static rather than dynamic, i.e., it valued the benefits of health and education in future years the same as current years. For example, no differential is given to the value of life according to the age at which life is lived. In addition, this model has no discount rate that reflects differing social values. The higher the discount rate, the more one is inclined to spend on near-term life expectancy improvements.

Not surprisingly, answering this question is not straightforward. Choices between, say, health, education, sanitation, and infrastructures depend on several factors that may be valued differently. How much the present is valued compared with the future will influence choices between sanitation interventions that have an immediate impact and education benefits that are manifested in a subsequent generation. There is also the question of how benefits are to be compared.

This will influence such decisions as whether to spend public money on a better road that leads to economic prosperity or on a food supplement program that decreases the risk of dying from infection. Ultimately, governments are forced, either implicitly or explicitly, to estimate the impacts of investments in different sectors to determine the opportunity costs or benefits per dollar invested. Such estimations must account for the various perspectives (in the form of discount rates, valuations, and explicit trade-offs), and incorporate them into the decision process.

THE VARIABILITY OF HEALTH STATUS

Despite the general gains in health and the regional improvements in equity in East Asia, there are still broad disparities between regions in Asia, between individual countries, and within individual countries. Across Asia, for example, UNICEF estimates that every year, more than seven million Asian children still die from common, preventable diseases such as diarrhea and pneumonia, mostly among the poorer countries in the region. (See UNICEF, 1996.) Measles alone accounts for more than 635,000 preventable deaths in Asia—most of them in South Asia. (See WHO, 1996i; Murray and Lopez, 1996.)

The differences between countries are often profound. In India, tetanus causes over 280,000 newborn deaths yearly that could be prevented with a simple vaccine. Maternal mortality, for which there are inexpensive solutions such as prenatal care and "walking blood banks," varies from 600 per 100,000 live births in Bangladesh and Bhutan, to around 500 in South Asia and parts of Southeast Asia, to less than 100 in China, Sri Lanka, and Malaysia. (See UNICEF, 1996.)

Finally, variations within individual countries in Asia are profound and striking. While approximately 90 percent of the urban residents in Asia and the Pacific have access to safe water and 70 percent have adequate sanitation, rural residents are 10 to 40 percent less likely to have safe water and 76 percent less likely to have appropriate sanitation. (See UNICEF, 1996.) In Papua New Guinea, life expectancy as a whole was 57 years in 1994; however, we find that life expectancy within the country varies by as many as 10 to 15 years between those in the Highland provinces and the longer-living residents of the Island provinces. (See Peabody and Maerki, 1995.) And in Laos, while the under-five mortality rate was 152 per 1,000 in the country as a whole in 1994, it was 250 among the poorest 20 percent of the population—three times as high as it is among the uppermost quintile. (See Loevinsohn, 1996.)

If disparities between countries could be explained by the variation in national income or education, we would expect to see less deviation when we examine expected health status indicators in Asian countries after factoring out income, education, and public spending. (For this discussion, we assume technology is the same for all countries.)

But the graph in Figure 1.5 from the *World Development Report 1993*, modified to be more Asia-specific, indicates that this does not seem to be true. The vertical axis shows how far (measured in standard deviations) life expectancy in a country differs from the value predicted by that country's income and average schooling, while the horizontal axis shows how far life expectancy in a country varies by total health spending from the value predicted by income and education. The lines that divide the vertical and horizontal axes at the halfway point represent "predicted" life expectancy and GDP spent on health, respectively. By using

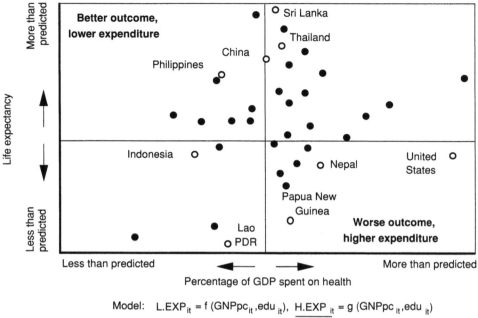

Model: $L.EXP_{it} = f (GNPpc_{it}, edu_{it})$, $\dfrac{H.EXP_{it}}{GDP_{it}} = g (GNPpc_{it}, edu_{it})$

SOURCES: World Bank, 1993a, b.

**Figure 1.5—Deviations from Estimated Life Expectancies and Total
Health Spending Controlling for Per Capita Income and Education**

regression to control for income and education, we can compare how much life expectancy varies by factors other than income, education, and health spending.

If income, education, and health care spending perfectly predicted health outcomes, we would expect countries to cluster around the center of the graph at zero deviation (the areas of predicted life expectancy and predicted GDP spent on health). Instead, what we see is a wide "scatter" among the countries. Countries in the upper left quadrant and lower right quadrant are particularly important. The upper left quadrant shows countries that spend less than predicted yet still have better-than-predicted life expectancy. Those in the lower right quadrant spend more than predicted but have lower levels of life expectancy than we would predict. These differences can be thought of in terms of a "performance gap" between observed life expectancy and predicted life expectancy based on income and education alone.

What we see from Figure 1.5 is that many countries in Asia reach levels of life expectancy far above those that would be dictated by pure economic determinism. Sri Lanka, with a 1994 per capita income of $640, has a life expectancy comparable to the most developed countries in the region. China, with roughly one-fifth the per-capita income of Thailand, has the same life expectancy (69 years). So variations in spending, holding income and education constant, do not explain all the differences in outcome. In contrast, the chart also

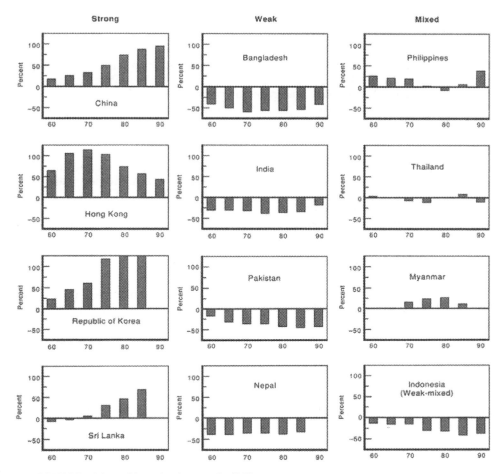

SOURCE: Adapted from Jamison et al., 1996.

Figure 1.6—Performance Gap of the Observed Minus the Expected Under-Five Mortality in Twelve Asian Countries, 1960–1990

shows that the Philippines and Lao PDR both spend about the same percentage of their GDP on health; however, the Philippines has significantly higher levels of expected life expectancy than does Lao PDR.

Figure 1.6 (above) compares the *expected* improvement in the under-five child mortality rate with the *observed* performance for 12 countries in Asia and the Pacific. China, for example, which spends just over 3 percent of its GDP on health, has an under-five mortality rate that is 93 percent better than expected when compared to other countries with the same income and level of education.

The performance gap between the observed and the expected has changed over time. Health outcomes in Nepal and Pakistan have never achieved the level expected given their national income. Underperforming countries, particularly those in South Asia and Indonesia, have begun to reverse their performance and move toward expected outcomes. Sri Lanka, China, and wealthier countries like South Korea and Hong Kong have continued to perform well.

The Philippines is a particularly interesting example, showing consistently good performance until the late 1970s and early 1980s, when political and economic instability negatively affected health-sector performance. When stability returned and health-sector reform began, increased health care to the poor and to rural residents of the country closed the performance gap, drastically improving health status. Health indicators have improved dramatically.

What all this tells us is that the four factors discussed above—economic growth, improvements in education, growth in medical technologies, and public spending on health—are necessary but not sufficient conditions for improving health status. The exceptional performance of many countries in Asia shows that it is possible to achieve the same outcomes despite enormous variations in per capita income and government spending.

GOVERNMENT INTERVENTIONS

How governments *implement* national health policy has an impact on improving health status. In terms of implementation, we are referring to "when" governments intervene, "how" they do the interventions, and "why" they intervene.

When Governments Intervene—Unique Roles

While the relationship between health and development explains government's interest in good policy and its will to participate, this does not in itself provide justification for government participation. (See de Ferranti, 1985; Hammer, 1997a.)

When governments intervene in the health sector, they do so with the general goal of trying to improve the health status of their people. While any intervention can theoretically fulfill this goal, governments generally intervene to fulfill unique roles. In general, governments have two such roles in the health sector: (1) preventing or correcting failures in health-sector markets, and (2) ensuring equity when poor and vulnerable patients cannot afford health care.

Preventing or Correcting Market Failures. There are three important types of market failures in the health sector. The first two have to do with providing or subsidizing something in the public market because the private market is incapable or unwilling to do so. The third has to do with insuring against catastrophic loss through health insurance.

Providing/Subsidizing Public Goods. From an economic point of view, a market can fail in the health sector when it does not provide enough needed medical goods or services, and a subsidy or production of the *public good* is needed. A public good is a health service in which one person's use or benefit does not exclude the use or benefit of another. For example, the national and international efforts to eradicate mosquitoes that cause encephalitides, malaria, and dengue are examples of a publicly financed service (provided publicly or privately through contracts) that benefits everyone. It would be unlikely that any person alone would be willing to shoulder the costs of spraying and removing resting water.

Water and sanitation projects are other obvious examples of public works projects that exist because the private market provides too little of the health infrastructure essential for improving health.

Private Goods With and Without Externalities. Private goods may or may not reflect their social value. When they do, the amount of a good or service produced is efficient; when they do not, a positive (or a negative) externality exists. This is a market failure because there are benefits beyond the private benefits that are not captured by the individual and thus are "external" to what one person would pay. For example, preventing a communicable disease in one person confers a positive benefit—has a positive externality—on everyone else in the community, because there is one less person who can transmit the infectious agent. This benefit is external to the individual who paid for the service and has value to all others who now have less of a chance of becoming infected.

Of course, there are also negative externalities. For example, if an individual does not value or is unwilling to pay for an immunization, there is an incremental chance that someone else will get the disease. Another example is when second-hand tobacco smoke or industrial pollution confers health risks to persons in proximity to the smoker or the polluter who does not own the smoke-free or clean air that is fouled. On a more general level, there are negative externalities to watching people suffer. Individuals and governments are willing to pay to decrease the suffering of others.

Clearly, preventing or correcting market failures like the ones described above has also been described in the medical paradigm. Public health campaigns have the same rationale as providing public goods (e.g., treating patients with sexually transmitted diseases and tracing their contacts); reducing the suffering of a malnourished child has the same rationale as eliminating the negative externality of starvation.

Beyond this overlap between economic and medical justifications, there are other clinical issues. Disease and illness represent an opportunity to restore a person to his original health or, at a minimum, a chance to limit the effects of the disease both on the individual and on others. Illness, therefore, is a biologic event that requires skilled intervention. For example, giving rifampin to a military recruit colonized with meningitis prevents a local epidemic and the sequellae of brain damage; properly treating a businessman for tuberculosis prevents the emergence of multidrug-resistant tuberculosis to passengers on an international flight.

Health status is clinically defined by multiple factors—genetics, the environment, individual hygienic behaviors, and clinical care. Therefore, medical interventions need to be properly timed and effectively coordinated on a broad societal scale by governments through their MOHs. This coordination is also a public good. As we will see in Chapters 3, 6, and 7, clinicians think of care as being of three types: preventive, promotive, and prescriptive (curative) care. Public subsidies or even public provisions should be contingent upon whether there is a market failure.

Failures in the Insurance Market. Market failures may exist within the health insurance market. From an economic viewpoint, these insurance market failures occur because of *cream skimming* by private insurers who have incentives to

**Box 1.4: The Complexities of Financing Health Reform:
A Case Study of Community Rating**

In countries with voluntary health insurance schemes, insurers attempt to attract only the best health risks to their plans. Often, this leads to the practice of "experience rating"—in which insurers charge higher premiums to individuals or small groups expected to have higher expenditures—or to "medical underwriting"—in which insurers require those with chronic or temporary conditions who may require expensive treatment to pay higher premiums. These practices, in turn, often lead to outcomes governments find objectionable: higher premiums for the chronically ill or for employees engaged in more-hazardous occupations, and a large population of uninsured people.

What can governments do to prevent these outcomes? One solution is to regulate price-setting behavior by insurers through "community rating," which requires insurance companies to charge the same premium to all individuals in a market. While such regulation appears desirable, how desirable is it? The answer to this question reveals the complexities governments face in implementing health reform.

Typically, community rating entails pooling risks over large geographic areas—including rural and urban populations—which may induce regressive transfers from poorer rural communities to more-affluent urban ones. The reasons for these transfers are twofold. First, once a regional pool sets a community rate, all households in the region pay the same amount for insurance. Implicitly, the poorer, rural households end up bearing part of the cost of care for the wealthier, urban households in the community pool. In diverse regions with heterogeneous communities, potentially large transfers could occur from low- to high-cost areas.

Second, with any standard benefits package, wealthier households tend to use more medical services than poorer ones. For a given increase in price, the wealthier households will change their consumption less than poorer ones. Furthermore, because they tend to live in urban areas, wealthier households pay higher prices for a given service than their poorer, rural counterparts. For example, wealthier individuals pay more for an appendectomy than poorer individuals because of where they live; if they are pooled together, the poorer individuals end up subsidizing the wealthier individuals' higher-priced care.

Policymakers might decide to pool only within urban areas, thereby mitigating the impact of price differentials between urban and rural areas. However, there may still be substantial transfers across income groups, with traditionally poorer neighborhoods subsidizing more affluent ones. For example, pooling across urban areas in Los Angeles could put people living in wealthy Beverly Hills in the same group with some of the city's poorest residents living in East Los Angeles.

Without explicitly adjusting premiums for income, community-rated areas cannot be constructed to completely eliminate this regressivity. Thus, policymakers might consider providing subsidies to poorer households to purchase health insurance. Unfortunately, such a policy would be difficult to implement, and thus the overall regressive consequences of community rating would be difficult to assess.

Clearly, governments do play an important role in regulating insurance markets to prevent inequities and market failures; unfortunately, as the case of community rating illustrates, successfully implementing regulations is fraught with complexities.

insure mainly healthy people who will not need care, because of *adverse selection* that arises when unhealthy people seek (or continue) insurance coverage more than healthy people, or because of the *moral hazard* of patients who do not respond to the true cost of care (because they are insured) and ask for additional diagnostic testing and treatment. We found in South Korea, for example, that the demand for care, which is provided by a private health care market, increased dramatically when universal coverage was introduced. (See Peabody et al., 1994.)

Just as failure may exist within the insurance market, market failures may also exist that prevent private insurance from being developed in the first place. For instance, very poor individuals will not buy insurance if they are not at financial risk. And insurers will not enter a market that is too competitive (and where prices are too low). They also will not enter if there is a dearth of individuals with sufficient income and low enough health risk in a market that is already dominated by public insurance. Capital markets also must be adequate to allow for insurance payments (premiums) to be invested. These investments generate returns that defray the costs of claims and yield profits. Given these factors, it is not too surprising that less than 1 percent of the Asian population is presently covered by private insurance. (See Newbrander, 1997.)

This moral hazard also applies to providers who, acting on behalf of their patients, advise them on treatments linked to their income and *induce demand* for more services than are warranted. Cream skimming, adverse selection, and moral hazard among patients and providers are examples where the private market can fail and where public intervention can mitigate adverse effects.

As was true in providing or subsidizing public goods, there are also health reasons to justify insuring against catastrophic loss. Certain diseases are catastrophic but ultimately treatable in a battle against limited resources and time. Medical intervention has a unique biologic moment that cannot be reversed if action is not taken immediately. For example, a trauma victim may need an emergency thoracotomy to relieve a punctured lung, or a child with pneumonia may need antibiotics. Without insurance against these catastrophic events, death may ensue—a death that is entirely preventable with appropriate technology.

Promoting Equity. Governments also intervene when there is a need to ensure that poor and vulnerable patients have access to health care. Most people (and countries) view health care as a basic need and view access to care as a fundamental right. Beyond this, health is a primary good that enables people to work and acquire the means for feeding, sheltering, and clothing themselves or their families.

Unfortunately, although routine health care is not usually a problem for those with sufficient income, it is a problem for the poor, for whom basic health may not be affordable or accessible. When asked to make choices about what to purchase, the poor are more likely to spend money on improving their health through non–health purchases, such as better sanitation, nutrition, and housing. As income goes down, the purchase of health care is jettisoned in favor of other primary goods, such as food or leisure.

This means that relatively richer people not only spend a greater amount on health, they spend a greater percentage of their income on health than do the poor. Stated another way, the less money people make, the less health care they use. Some of that care, however, is necessary for survival. Thus, one means to improve equity and alleviate poverty is through direct government intervention to subsidize or provide health services.

It is important to distinguish between subsidizing or providing health care for the poor and insuring against catastrophic illness. Paying for catastrophic health care is beyond the financial capacity of most families except for the wealthy and is a problem for almost all income groups. Care for the poor refers to government subsidy or provision of low-cost highly effective care. But the distinction between care for the poor and the need for insurance should not be made too finely: Doing without the low-cost care still means that an avoidable death or disability might occur. Viewed in this way, medical indigence is no different from poverty. Government participation in health for the poor is an intervention in the private market for health care justified on the grounds that the poor are unable to afford such care.

The two unique roles of correcting market failures and ensuring equity often overlap. For example, not only is the treatment of tuberculosis more likely to be a service needed by the poor, but successful therapy produces a positive externality benefiting others. Moreover, this additional benefit leads to overpricing the cost of the service to the poor but underpricing the aggregate (potential) benefit to everyone else—it is free. An untreated case and the resulting spread of tuberculosis hurts everyone: The disease can spread, it can potentially lead to multidrug resistance if partially treated, and it can lead to death in the index patient, since over 70 percent of patients with untreated tuberculosis will be dead in 10 years.

Thus, the question of "when" governments get involved in providing health care must be carefully decided to provide a greater benefit than would be possible if the government did not participate at all. (See Musgrove, 1996.) Deciding when participation is appropriate, therefore, lies at the core of good policy to improve health status.

How Governments Intervene—Approaches to Correct Market Failures and Improve Equity

Governments have five basic ways to correct market failures and improve equity. They can inform, regulate, mandate, finance, or deliver. Although these approaches are not unique to health care and are typical of government involvement in other sectors, the involvement in health is typically extensive and employs all five of these approaches. (See Musgrove, 1996.)

Inform. Governments inform by providing information about health promotion campaigns or disseminating health services research findings that report on the effectiveness of, say, a pilot immunization-outreach program into a rural area. In the first example, governments are correcting information asymmetries by providing information to the general population, while in the latter, they are improving access to medical care for peasant farmers by informing local health providers of a potentially better strategy.

Regulate. Governments generally regulate by legislation or executive order, for example, by restricting antibiotic availability to correct negative externalities such as microbial drug resistance, or by licensing providers and insurers to reduce induced demand from unscrupulous providers doing unnecessary tests.

Mandate. Mandates are also specified by law, but unlike regulations, they involve performance. Epidemiologic surveillance reporting by hospitals and employee insurance benefits are examples of mandates designed to promote the public interest.

Finance. Financing public health campaigns, such as for diagnosing tuberculosis and providing treatment for immunizations, is an example of correcting externalities as already discussed. Research and development (R&D) is another type of public good (often an international one) that is generally financed with public funding. The technological advance cannot be "rebottled" and, once discovered or analyzed, is potentially of benefit to everyone.

Pharmaceutical research for orphan drugs—compounds for which there is not sufficient potential for corporate profit but for which there is an unmet need for effective treatment—is an example. Basic science discoveries—which, while they may lead to future advances in diagnosis and therapy, have no commercial value—are another example. These possibilities serve as the basis for public investment in scientific investigations.

Financing or subsidizing care for equity reasons should begin with the most cost-effective care *and* care that is a public good. In poor countries, these alone may exhaust public financing. If more resources are available, the next level of public spending should be for clinical services needed by the poor that, although curative and a private good, should be included as a part of a basic benefits package. The reason for this ranking is that it is not possible to completely exclude the nonpoor from using these services, and government participation in the name of equity will necessarily make some trade-offs in efficiency. A more thorough discussion of cost effectiveness and resource allocation issues is presented in Chapters 3 and 4, respectively.

Deliver. Once a government decides to finance a health service, the subsequent choice is whether it also will deliver or provide the service. The government can potentially deliver a whole range of services from public health to curative care. But, as we have argued above, if the government is to act as a provider, it should provide care only if it can do so more effectively than the private sector. Government provision often occurs when there is no alternative source of delivery, for example in remote rural areas where it is unlikely that there will be enough private capital or demand to support private initiatives. Direct government provision of services is often the most expensive approach, because it eliminates incentives for efficiency, distorts the parallel private sector, often prevents the private market from entering, and is subject to fraud and waste. (This issue is discussed in more detail in Chapter 7.)

Governments, therefore, must marshal a combination of strategies to correct market failures and/or subsidize poor and vulnerable populations. However, the five approaches discussed above should not be viewed as discrete points along a continuum of government intervention; good policy involves the right combination of approaches, and bad policy involves too much of some approaches and not enough of others.

Why Governments Intervene—Multiple Strategies Based on Different Values

Whether it is to correct market failure or improve equity, whatever approach governments take, they are influenced by many groups. Consensus statements (and accompanying policy delineations) such as WHO's *Health For All* and the World Bank's *World Development Report 1993: Investing in Health* have focused the debate, but their several approaches attest to the lack of unanimity about why reform should be undertaken. The lack of consensus describes the reality: There is no simple prescription for health policy interventions—no one-time injection that will vaccinate the health sector against the ills that continue to plague economies or societies. Some of this is explained by the absence of an approach that is successful enough to become the dominant paradigm, but many complexities lie at the heart of the debate.

Although the health care debate is often framed in political and economic terms, the main difficulty is a disagreement about values. In fact, discussions about how to accomplish health-sector reform are often misplaced debates over the values of reform. In Taiwan, for example, incremental steps toward health reform, rather than sweeping structural changes, helped to define a social value (health for all), which, in turn, was translated into public policy (national health insurance). (See Peabody, 1995.)

Thus, while health-sector reform attracts broad support, specific approaches are not always met with the same unanimity. Even with the single goal of improving people's well-being, no set of values is suitable for all countries. Nevertheless, three sets of values can be laid out that summarize the debate over policy reform. (See Hammer and Berman, 1995.) Specifically, governments can seek to (1) value the most health for the least cost; (2) guarantee a minimum amount of health service for everyone; or (3) provide the most overall welfare, including health, for individuals and society.

Value the Most Health for the Least Cost. On its face, improving health status through the best use of national resources is a reasonable and commonly advocated approach. Often referred to as *procedural justice*, this approach says that with a limited budget, governments should value and pay for efficient services. The priority is placed on what works: Thus, resources may be targeted toward public goods that are undervalued and likely to improve everyone's health, such as immunizations, nutritional supplements, supervised deliveries, public health campaigns for family planning, and preventive programs for tobacco and other drugs. Resources may also be provided for funding private goods, such as coverage for all fractures, minor trauma, and acute illnesses such as pneumonia or a myocardial infarction (heart attack). While appealing, the approach of valuing the most health for the least cost does not take into account who needs help the most, referred to as *distributional justice*. The poor and the elderly might not get care without subsidies under an approach that prioritizes efficiency. But providing health care services based on the most health for the least cost often amounts to "subsidizing" the middle and upper classes because they use more health care services. It also does not take into account the dimensions of well being beyond health that we refer to as overall welfare. We take up the subjects of subsidies, allocation, and social welfare in detail in Chapter 4.

Guarantee a Minimum Amount of Health Service for Everyone. One way around this problem is to target services that are commonly used by the poor alone. Such an approach values equity by emphasizing that individuals do not have the same opportunities. Based on the concept of *distributional justice*, this approach argues that governments can more effectively reduce poverty and improve equity by targeting health care services for the poor rather than paying for services for everyone. While there are a number of ways to do this, targeting geographically—i.e., putting up clinics in areas inhabited by the poor—or targeting by disease or medical conditions—i.e., providing subsidized care for things like infectious diseases, which are more likely to afflict the poor—are two ways to redistribute and improve equity. (This subject is taken up in detail in Chapter 5.) Governments following this strategy, such as Sri Lanka, provide universal primary care with a guaranteed basic package of benefits targeted toward pregnant women, who are likely to be younger, live in the countryside, and have less income.

In targeting by type of service, governments must avoid targeting those services likely to be used by everyone no matter what the price. Studies of prenatal care in Jamaica, for example, have shown that even women in the lowest income quintile were still willing to pay for prenatal care from private providers, but virtually none sought care for immunizations outside the public sector.

Whatever services are targeted, they need to be paid for from public monies that originate from taxes, which disproportionately affect the poor. Tax policy, therefore, is another perspective on equity to consider. A progressive income tax scheme, where a larger percentage of taxes are paid by those with larger incomes, is one obvious means to redistribute resources. In developing countries, workers in the formal sector tend to have higher-paying jobs and are identified as having a regular salary or wage; thus, they are easier to assess with taxes. This is a potentially effective redistribution strategy when combined with targeting strategies.

Provide the Most Overall Welfare, Including Health, for Individuals/Society.
The first two sets of values are primarily concerned with the public provision of health services to improve health status. However, beyond the public provision of health services, there are other means to achieve the goal of improving people's well-being. The total-welfare approach looks at more than health status and values people's total welfare, of which health is just one component that individuals value. Consider prenatal care: The total-welfare approach presumes that a woman values her health and the health of her child; however, she also values other things like nutrition and education, all of which may lead to better health and better welfare in the aggregate for her and her baby. Thus, she would seek care when it was needed and when it was not superseded by another need.

If she needs care but does not seek it, the government can lower costs, provide information (to change her priority), or correct other market failures. The total-welfare approach means governments take into account externalities, such as preventing communicable disease, and merit goods, such as ensuring that all deliveries are medically supervised. Policy can also mandate services that lower costs or provide care for random, catastrophic illness. (This is an extension of the argument by Hammer and Berman.) Thus, the argument for government as the agent to reduce risk and improve welfare has both an economic value to society—to maintain household productivity—and a humanitarian value—to help the disadvantaged.

Box 1.5: When Simple Technical Solutions Are Not Enough: Treating Neonatal Hypothermia in Eastern China

During winters in Zhejiang Province, Chinese and foreign physicians noted a higher incidence of children, particularly neonates, who appeared hypothermic. Subsequent temperature readings by a team of Project HOPE researchers using low-reading thermometers confirmed the diagnosis. There was no mystery about the diagnosis: Throughout China in the 1980s, no external heat was available to hospitals (including delivery rooms) or homes south of the Yellow River, babies were often not dried after birth, skin-to-skin contact between mother and child was not a common cultural practice, and parents (and health care workers) were unaware of the danger of cold exposure. Clinical treatment was equally straightforward: Early diagnosis upon admission, treatment of concurrent conditions, and external rewarming.

However, translating clinical treatment into policy proved hard. The initial clinical assessment generated interest in treating the problem inside the Children's Hospital in Hangzhou where researchers addressed the general problem of underdiagnosis, but it did not consider the problems of incidence, severity, and financial and personnel constraints. The Bureau of Public Health (BOPH) and the Provincial Government to whom researchers turned were supportive but lacked information on how severe and widespread the problem was in the province. Interwoven with these clinical and epidemiological concerns were specific cultural and social issues related to policy in Eastern China (e.g., questions about birthing practices, postpartum beliefs, and family preferences).

Addressing these broader concerns required looking beyond clinical aspects to epidemiological and sociocultural aspects as well. Researchers used a series of hypotheses—clinical and clinical/epidemiologic hypotheses (e.g., the method of rewarming would affect survival), epidemiologic/sociocultural hypotheses (e.g., transportation resources were limited and most referrals would be from areas immediately around the hospital), and sociocultural/clinical hypotheses (e.g., there would be a preponderance of boys admitted to the hospital)—to limit the amount of investigation needed in each discipline and to investigate operationalizable issues with known public health solutions.

The results of the analysis yielded a policy story that changed the perspective and initial orientation of solutions—away from acute-care interventions and toward more-practical, accomplishable public health solutions. For example, the approach revealed that the problem's scope was broader than originally believed, and the discovery that rewarming was not affected by method or rate of rewarming suggested that available rewarming techniques might suffice.

Armed with these findings, researchers focused on three approaches to provide solutions. First, they introduced neonatal hypothermia as a significant medical problem to the medical profession, at both the Children's Hospital and at the national level. Today, a few years later, there is evidence that the general awareness of hypothermia has increased in China. Second, with the realization that hypothermia was a province-wide problem, researchers embarked on an outreach education program (starting with a BOPH-promoted pilot program to secondary-level hospitals province-wide) to delivery-room obstetricians and nurses and to parents. Third, to operationalize the treatment and prevention of hypothermia, researchers focused on preparing a series of self-instruction modules that addressed hypothermia in the context of other common newborn problems, such as hypoglycemia and hypoxia. The modules proved so successful they were expanded by the BOPH throughout Zhejiang Province and included by the MOPH early on in its three-year "rural physician" training program.

HEALTH POLICY IMPLEMENTATION AT THE MINISTRY LEVEL

Although governments drive when and how interventions should occur and struggle with what values justify why they should be done, the actual implementation of the health programs occurs at the Ministry of Health (MOH) level.

Deciding on these actual interventions at the MOH level is the focus of this book. Specifically, in Chapter 3, we look at the clinical medical practices that cannot be ignored and that the MOH should pursue to ensure that a minimum package of services are universally available. In Chapter 4, we examine the best policy options for the MOH to finance and allocate health care resources. In Chapter 5, we look at how MOH policies can target poor and vulnerable populations. Chapter 6 describes how the MOH can promote policies that encourage healthier individual behaviors and better provider care. And Chapter 7 considers how the MOH can organize and structure itself to efficiently and effectively deliver health care services and how to make sure that there are no discontinuities between national-level health values, objectives, and goals and actual health care programs.

When MOH policymakers implement specific health interventions, they do so based on what the evidence tells them needs to be addressed (e.g., when there are equity concerns among certain groups of people in different regions) and on what the evidence tells them about the efficiency and effectiveness of the interventions to improve health status. Efficiency matters because governments have limited resources to invest in policies to help improve health status, so it is important to spend those resources on the right groups of people and for policies where the evidence shows they work. Policies should be evidence-based, since the effectiveness of the intervention also matters. When resources are devoted to health policies that do not work or work less well than others, people will not get better and many others may die because they were excluded from effective care.

Given the critical importance of evidence-based health policy, we devote all of Chapter 2 to examining the issue across the Asian region, looking specifically at what kinds and types of data policymakers need and at what the overall status and quality of those data are. It is important to clarify that evidence means more than just clinical evidence. Health policy must be based on both clinical and nonclinical evidence—that is, on evidence from studies done in such disciplines as health care financing, political science, management science, and behavioral science. This argues for the need to use multiple paradigms to solve sectoral problems. In some cases, health researchers already use these approaches, as well as paradigms from economics, organizational analysis, operations research, and law. (See Peabody, 1996a; WHO, 1995d.)

The question of data quality and multiple disciplines infuses the entire book. Specifically, evidence is critical for determining what clinical interventions to choose (Chapter 3), how to finance and allocate resources for health economic interventions (Chapter 4), how to determine the right policies to ensure better social equity (Chapter 5), how to motivate individuals and providers to change behavior so that interventions will be used and sustained (Chapter 6), and how to organize the MOH to manage health care services most effectively and efficiently (Chapter 7).

CHAPTER 2: SUMMARY OF POLICY QUESTIONS, FINDINGS, AND IMPLICATIONS

ISSUES	EVIDENCE
• What kinds of data are needed to make informed health care policy?	• Because so many factors affect health outcomes, policymaking requires many types and sources of data.
• What is the status of these types of data for Asian countries?	• Significant data gaps exist; existing data may have problems that limit their usefulness unless the data are well explained.
• What other data issues affect the ability of policymakers to make evidence-based health care policy?	• Discontinuities between policymakers and researchers occur because of study design, data analysis, and policy issues.

POLICY IMPLICATIONS
• Implementing health policy interventions—whether clinical, management, or financing—should be based on the best available evidence and analysis.
• Where evidence does not yet exist and policy must be implemented, data should be collected using the most rigorous studies/research design possible.
• Implemented policies, particularly if enacted without rigorous evidence, need to be evaluated to determine their benefit, harm, and cost-effectiveness.
• Data are a public good; thus, funding data collection is a responsibility of government and international donors.

EVIDENCE-BASED POLICY: USING DATA TO INFORM POLICY AND IMPROVE HEALTH OUTCOMES

OVERVIEW

In Chapter 1, we argued that good health policy can have a direct impact on improving health outcomes. Exactly which policy to pursue is decided from a complicated mixture of politics, available funding, and technical expertise. The technical elements of this mixture are determined, to varying degrees, by the evidence available for policymaking. Ideally, policy should always be evidence-based, but this is obviously not always the case. Oftentimes, policy is made without evidence—a situation that demands that policy be evaluated *in vivo* to determine if it is having its intended impact. Other times, policy is made that ignores the available evidence. Creating evidence-based policy, therefore, faces twin challenges: high-quality data must be used during the policymaking (or policy revision) process, and policy made in the absence of evidence must be implemented cautiously until its impact is properly understood.

Data are important for policy analysis for a simple reason: Better data should generate or lead to better policy. Better policy, in turn, is expected to lead to better health outcomes—the ultimate goal of health policymakers.

Do better data actually guide policymaking? It is not hard to demonstrate that information and scientific investigation are used to inform health policy, and there are many examples of this relationship in Asia. For example, data from observational studies have shown that sexually transmitted diseases (STDs) are associated with cervical cancer and the spread of HIV. Establishing this link has led policymakers to expand publicly funded STD clinics throughout Asia and the Pacific. Another example: Epidemiologic studies have uncovered that neonatal tetanus kills more children than any other vaccine-preventable illness except measles. Based on this information, WHO and UNICEF have expanded immunization campaigns to every country in Asia. Today, these programs have reached 80 percent of the world's children, and 700,000 deaths were prevented in 1995 by immunizing women against tetanus. Such impressive results argue that better data and better information lead to more informed policies.

But can better data lead to policy choices that produce greater improvements in health outcomes? Although there is less evidence of this, there are some examples. For example, data proved critically important in choosing between two competing contraceptive service programs to reduce fertility rates in rural Bangladesh. One group contended that contraceptive programs only work when there is an existing demand (i.e., a perceived need for fertility control), whereas a second group contended that introducing contraceptive services could itself initiate a fertility change.

To test these two policy positions, a field experiment was conducted in Matlab, Bangladesh; the experiment set up a control group where contraceptive programs were not developed and implemented and a treatment group where they were.

The two groups were then followed and the fertility rates of the two groups were compared over time between 1977 and 1981. The results showed that the fertility rates of the treatment group were lower.

Based on these results, policymakers initiated family planning programs in 1982 and reinforced them to include maternal and child health (MCH) services. By the end of 1984, there had been a sustained increase in contraceptive use to levels unprecedented in the history of the Matlab area, reaching nearly 46 percent of the currently married women of reproductive age. (See DeGraff et al., 1986.) This increase, in turn, reduced the quarterly fertility rate, from more than 240 births per 1,000 women age 15–29 and 160 births per 1,000 women age 30–44 in 1974 to fewer than 80 and 60 births, respectively, in 1986.

The Bangladesh example shows the full linkage between studies, data, health policy, and improved health outcomes. Figure 2.1 illustrates this more extended relationship, showing the various roles health policymakers and health researchers play in the process.

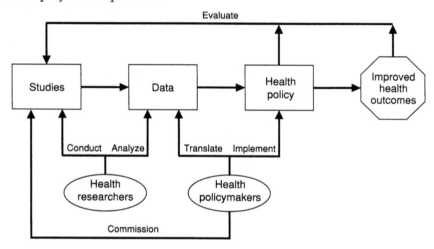

Figure 2.1—The Relationship Between Studies, Data, Health Policy, and Improved Health Outcomes

The figure shows that health policymakers have three roles in the process. Aside from the obvious role of implementing health policy (the role discussed in Chapter 1 and shown in Figure 1.1), policymakers are also directly involved early in the process by commissioning the studies researchers conduct and by interpreting the data researchers generate and analyze.

Policymakers bear a responsibility not only for understanding how researchers do their jobs but also for understanding the types and quality of studies researchers conduct, as well as the meaning and value of the data such studies generate. The role of the policymaker is to interpret the data researchers collect and analyze; the data then become *evidence* for policymakers to use in implementing health interventions. This is the critical issue: Policy decisions should be evidence-based, and the evidence should use the best available data.

Given the critical value of data and the roles and relationships of researchers and policymakers, we can formulate three policy questions that need to have answers:

1. What kinds of data are needed to make informed health care policy?

2. What is the status of these types of data for Asian countries?

3. What other data issues affect the ability of policymakers to make evidence-based health care policy?

The answers to these questions form the basis for the rest of this chapter. In turn, this chapter, with its focus on data, underlies the evidence-based approach that is the foundation for examining the policy areas discussed in the rest of the book.

DATA SOURCES REQUIRED FOR POLICYMAKING

What kinds of data do policymakers need? Several examples are illustrative. Walsh and Simonet describe how the Thai Ministry of Health set up an expert panel, the National Epidemiology Board, to provide expert technical advice in policy and planning (see Walsh and Simonet, 1995a). The general strategy was to use the literature, evaluation strategies, and biomedical, epidemiologic, economic, and social science research to address policymaking needs. Where policies were needed, studies were commissioned in consultation with policymakers. As a result of this effort, the board has had a substantial impact on varied policies that address iodine deficiency, essential drugs, vaccination programs, and auto immune deficiency syndrome (AIDS).

In Papua New Guinea, the planning process has been accompanied by an in-depth review of the burden of disease and availability of resources. The preponderance of budgetary expenditures on personnel and the dramatically higher IMR in rural areas shifted policy priorities in the plan. Data also showed that decentralization to provinces did not improve targeting or resource allocation. This led to an evaluation of the budget allocation process, which was completely revised in 1996. (See Campos-Outcalt et al., 1995.)

As these examples clearly show, intervening in the health sector requires policymakers to make use of many types and sources of data from multiple disciplines. But what specifically should these types and sources be? We discuss this question below.

Categories of Data

To a policymaker, there may seem to be a cacophony of data espoused by a legion of informed experts. So categorization of data may prove useful as policymakers attempt to commission studies and interpret data. We propose a straightforward method of categorization.

To guide our discussion, we have constructed a simplified model that captures the main factors that influence the health status of the population (Figure 2.2).

We start by assuming that for a given population group, factors such as geographic location, level of income, and composition in terms of sex and age (i.e., demographic factors) determine the level of access to a set of basic needs—adequate nutrition, sanitation, safe water, education, and health services. These demographic factors, in conjunction with the cultural and social characteristics of

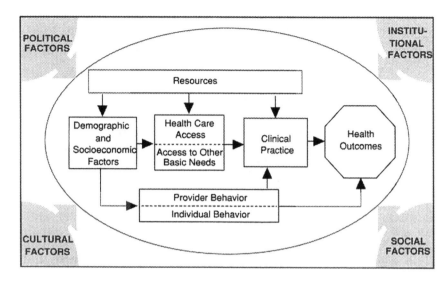

**Figure 2.2—Types of Data: A Simplified Model of Factors
Affecting Health Outcomes**

the population, influence the behavior of individuals and thus the type of actions they undertake daily that affect their health status (e.g., washing their hands, boiling water for drinking, and seeking professional advice or follow-up medical prescriptions). Once the access to health services has been realized (for preventive or curative purposes), improvements in health status depend on the quality and effectiveness of clinical practice. These, in turn, are affected both by the amount of resources allocated to the health sector and by the behavior of providers. Finally, the overall performance of the health system will be influenced by both political and institutional factors, such as how governments organize their institutions and what management styles they use.

Based on the model depicted in the figure, we have grouped the types of data needed for health policy analysis into seven categories:

1.   Demographic and socioeconomic data (e.g., age, sex, income);

2.   Measures of access to health care and other basic needs (i.e., nutrition, education, safe water, and sanitation);

3.   An inventory of public and private resources (e.g., infrastructure, manpower, and money);

4.   An estimation of individual behavior and provider preferences, which motivate access to, and provision of, better care;

5.   An assessment of clinical practice, focusing on the estimation of the costs and on the effectiveness of alternative treatments and technologies;

6.   An assessment of the political, social, institutional, and managerial environment in which health policy is made;

7.   Measures of health outcomes (typically, morbidity and mortality).

Below, we look at each data type and show how it is used in health care policymaking.

Demographic and Socioeconomic Factors. This data type refers to the geographic distribution of the population, its composition in terms of age and sex, its growth rate, and level of income. Changes in the composition of the population in terms of age and sex necessarily produce changes in morbidity and, therefore, in health priorities. This affects the allocation of resources among policy interventions, population groups, and geographic regions. In the discussions of equity and access (Chapter 5), we will show how useful such data are.

Measures of Access to Health Care and Other Basic Needs. Access to adequate nutrition, education, sanitation, and preventive and curative health services is an essential determinant of health status. For example, we will see in Chapter 3 that malnutrition causes a burden of 10.5 Disability Adjusted Life Years (DALYs) per 1,000 population (computed on the basis of DALYs per region and population per region) in Asia, and the estimated burden of disease caused by a poor household environment amounts to a staggering 338 million DALYs per year. Hence, to identify and target those in the population exposed to a high risk of morbidity, policymakers require measures of access to these basic needs for different population groups.

An Inventory of Private and Public Resources. The amount of private resources and government allocations to the health sector, as well as the distribution of th0se public resources between regions, socioeconomic groups, health interventions, and types of research and technologies, may seem like an obvious type of data, but in practice it is very hard to obtain accurate estimates. An important component of any project of health-sector reform relates to mobilizing and reallocating these resources (as we discuss in Chapter 4). Thus, health-sector resources are ultimately related to financial resources (public subsidies and private health expenditures), infrastructure (number of hospital and clinics), and human capital (number of physicians and nurses).

Several factors influence the amount of financial resources available for the health sector. Among the most important are the level of production per capita, the level of employment, the size of the formal wage sector, the level of wages, the size of the public budget, general tax rates (and the rate of tax evasion), the social security system, and the flows of foreign assistance.

An Estimation of Individual and Provider Behavior. Individual prices, preferences, and behaviors affect the availability of resources, the response to policy, and, ultimately, health status. For example, as we discuss in Chapter 4, individual preferences will affect how individuals behave when user fees are introduced. These fees, depending on consumer response, can reduce utilization so much that the increase in unit revenue is offset by the decline in unit volume, thus reducing the amount of resources available. From a health perspective, utilization of services is highly sensitive to price; consequently, an increase can have important negative effects on a population's health status.

As a result of these uncertainties, understanding individual and provider behaviors is one of the priorities of health policy analysts; this is the focus of Chapter 6. Only when information describing individual behaviors is available can policymakers answer such questions as: How do individuals change their utilization of health services when faced with changes in price? How does an increase in income affect their health status? How does education induce preventive behavior or compliance with an antibiotic regimen? The same kinds of questions arise on the provider behavior side: How is the quality of services affected by the mechanism of payment? Are medical practice guidelines effective in changing providers' behavior about the prescription of tests, drugs, and treatments?

An Assessment of Clinical Practice. How well preventive and curative interventions improve health will affect resource allocation. These data come from studies that test for the effectiveness of such everyday practices as drugs, diagnostic tests, or the timing of surgical interventions. Policymakers continually require data to answer questions about new therapies, expensive therapies such as post-traumatic rehabilitation and fiberoptic surgery, or new tests such as digitalized radiographs. These interventions and practices come with a cost and may fuel an acceleration of medical expenditures that policymakers need to understand. As we discuss in Chapter 3, the correlation between medical therapy and outcome is mediated by the quality of care and the effectiveness of current clinical practice.

An Assessment of the Political, Social, and Institutional Environment. The functioning of the health system is influenced by the political environment and by the organization and management style of its institutions. As we discussed in Chapter 1 and examine in more detail in Chapters 6 and 7, any reform of the health sector requires characterizing the players in the process, their role, their political power, their social support, and their interests. Thus, policymakers need data and information describing the distribution of political forces, the organic structure of the health sector, and the managerial styles of its institutions.

Measures of Health Outcomes. Measures of health outcomes are used to respond to such questions as: Which diseases cause the major burden? And what population groups are more exposed to the risk of disease or death? Such data are crucial in providing policymakers with baseline information to construct the agenda of future policy interventions. These measures are also used to evaluate clinical interventions (like those discussed in Chapter 3), answering such questions as: Which public health interventions are more effective at reducing infant mortality or the general burden of disease?

Traditionally, mortality rates and morbidity measures have been used as the key outcome measures. While nobody would argue that mortality rates are not an important measure of outcomes, the fact that much disease does not result in death make them difficult to use. Moreover, the multidimensional causes of death make it very difficult to isolate the effects of policy interventions on mortality rates from the effects of other factors, ranging from climate to genetics. Morbidity measures, such as disease incidence or prevalence, reduce the problem of infrequency and etiology. However, it is inherently difficult to establish the clinical factors associated with disease by using traditional mortality or morbidity indicators. The indicators also do not account for the effect that different types of disease have on the quality of life.

One of the most important shortcomings is not having an aggregate indicator of morbidity and mortality. For example, how do we compare the mortality from measles with morbidity from manic depression? This inability can result in an arbitrary distribution of resources between health programs designed for mortality reduction and health programs designed for morbidity reduction. If outcome indicators are used to define health priorities and to identify disadvantaged groups, policymakers are establishing an ethical dimension for receipt of public resources. Any combined indicator of health status should explicitly incorporate a set of social values and preferences.

DALYs and HeaLYs. This issue is not new to researchers and policymakers. Over the last few years, new indicators have been developed, known as DALYs and Health Adjusted Life Years (HeaLYs). These indicators simultaneously consider both premature death and nonfatal health consequences of disease and injury. (See Morrow and Bryant, 1995.) The indicators are based on an incidence perspective and provide an estimate of the number of years of life lost from premature death and the number of years of life lived with a disability arising from new cases of disease or injury. (See Murray and Lopez, 1994; Hyder et al., 1998.) DALYs and HeaLYs in relation to morbidity and mortality are discussed in detail in Chapter 3.

While DALYs and HeaLYs represent a major advance, they are not without problems (again, discussed in more detail in Chapter 3). DALYs, for example, do not include social costs and do not weigh such quality of life (QOL) measures as emotional and social well-being. QOL measures are now available for a wide range of conditions (e.g., in arthritis patients) and have proven to be reliable measures of well-being.

Measures of Process. Given these concerns, process measures—which are particularly valuable for evaluating the quality of care—are an alternative indicator to simply measuring outcomes. Process measures can show whether the right diagnosis was made, whether the correct advice was given, or whether the appropriate disease was excluded. For process measures to be useful, they must be closely linked to outcomes. This is less common than the nonphysician might think. For example, internal-external carotid bypass operations to treat cerebrovascular illness were performed for years in the United States (and presumably done quite well in leading medical centers), until a longitudinal clinical trial showed not only that operations did not help but that patients actually died sooner than their matched controls.

However, if processes (such as the correct choice and dose of antibiotics for pneumonia) are linked tightly to better outcomes, there are three advantages of measuring processes instead of just outcomes. First, processes occur more commonly and are easier to observe. Second, better processes using the same resources can more efficiently produce better health. Third, better processes can produce the same health at less cost, leading to a cost savings.

Kinds and Sources of Data

So far, we have argued that to make informed health care policy interventions, policymakers can use a simple system to categorize the types of data they need. It is also useful to briefly distinguish the kinds of data that are commonly used for policymaking and the sources of these data.

Qualitative Versus Quantitative Data. Data are often described as qualitative or quantitative. While helpful in describing what data are being gathered, such a categorization generates an unfortunate and unnecessary schism between the two kinds of data—a schism that reflects differences between data collectors more than the relative importance of the data in policymaking. For example, institutional analyses and detailed descriptions of a hospital system are more qualitative and are typically done by political scientists and policy analysts.

**Box 2.1: Implementing Continuing Medical Education:
An Illustration of Evidence-Based Health Policy**

Changing physicians' behavior is very difficult to accomplish. A potential approach is to use continuing medical education (CME) to affect the way physicians treat their patients, thus improving physician competence and performance and, ultimately, patient health outcomes. CME entails several types of methods: comprehensive clinical management of general medical conditions, including investigation, diagnosis, and treatment; the use of laboratory and radiological investigations; prescribing practices; patient counseling; and primary prevention activities. Although such CME methods have been a part of health policy for decades, policymakers have been concerned about how effective CME actually is in improving physician capabilities and patient outcomes.

The only way to answer the effectiveness question is to understand the link between the studies conducted, the evidence they produce, the policies implemented based on that evidence, and the results in terms of process outcomes (improvements in how physicians practice) and patient outcomes (improvements in the health of the individuals treated). In a 1984 literature review, Haynes and Davis examined several randomized control trials (RCTs) of CME. (See Haynes and Davis et al., 1984.) These analyses provided strong evidence that some CME interventions improved physicians' ability to perform in the test situation and some evidence that interventions actually improved physicians' clinical performance. However, the analyses clearly showed only weak evidence that CME changed health outcomes. Research to find ways to make CME more effective continued beyond 1984. A more recent literature survey (see McLaughlin and Donaldson, 1991) examined CME interventions between 1984 and 1991 and found that CME effectiveness had increased compared with the results a decade earlier, especially in terms of improving patient outcomes. This finding was confirmed by a 1992 meta-analysis that examined the evidence from 50 RCTs (out of over 700 reported studies on CME). (See Davis et al., 1992.) The RCTs focused on improving the performance of internists, general practitioners, and family physicians and on the resulting improvements in patients' outcomes. Eighteen of the 50 RCTs measured the effect of CME interventions on patient outcomes; of these 10 were inconclusive, and 8 showed positive changes in at least one measure.

Several factors were found to lead to better outcomes. Vinicor and associates showed that facilities that implemented didactic presentations, protocols, physician reminders, and patient education strategies significantly improved diabetic outcomes—specifically, physiological parameters of glycosylated hemoglobin, fasting plasma glucose, diastolic blood pressure, and body weight. (See Vinicor et al., 1987.) Another RCT showed that in an emergency department, a combination of protocols, feedback, and traditional teaching methods improved patient outcomes, as measured two weeks after discharge and again at three months. (See Linn, 1980.) A third RCT (see Rogers, 1982) demonstrated that computerized medical records for prompting physician activities led to positive patient outcomes in mitigating obesity and renal disease.

Besides contributing to an understanding of the effects that CME has on physician behavior and patient outcomes, the continuing analysis of CME effectiveness has also allowed policymakers to identify which forms of CME produce better results. (See Davis et al., 1995.) The evaluation of CME is a good example of policy that was implemented and later refined even though data were not initially available. The "post policy" research showed that simply publishing and disseminating clinical policies or practice guidelines does not have positive effects on physician performance or patient outcomes. But more-specific practice protocols and clinical algorithms—coupled with printed materials, workshops, and "practice rehearsals"—improve physician performance and patient care outcomes.

As policymakers have understood the implications of these study results, the CME programs they implement have evolved over time to take advantage of what has been shown to work.

Measuring health conditions, which relies on inpatient registrations, and utilization, which relies on discharge figures or medical records from clinics, are usually done by health services researchers. Both types of data would obviously be useful to policymakers trying to shift care to the outpatient setting.

Qualitative data typically are derived from case studies that provide in-depth analyses and focus on the interrelationships between factors—factors that are likely to be perceptions and subjective evaluations. (See Yin, 1994.) They also come from focus groups, which are often used, for example, to review advocacy programs or to test survey instruments, and from ethnographic studies, which are particularly important in evaluating cultural perceptions of disease. For example, when researchers in China found that a third of all newborns admitted to a tertiary hospital in the winter suffered from hypothermia, qualitative ethnographic research showed that fathers, who cared for newborns while mothers were confined to bed for weeks following delivery, were critical in preventing the problem; thus, an education program targeted at men was required. (See Peabody et al., 1996a.)

Quantitative data and analysis are more extensive, more familiar to most analysts, and more commonly used. This is partly because, in addition to such quantitative items as price and staffing levels, many qualitative measures, such as alive or dead or rich or poor, can be presented as counts, rates, or proportions. It is also because quantitative information easily summarizes large amounts of data in a very brief format, such as a single figure or percentage. Thus, the use and interest in quantitative data and quantitative reasoning is quite broad.

Routinely Collected Data Versus Specially Commissioned Studies. Another way to categorize the data is by how they are collected. Many of the data policymakers use are gathered through routinely collected information systems, such as vital registries, national health accounts (NHAs)—which are discussed in Chapter 4—ministry of health budgets, national household surveys, national provider and patient surveys, insurance rolls, medical discharge data, medical records, surveillance systems, and regulatory commissions (e.g., drugs and facility licensing).

Some routinely collected data, such as information on management or licensing from institutions, are descriptive and, when available, of enormous value to other analysts and policymakers. However, researchers find that many routine data sources, such as registries, vary significantly in how complete they are. As a result, secondary data analysis, which relies on data collected for one purpose (e.g., insurance claim forms) to be used for another purpose (e.g., information on cost of services), needs to be supplemented by specific surveys. Another problem of routinely collected data is the cost (in equipment and personnel) to establish and maintain a health information system (HIS). Enormous resources have been spent on HISs in developing countries—resources that have produced poor-quality data and little information for policy. (See Cibulskis and Izard, 1996.)

The need for supplementary information is vital to health reform and policy evaluation. External agencies have assisted in conducting specialized household surveys. The United States Agency for International Development (USAID), the United Nations Fund for Population Affairs (UNFPA), and specific countries sponsored the World Fertility surveys from 1974 to 1982 in 43 countries. The World Bank's Living Standards Measurement Surveys (LSMS) have been implemented in 19 countries, and nine additional studies are in the field. These surveys collect detailed economic information, as well as demographic and health data, and have results available within a year. Since 1984, USAID, countries, and other donors have completed 58 demographic and health surveys (eight in Asia).[1]

Population-based surveys are particularly valuable for policymaking. They provide three key pieces of information. First, they provide information on nonusers of health care—typically, the poor and marginalized—who would be overlooked in facility-based surveys. Second, they provide weights or corrections for data collected from unrepresentative samples, such as hospital discharges. Third, they get at determinants of the demand for types of health care, such as the use of private practitioners, that are typically hard to measure.

Other Sources of Data. Beyond routinely collected data and specially designed studies, another large source of data is published studies in the academic and scientific literature. In health, this literature is often focused on medical specialty areas, but there are a growing number of journals dedicated to policy, international health issues, and development; journals such as *Social Science and Medicine* and the newly released *Journal of Health Services Research and Policy* are beginning to bridge this gap. The scientific literature tends to be the source for advances in clinical care. It is here that RCTs are presented and case series of new diseases and syndromes are first reported. These publications, however, target academic audiences generally; as such, they are often more concerned with internal validity than external generalizability. Although less abundant, there are also journals centered on other disciplines, such as demography, economic development, and political science.

In addition, data from routinely collected systems are often modeled by researchers as a way to generate more useful data or measures. For example, national census data are modeled to enable researchers to calculate measures of life expectancy. Data are also sometimes provided by expert judgment. One example is the Delphi method, which is a formalized process designed to help coalesce expert opinion; another example of expert judgment is review articles prepared by self-selected experts or a group of experts to canvas a subject or area and report on their opinion of the current state of knowledge.

The meta-analysis is an increasingly popular way to report on the accumulated evidence. This technique uses a collection of statistical methods and combines quantitative information from several sources to give a summary figure with uncertainty. Once available, it provides clinicians, analysts, or policymakers state-of-the-art information. Often, when no single study is compelling by itself because it is too small, aggregated findings provide clear evidence in favor of a policy or clinical intervention.

Table 2.1 summarizes the types, collection processes, and typical sources for the seven categories of data discussed earlier. As can be seen, with the exception of data for individual and provider behaviors and for the political, social, cultural, and institutional environment, most of the needed data are quantitative; moreover, while routinely collected data are needed throughout, specially commissioned studies are also needed to fill gaps.

---

[1]The eight in Asia were in Bangladesh, Indonesia, Kazakhstan, Kyrgyz Republic, Nepal, Philippines, Sri Lanka, and Thailand.

Table 2.1

Categories of Data, Process of Collection, and Typical Sources

Category of Data	Types of Data	Data Process	Typical Sources
1. Demographic and socio-economic factors	Primarily quantitative	• Routinely collected public information systems (HIS) • Surveys • Models	• National census • National household surveys • LSM surveys • RAND surveys • DHS surveys
2. Access to basic necessities/ access to health care	Primarily quantitative	• Surveys • Routinely collected public information systems (HIS) • Private information systems	• National census • National household surveys • National provider surveys • Hospital discharge data • Insurance rolls • LSM surveys • DHS surveys • United Nations Educational, Scientific and Cultural Organization (UNESCO) • WHO
3. Public and private resources	Primarily quantitative	• Surveys • Routinely collected public information systems (HIS) • Private information systems	• National household surveys • National providers surveys • Ministry of health budget • National health accounts • Microaccounting systems • Hospital discharge data • Hospital invoice data • LSM surveys • DHS surveys
4. Individual and provider behaviors	Primarily qualitative	• Surveys • Social experiments	• National household surveys • National providers surveys • LSM surveys • DHS surveys • Academic literature • Interviews • Case studies
5. Clinical practice	Primarily quantitative	• Experiments • Surveys • Expert judgment • Meta-analyses	• National providers surveys • National patients surveys • Literature and research reports • Case studies • Disease reporting
6. Political, social, and institutional environment	Primarily qualitative	• Surveys • Social experiments	• Media • Interviews • Case studies
7. Health outcomes	Primarily quantitative	• Surveys • Experiments • Expert judgment • Models • Routinely collected public information systems (HIS)	• National household surveys • Hospital discharge data • LSM surveys • DHS surveys • Vital registration systems • Surveillance systems

SIGNIFICANT DATA GAPS

What is the status of data in Asia? We examined the current state of data availability in each data category for 44 selected countries in Asia and the Pacific[2]

[2]Of the 44 countries, 36 are designated by the Asian Development Bank as developing member countries (DMCs): Afghanistan, Bangladesh, Bhutan, Cambodia, China, Cook Islands, Fiji, Hong Kong, India, Indonesia, Kazakhstan, Kiribati, Democratic People's Republic of Korea (North Korea), Republic of Korea (South Korea), Kyrgyz Republic, People's Democratic Republic of Lao, Malaysia, Maldives, Marshall Islands, Federated States of Micronesia, Mongolia, Myanmar, Nauru, Nepal, Pakistan, Papua New Guinea, Philippines, Singapore, Solomon Islands, Sri Lanka, Taipei China (Taiwan), Thailand, Tonga, Tuvalu, Vanuatu, and the Socialist Republic of Viet Nam.

and focused, where possible, on the developing countries in Asia. Despite this focus, here and throughout the rest of the book, we draw on examples from all Asian countries and from countries around the world if a better example or a more relevant piece of information was available.

We have divided the 44 countries into six geographic regions:

1. **South Asia**—Afghanistan, Bangladesh, Bhutan, India, Maldives, Mauritius, Nepal, Pakistan, Seychelles, Sri Lanka;

2. **Southeast Asia**—Cambodia, People's Democratic Republic of Lao, Myanmar, Philippines, Seychelles, Socialist Republic of Viet Nam;

3. **East Asia**—China, Mongolia, and Democratic People's Republic of Korea;

4. **Central Asian Republics**—Kazakhstan, Republic of Kyrgyz, Uzbekistan;

5. **Pacific Islands**—Cook Islands, Fiji, Kiribati, Marshall Islands, Federated States of Micronesia, Nauru, New Caledonia, Niue, Papua New Guinea, Solomon Islands, Tokelau Island, Tonga, Tuvalu, Vanuatu, Wallis and Futuna Islands, Western Samoa;

6. **High-Performing Asian Economies**—Hong Kong, Indonesia, Republic of Korea, Malaysia, Singapore, Taipei China (Taiwan), Thailand.

The tables that follow would typically belong in an appendix; however, our intent is to highlight the overall patterns in data availability—something that the holes in the tables convey rather easily. We also want to emphasize the link between data—whether they be available or missing—and policymaking. We have put the source information, a glossary, and category definitions for the tables discussed below into an appendix. But the tables, placed within the text, underscore the importance policymakers should attach to using the best available information to develop policy.

Status of Data for 44 Selected Asian Countries

When we examine the status of the data for the selected countries, we generally find significant gaps. The gaps vary by category and by source of data. The issue of data variability underscores two points made earlier. First, policy must be made, and will continue to be made, even in the absence of reliable information. Second, some countries, many of them very poor, have made remarkable progress in filling the data gaps—suggesting that more can be done. After discussing the data available for policymaking in Asia, we turn to four important steps that can be taken to improve this situation.

Demographic and Socioeconomic Factors. Tables 2.2, 2.3, and 2.4 contain data for the population structure and dynamics (Table 2.2), population distribution by region (Table 2.3), and distribution of income (Table 2.4). As Table 2.2 shows, most countries in Asia (and, for that matter, around the world) collect basic information about the size of their populations and their structure by sex and age. In fact, all the countries on our list have this information. A few countries do not have projected population figures, but these can be inputed without great expense from national census data.

Table 2.2

Population Structure and Dynamics in 44 Asian Countries

	Population in Millions			Average Annual Pop. Growth (%)	Crude Birth Rate (per 1000)	Crude Death Rate (per 1000)	Fertility Rate	Age Structure of Population (%) and Projection in 2025					
	Projected Population							0-14 years		15-64 years		65+ years	
Country	1995	2000	2025	1991-2000	1993	1993	1995	1991	2025	1991	2025	1991	2025
South Asia													
Afghanistan	23.50	26.70	41.6	2.8	4.8e	2.8e	6.9	42	37.2	55.2	59.1	2.8	3.7
Bangladesh	119.80	131	180	1.9	29	10	3.5	42.3	26.2	56.8	69	0.9	4.8
Bhutan	0.70	2	3	2.4	40	9.0	5.7	40.6	34.3	55.8	61.7	3.6	4
India	929.40	1017	1365	1.8	28	9	3.5	35.8	23.9	60.2	68.1	4	8
Maldives	0.30	0.28	0.46	2.4	27	5	6.7	44.6	33.7	52.1	62.2	3.3	4.1
Mauritius	1.10	1	1	1.1	21	7	2.2	29	20.4	67.5	66.7	3.5	12.9
Nepal	21.50	24	38	2.5	39	13	4.6	43.4	30.8	53.7	64.7	2.9	4.5
Pakistan	129.90	148	244	2.8	40	9	5.3	44	29.6	53.5	65.5	2.5	4.9
Seychelles	0.10	0.08	0.08	0.9a	...	...	2.5	...	...	...	...	...	...
Sri Lanka	18.10	19	24	1.1	20	6	2.4	31.7	21.3	64.2	66.1	4.1	12.6
Southeast Asia													
Cambodia	10.00	10.50	15.5	2.5	41.4	16.6	4.7	40.6	37.7	56.2	58.4	3.2	3.9
Lao, PDR	4.90	6	10	2.9	44	15	6.5	44.5	37.1	51.7	59.3	3.8	3.6
Myanmar	45.10	51.50	71.3	2.1	28	8.6	3.5	37.9	28.6	58.1	66.2	4	5.2
Philippines	68.60	74	102	1.9	30	6	3.8	39.2	24	59.1	68.5	1.7	7.5
Viet Nam	73.50	81.50	110	2.0a	30	8	3.1	38.5	26.4	56.8	68	4.7	5.6
East Asia													
China	1203.30	1290	1569	1.3	19	8	1.9	27	21.2	66.4	67.1	6.6	11.7
Korea, DPR	23.92	25.90	31.9	1.9	20.4	5.3	2.2	28.6	21.9	67.3	69.8	4.1	8.3
Mongolia	2.50	2.80	4.2	2.6	27	7	3.4	41.2	31.2	55.6	63.5	3.2	5.3
Central Asian Republics													
Kazakhstan	16.60	18	22	0.7	20	7	2.3	31.6	22.3	62.4	64.6	6	13.1
Kyrgyz, Rep.	4.50	4.9	6.8	0.4	28	7	3.3	...	...	...	...	...	...
Uzbekistan	22.84	26	42	2.4	31	6	3.7	41.6	27.5	53.9	65.5	4.5	7
Pacific Islands													
Cook Islands	0.02	0.02	0.02	0.2b	28.4	6.1	1.2d	27.4	19.3	66.9	69.6	5.7	11.1
Fiji	0.78	0.80	0.9	1.1a	23.6	4.6	2.8	38	24.6	58.7	66.8	3.3	8.6
Kiribati	0.08	0.09	0.12	2.2a	29.4	9.2	3.8	40.8	...	55.8	...	3.4	...
Marshall Islands	0.05	0.07	0.12	3.6a	49.2	4.3	7.2	51.5	...	...	...	...	...
Micronesia, FS	0.12	0.15	0.26	3.5a	37.9	8	4.6	46.1	...	50.3	...	3.6	...
Nauru	0.01	...	...	2.6a	24	5	7.5	41.8	...	55.4	...	2.8	...
New Caledonia	0.18	0.2	0.25	1.8a	24.9	5.3	2.5	30	...	...	...	...	...
Niue	2.2f	...	...	2.1	31.1	7.8	3.5f	36.7	...	56.1	...	7.2	...
Papua New Guinea	4.30	5	7	2.3	33	11	4.8	40.3	29	57.2	66.5	2.5	4.5
Solomon Islands	0.38	0.44	0.76	3.3a	37	4	5.2	45.9	36	51.3	60.1	2.8	3.9
Tokelau Island	0.002	...	...	3.0	31	8.2	13.0f	46.3	...	46.3	...	7.4	...
Tonga	0.10	0.10	0.12	0.6a	24.3	3.9	3.3	40	...	55.7	...	4.3	...
Tuvalu	0.01	...	...	1.6	25.5	9.1	3	26.1	...	69.4	...	4.5	...
Vanuatu	0.17	0.19	0.31	2.5a	37	9	5.0	44	...	52.8	...	3.2	...
Wallis and Futuna Islands	0.014	...	...	2.3f	31	6	4.6d	41.9	...	...	...	...	...
Western Samoa	0.17	0.16	0.18	0.2a	25.9	4.9	4.3	41	...	53	...	6	...
High-Performing Asian Economies													
Hong Kong	6.2	6	7	0.8	11	6	1.2	20.6	15.4	70.3	61.4	9.1	23.2
Indonesia	193.3	206	265	1.4	25.3	7.5	2.7	35.8	26.6	60.2	68.4	4	5
Korea, Rep.	44.9	47	53	0.8	16	6	1.8	25.1	18.2	71	66.6	3.9	15.2
Malaysia	20.14	22	31	2.2	28	5	3.4	38.6	23.9	58.5	67.6	2.9	8.5
Singapore	3.0	3	4	1.5	16	6	1.7	22.9	18.3	70.7	63.5	6.4	18.2
Taipei, China	21.1	21.9	25.4	0.8	16d	5d	1.8	...	...	...	...	6.5c	13.0c
Thailand	58.2	65	82	1.4	16.3	5.5	2.1	32.4	21.8	65.9	68.5	1.7	9.7

MAIN SOURCES: WHO, 1994a, 1995a, 1995b, 1995c, 1997b; World Bank, 1996a, 1997a. OTHER SOURCES: (a) WHO, 1994a, period 1990-95; (b) WHO, 1994a, period 2000-2005; (c) Hsiao et al., 1989; (d) Peabody, 1995; (e) WHO, 1996b; (f) WHO, 1995a, natural rate, different years (1980-1990, 1992, 1993).
Note the following abbreviations: China - People's Republic of China; Korea, DPR - Democratic People's Republic of Korea (North Korea); Lao, PDR - People's Democratic Republic of Lao; Viet Nam - Socialist Republic of Viet Nam; Kyrgyz, Rep. - Republic of Kyrgyz; Micronesia, FS - Federated States of Micronesia; Korea, Rep. - Republic of Korea (South Korea); China, Taipei - Republic of China (Taiwan).

Table 2.3 presents data about the distribution of the population in urban areas and rural areas. Data for 1995 on the percentage of the total population that is urban are available for 40 of the 44 countries. Growth rate data are less available. The urban population is expanding rapidly in Asia, producing epidemiological changes with important impacts for services, planning, and allocation. This is often viewed as an alarming trend, but only 57 percent of the countries have data about their 1990–1994 urban growth rates and only 43 percent have data about the percentage of their populations living in capital cities.

The overall population growth rates shown in Tables 2.2 and 2.3 have generally declined and a rapid process of urbanization is in progress. The composition of the Asian populations is also changing. According to population projections for the years 1995–2025, as shown in Table 2.2, the percentage of the population between 0 and 14 years of age is decreasing, while the percentage of the population 65 years and older is increasing.

Table 2.4 charts a standard distribution of income or expenditure (consumption), by share of population quintiles. Despite its primary impact on health, poverty is characterized (by income quintiles) for only 14 of the 44 countries. The table shows that distribution of income is highly concentrated in Asian countries. Typically, the poorest 10 percent of the population controls between 2.5 percent and 4.2 percent of total income, whereas the richest 10 percent controls between 24 percent and 37 percent. In countries with rapid economic growth (e.g., Thailand), this concentration has been significant. In China, after seven years of economic liberalization, the richest 20 percent of the population already controls more than 40 percent of the total national income. In Chapter 5, we will look at how poverty levels and income distribution relate to poor health.

Measures of Access to Health Care and Other Basic Needs. Tables 2.5 and 2.6 capture the levels of access to basic needs and health care in the 44 countries. Table 2.5 provides data for three measures of basic needs—child malnutrition, adult literacy rate, and sanitation. In terms of child malnutrition, we have data for 39 out of 44 countries. For countries such as Bangladesh, Nepal, and India, the data paint a dramatic picture. Widespread protein-energy malnutrition in children there inhibits their growth, increases their risk of morbidity, affects their cognitive development, and reduces their subsequent school performance and labor productivity. Short-term interventions, such as micronutrient supplementation, are still on the policy agenda, but such high malnutrition levels command that sustainable policies be devoted to improving the level of income of the poor population and the productivity of the agricultural sector. Unfortunately, these types of interventions often escape the attention of health policymakers. This might be because such data are not typically used in health, either because interventions are outside health policymakers' jurisdiction or because formal mechanisms are not set up for intersectoral collaboration.

For education, the adult literacy indicator is available for 31 of the 44 countries. It is not available for the Central Asia Republics (although it is well known that in the past these areas had high literacy rates) and for countries like Nauru or Micronesia. In South and Southeast Asia, adult literacy rates are still low in most countries, the problem being more serious for women. Overall, access to education for women is, on average, 18 percent lower than for men.

Table 2.3

Population Distribution by Region in 44 Asian Countries

| | Urban Population | | | | | Concentration in Capital | |
| | As a Percentage of Total Population | | | Average Annual Growth Rate % | | As a Percentage of Urban | As a Percentage of Total |
Country	1980	1990-1992	1995	1980-1990	1990-1994	1990	1990
South Asia							
Afghanistan	15.0	18.2	20	4.0	...	...	...
Bangladesh	11	16.4	18.3	5.9	4.9	39	6
Bhutan	3.9a	5.3a	6.4a	5.3a	6.0a	...	...
India	23	25.5	26.8	2.2	2.9	4	1
Maldives	22.3a	29.6	26.8	5.8a	5.5a	...	...
Mauritius	42	40.6	41	0.4	1.4	37	15
Nepal	6	10.9	13.7	8	7.4	17	2
Pakistan	28	32	34.7	4.5	4.7	1	0
Seychelles	...	...	54.5	...	...	...	...
Sri Lanka	21.6a	21.4a	22.4a	1.4	2.2	17	4
Southeast Asia							
Cambodia	...	11.6	20.7	...	...	...	...
Lao, PDR	13	18.6	21.7	6.2	6.4	52	10
Myanmar	24	24.8	26.2	2.5	3.3	32	8
Philippines	38	42.7	54.2	5.2	4.4	29	14
Viet Nam	19	19.9	20.8	2.5	3	24	5
East Asia							
China	17	26.2	30.3	3	4.3	4	1
Korea, DPR	56.9a	59.8	61.3	2.2a	2.4a	...	...
Mongolia	52	57.9	60.9	3.9	2.9	37	22
Central Asian Republics							
Kazakhstan	54	...	59.7	1.9	0.9	...	...
Kyrgyz, Rep.	38	...	39	1.9	0.8	...	...
Uzbekistan	41	...	41.3	2.5	2.6	...	...
Pacific Islands							
Cook Islands	...	58.0	60.4	...	...	...	...
Fiji	...	39.3	40.7	...	...	...	...
Kiribati	...	34.8	35.7	...	...	...	...
Marshall Islands	...	...	69.1	...	...	...	...
Micronesia, Fed. States of	...	59.7	28	...	...	...	...
Nauru	...	...	100	...	...	...	...
New Caledonia	...	...	60a	...	...	...	...
Niue	...	30.5	...	...	...	...	...
Papua New Guinea	13	15.8	16	3.6	3.7	35	5
Solomon Islands	...	14.7	17.1	...	...	...	...
Tokelau Island	37	...	...	...	...	...	...
Tonga	...	...	41.1	...	...	...	...
Tuvalu	...	42.5	46.2	...	...	...	...
Vanuatu	...	17	19.3	...	...	...	...
Wallis and Futuna Islands	...	...	...	...	...	...	...
Western Samoa	...	...	21	...	...	...	...
High-Performing Asian Economies							
Hong Kong	92	95.2	95a	1.6	1.7	100	95
Indonesia	22	28.8	35.4	5.3	3.8	17	5
Korea, Republic of	57	74.4	81.3	3.8	2.9	35	26
Malaysia	42	43	53.7	4.4	4	19	10
Singapore	100	100	100	1.7	2	100	100
Taipei, China	...	...	...	...	...	...	...
Thailand	17	...	20	2.8	2.4	69	13

MAIN SOURCES: World Bank, 1993a and 1996a. OTHER SOURCES: (a) WHO, 1995a.
Note the following abbreviations: China - People's Republic of China; Korea, DPR - Democratic People's Republic of Korea (North Korea); Lao, PDR - People's Democratic Republic of Lao; Viet Nam - Socialist Republic of Viet Nam; Kyrgyz, Rep. - Republic of Kyrgyz; Micronesia, FS - Federated States of Micronesia; Korea, Rep. - Republic of Korea (South Korea); Taipei, China - Republic of China (Taiwan).

Table 2.4

Distribution of Income in 44 Asian Countries

Country	GNP Per Capita 1995 ($US)	Year Reported	Gini Index (%)	Lowest 10%	Lowest 20%	Second Quintile	Third Quintile	Fourth Quintile	Highest 20%	Highest 10%	Poverty % people living on <$1/day (PPP) 1981-1985
South Asia											
Afghanistan	160	...	...	...	...	...	...	...	...	...	...
Bangladesh	240	1992	28.3	4.1	9.4	13.5	17.2	22	37.9	23.7	...
Bhutan	420		...	...	...	...	...	...	...	...	...
India	340	1992	33.8	3.7	8.5	12.1	15.8	21.1	42.6	28.4	52.5
Maldives	990		...	...	...	...	...	...	...	...	...
Mauritius	3380		...	...	...	...	...	...	...	...	...
Nepal	200	1984/85	36.7	4	9.1	12.9	16.7	21.8	39.5	25	53.1
Pakistan	460	1991	31.2	3.4	8.4	12.9	16.9	22.2	39.7	25.2	11.6
Seychelles	6620		...	...	...	...	...	...	...	...	...
Sri Lanka	700	1990	30.1	3.8	8.9	13.1	16.9	21.7	39.3	25.2	4.0
Southeast Asia											
Cambodia	270		...	...	...	...	...	...	...	...	...
Lao, PDR	350	1992	30.4	4.2	9.6	12.9	16.3	21	40.2	26.4	...
Myanmar	220		...	...	...	...	...	...	...	...	...
Philippines	1050	1988	40.7	2.8	6.5	10.1	14.4	21.2	47.8	32.1	27.5
Viet Nam	240	1993	35.7	3.5	7.8	11.4	15.4	21.4	44	29	...
East Asia											
China	620	1992	41.5	2.6	6.2	10.5	15.8	23.6	43.9	26.8	29.4
Korea, DPR	436		...	...	...	...	...	...	...	...	...
Mongolia	310		...	...	...	...	...	...	...	...	...
Central Asian Republics											
Kazakhstan	1330	1993	32.7	3.1	7.5	12.3	16.9	22.9	40.4	24.9	...
Kyrgyz, Rep.	700		...	...	...	...	...	...	...	...	18.9
Uzbekistan	970		...	...	...	...	...	...	...	...	...
Pacific Islands											
Cook Islands	350a		...	...	...	...	...	...	...	...	...
Fiji	2440		...	...	...	...	...	...	...	...	...
Kiribati	920		...	...	...	...	...	...	...	...	...
Marshall Islands	1600a	1988	...	...	...	...	...	...	...	...	...
Micronesia, FS	2010	1985	...	...	...	...	...	...	...	...	...
Nauru	8070a		...	...	...	...	...	...	...	...	...
New Caledonia	13400a		...	...	...	...	...	...	...	...	...
Niue	3100a		...	...	...	...	...	...	...	...	...
Papua New Guinea	1160		...	...	...	...	...	...	...	...	...
Solomon Islands	910		...	...	...	...	...	...	...	...	...
Tokelau Island	3550a		...	...	...	...	...	...	...	...	...
Tonga	1630		...	...	...	...	...	...	...	...	...
Tuvalu	400a		...	...	...	...	...	...	...	...	...
Vanuatu	1150		...	...	...	...	...	...	...	...	...
Wallis and Futuna Isl.	1400a		...	...	...	...	...	...	...	...	...
Western Samoa	1120		...	...	...	...	...	...	...	...	...
High-Performing Asian Economies											
Hong Kong	22990	1980	...	...	5.4	10.8	15.2	21.6	47	31.3	...
Indonesia	980	1993	31.7	3.9	8.7	12.3	16.3	22.1	40.7	25.6	14.5
Korea, Rep.	8260		...	...	...	...	...	...	...	...	5.6
Malaysia	3890		...	...	...	...	...	...	...	...	
Singapore	26730	1982/83	...	...	5.1	9.9	14.6	21.4	48.9	33.5	...
Taipei, China	12790	1993	...	...	...	...	...	...	...	...	
Thailand	2740	1992	46.2	2.5	5.6	8.7	13	20	52.7	37.1	0.1

MAIN SOURCE: World Bank, 1996a, 1996b, 1997a. OTHER SOURCES: (a) WHO, 1995a, years 1989-1991.
Note the following abbreviations: China - People's Republic of China; Korea, DPR - Democratic People's Republic of Korea (North Korea); Lao, PDR - People's Democratic Republic of Lao; Viet Nam - Socialist Republic of Viet Nam; Kyrgyz, Rep. - Republic of Kyrgyz; Micronesia, FS - Federated States of Micronesia; Korea, Rep. - Republic of Korea (South Korea); Taipei, China - Republic of China (Taiwan). PPP = purchasing power parity.

In Afghanistan, Bangladesh, Bhutan, Nepal, Pakistan, and the Solomon Islands, the situation is particularly critical, with less than 50 percent of the adult population literate. Such levels of literacy severely limit any policy effort to improve health status.

Table 2.5 provides two measures of sanitation—access to safe water and access to sanitation facilities—with safe water data available for 41 of the 44 countries and sanitation data available for 40 of the 44 countries. As a rule, residents are more likely to have access to safe water than quality sanitation; the major exceptions to this rule are China and Malaysia.

Table 2.6 captures the available data on four measures of health care—access to health care services within one hour, prevalence of contraceptive use in families, prenatal care utilization, and immunization rates. These four measures are linked to clinical interventions characterized as highly cost-effective (discussed in Chapter 3). The recognized utility of these measures is reflected in their general availability—for example, 86 percent of the 44 Asian countries report data on access to basic health care.

Data on contraceptive methods are less frequently reported—by about 61 percent of the 44 countries. Contraceptive methods are slowly becoming popular in Asian populations; still, in five Asian countries, the percentage of women using some type of contraception is less than 20 percent.

The prenatal care indicator is also generally available, with 73 percent of the 44 countries reporting these data. In Afghanistan and Nepal, only 8 and 9 percent of the women, respectively, receive prenatal care, whereas in Singapore, Fiji, and the Cook Islands, level of access to prenatal services is above 90 percent. On average, the percentage of Asian women who receive prenatal care fluctuates between 40 percent and 60 percent. An increase in the level of access to contraceptive and prenatal services should be one of the primary concerns of policymakers.

Finally, information on immunization coverage is almost universally available (only 3 of the 44 countries do not report data) through the Expanded Program on Immunization (EPI) Information System. (See WHO, 1996a.) The data themselves tell a fairly optimistic story. Except for Afghanistan and Lao, immunization coverage has considerably expanded in Asia, primarily due to EPI programs implemented by WHO and UNICEF.

Looking across Tables 2.5 and 2.6, we see significant variation between countries. In countries such as Hong Kong, Cook Islands, Singapore, or the Democratic People's Republic of Korea, access to health care, prenatal care, safe water, and sanitation is nearly universal. As we discussed in Chapter 1, the level of income per capita alone does not explain this variation. Indeed, China has an average performance close to the Republic of Korea, although the Republic of Korea has a per capita GDP 15 times greater. This shows the importance of coupling policies to promote growth with ones that redistribute the gains ensuing from this growth.

An Inventory of Public and Private Resources. Table 2.7 compiles health expenditure data. It is immediately apparent how little is known about private expenditures. Where data are available, the level of private spending is quite high, even in poorer countries. Many analysts believe that in the absence of household expenditure data, out-of-pocket expenses are significantly underestimated.

Table 2.5

Access to Basic Necessities in 44 Asian Countries (%)

Country	Child Malnutrition (% children with <80% standard weight for age) 1985-1995	Adult Literacy Rate		Sanitation	
		Both Sexes 1995	Females 1995	Access to Safe Water 1985-1996	Access to Sanitation 1994-1996
South Asia					
Afghanistan	40	31.5	15	10	8
Bangladesh	68	38.1	35.9	49.1u, 96r	41.1u, 36r
Bhutan	38	54	28.1	74u, 58r	90u, 70r
Maldives	39	98.9	98.78	94u, 78r	98u, 26r
India	53	52	37.7	84u, 82r	50u, 3.7r
Mauritius	15	...	...	100	100
Nepal	49	40.0	23	59	23
Pakistan	40	37.8	24.4	60	30
Seychelles	6	...	...	98.5c	65.1b
Sri Lanka	38	87	87.9	70	75
Southeast Asia					
Cambodia	38	...	...	13	...
Lao, PDR	40	56.6	44.4	41	30
Myanmar	31	83.1	77.7	59.7	42.7
Philippines	30	94.6	94.3	84	75
Viet Nam	45	93.7	91.2	38	21
East Asia					
China	16	81.5	72.7	46	96.4b
Korea, DPR	5	100c	100c	100	100
Mongolia	12	82.9	77.2	54	75.5a
Central Asian Republics					
Kazakhstan	1	...	...	...	...
Kyrgyz, Rep.	...	...	...	75	53
Uzbekistan	4	...	...	...	18
Pacific Islands					
Cook Islands	1.0	100c*	85	95e	95e
Fiji	8	91.6	89.3	77	74b
Kiribati	3.01	90.0d	...	99	100
Marshall Islands	9.0	90.7d	...	67.5e	36.5e
Micronesia, FS	31	...	...	21.6e	39e
Nauru	...	...	...	...	...
New Caledonia	8.6	...	...	76e	72e
Niue	2.2	...	...	100e	100e
Papua New Guinea	30	72.2	62.7	31	26
Solomon Islands	21	30.0d	...	80a	u=73,r=21a
Tokelau Island	10	...	...	94e	64e
Tonga	2	100.0 d	...	100	100
Tuvalu	3.3	...	...	100	85
Vanuatu	7.4	70.0	...	72e	u=90,r=88c**
Wallis and Futuna Islands	3.0	...	...	100e	47.5e
Western Samoa	4.0	70.0d	...	81.8a	93.9
High-Performing Asian Economies					
Hong Kong	...	8	...	99e	99e
Indonesia	40	86.3	81.4	87u, 54r	80u, 61r
Korea, Rep.	...	98	96.7	89e	100
Malaysia	23	83.5	78.1	90	94
Singapore	14	91.1	86.3	100	100
Taipei, China	...	93.0	...	86	...
Thailand	13	93.8	91.6	89.3	95.7

MAIN SOURCES: WHO, 1996a, 1997b; World Bank, 1996a, 1997a. OTHER SOURCES: (a) WHO, 1994a, 1989-90 data; (b) WHO, 1994a, 1986-88 data; (c) WHO, 1995a, 1995b; (d) World Bank, 1994a; (e) WHO, 1995c. *Data are not consistent between alternative publications. **1988 data. u=urban. r=rural.
Note the following abbreviations: China - People's Republic of China; Korea, DPR - Democratic People's Republic of Korea (North Korea); Lao, PDR - People's Democratic Republic of Lao; Viet Nam - Socialist Republic of Viet Nam; Kyrgyz, Rep. - Republic of Kyrgyz; Micronesia, FS - Federated States of Micronesia; Korea, Rep. - Republic of Korea (South Korea); Taipei, China - Republic of China (Taiwan).

Table 2.6

Access to Health Care in 44 Asian Countries (%)

Country	Access to Health Care 1985-1995	Contraceptive Prevalence 1986-1996	Prenatal Care 1980-1990	Immunization: % Children 12-23 Months (1994-1996) [g]			
				BCG	DTP	Polio	Measles
South Asia							
Afghanistan	29	...	8c	15	12	8	19
Bangladesh	74	40f	40	100	91	92	96
Bhutan	65	22	63	98	87	86	86
India	85	40.6	70	97	92	48.3	32.7
Maldives	75c	23.4	47d	99	94	94	96
Mauritius	99	45b	90	94	90	90	85
Nepal	10a	28.8	9.4c	85	77	78	78
Pakistan	85	12f	70	65	55	55	53
Seychelles	99b	47	99	98	82	82	92
Sri Lanka	90	66.1	86.3	89	91	92.4	87.5
Southeast Asia							
Cambodia	53	...	...	95	79	80	75
Lao, PDR	67	18e	...	57	51	60	65
Myanmar	60	...	90.1	74	69	83.5	82
Philippines	76	40f	76.7	91	85	86	86
Viet Nam	97	53f	72.8	93	93	94	95
East Asia							
China	92	83f	u=98/r=72d	94	93	94	89
Korea, DPR	100	67	...	99	96	99	99.7
Mongolia	100	...	98.4	94	88	86	85
Central Asian Republics							
Kazakhstan	...	59d	...	86	80	75	72
Kyrgyz, Rep.	...	...	...	...	...	...	89
Uzbekistan	...	...	...	93	65	79	71
Pacific Islands							
Cook Islands	100b	45	100	96	93	93	96
Fiji	99c	32.2	100a	100	97	99	93
Kiribati	100	27.8	60.2	60	100	100	89
Marshall Islands	...	...	47	96	67	62	59
Micronesia, FS	75b	...	90	50	83	81	76
Nauru	...	...	...	93	74	74	...
New Caledonia	98e	...	100e	...	...	...	...
Niue	100e	...	...	92	100	100	34
Papua New Guinea	96	2.8	67.5	75	50	55	35
Solomon Islands	80c	41	92	77	69	68	76
Tokelau Island	100e	...	...	99	99	99	76
Tonga	100b	38.9	95	99	95	93	87
Tuvalu	...	...	...	88	87	92	94
Vanuatu	80b	12	98b	86	74	74	66
Wallis and Futuna Islands	...	...	...	100	98	94	95
Western Samoa	100b	20e	100e	98	95	95	81
High-Performing Asian Economies							
Hong Kong	99	81f	...	100	83	84	42
Indonesia	77	68.9	46.6c	95	91	86.6	89
Korea, Rep.	100	79f	96b	93	93	93	92
Malaysia	88	48f	83.8	100	90	90	81
Singapore	100	74f	95d	97	95	93	88
Taipei, China	97	...	...	...	...	...	...
Thailand	83	75	53.4	98	93	96	92

MAIN SOURCES: World Bank, 1993a, 1993c, 1997a; WHO, 1997b. OTHER SOURCES: (a) Peabody, 1995;
(b) WHO, 1994a, years 1989-90; (c) WHO, 1994a, years 1986-88; (d) WHO, 1994a, years 1983-85; (e) WHO,
1995c, year 1994; (f) United Nations, 1994; (g) WHO, 1996h, 1996i, 1996j (EPI program, percent insured).
u= urban. r=rural.
Note the following abbreviations: China - People's Republic of China; Korea, DPR - Democratic
People's Republic of Korea (North Korea); Lao, PDR - People's Democratic Republic of Lao; Viet Nam -
Socialist Republic of Viet Nam; Kyrgyz, Rep. - Republic of Kyrgyz; Micronesia, FS - Federated States of
Micronesia; Korea, Rep. - Republic of Korea (South Korea); Taipei, China - Republic of China (Taiwan).

Table 2.7

Health Expenditures in 44 Asian Countries

Country	Population 1995 Millions	GNP Per Capita 1995 ($US)	Per Capita Expenditures on Health 1990-1991 $US				Health Expenditures as Percentage of GDP, 1990-1995 (most recent)		
			Total*	Public (includes social security)	Private	Social Security	Total	Public	Private
South Asia									
Afghanistan	23.5	160	4.8	4.8	...	...	3.0f	3.0f	...
Bangladesh	119.8	240	7	3	4	3	3.04	1.22	1.82
Bhutan	0.7	420	7	4	3	14	1.7	1.0	0.7
India	929.4	340	21	5	16	4	5.6	1.2	4.4
Maldives	0.3	990	55	28	27	...	11.7	5.9	5.8
Mauritius	1.1	3380	160	4	...	156d	3.4	2.1	1.3
Nepal	21.5	200	8	4	4	...	12.4	1.0	11.0
Pakistan	129.9	460	12	6	6	3	3.5	0.8	2.7
Seychelles	0.1	6620	...	...	...	...	...	...	...
Sri Lanka	18.1	700	18	9	9	33	1.9	1.4	0.5
Southeast Asia									
Cambodia	10.0	270	2	...	...	...	7.2	0.7	6.5
Lao, PDR	4.9	350	9	4	5	...	2.6	0.8	1.8
Myanmar	45.1	220	6	6	...	...	1.7	0.45	1.25
Philippines	68.6	1050	14	7	7	7	2.4	1.3	1.1
Viet Nam	73.5	240	5e	2.6e	2.4e	...	5.2	1.1	4.1
East Asia									
China	1203.3	620	11	9	6	0.10d	3.8	1.8	2.0
Korea, DPR	22	479	...	...	...	...	4.6	...	...
Mongolia	2.5	310	68	50	18	15d	4.7	4.4	0.3
Central Asian Republics									
Kazakhstan	16.6	1330	96	60	36	...	4.4	2.8	1.7
Kyrgyz, Rep.	4.4	700	...	...	...	...	...	3.7	...
Uzbekistan	21	970	58	42	16	...	5.9	4.3	1.6
Pacific Islands									
Cook Islands	0.02	350b	30	...	...	...	8.5	...	...
Fiji	0.8	2440	70	42	28	...	3.4	2.0	1.4
Kiribati	0.1	920	69	...	...	...	14.6	...	...
Marshall Islands	0.05	1600a	...	...	...	...	...	...	...
Micronesia, FS	0.10	2010	135	...	...	...	9.0	...	...
Nauru	0.01	8070a	...	...	...	...	...	...	...
New Caledonia	0.182	13400a	...	...	...	...	...	...	...
Niue	0.002	3100c	287	...	...	...	9.3	...	...
Papua New Guinea	4.3	1160	36	23	13	11	4.4	2.8	1.6
Solomon Islands	0.4	910	28	6	21	...	5.6	3.3	2.2
Tokelau Island	0.002	3550	114	...	...	...	5.7	...	...
Tonga	0.09	1630	50	50	...	...	4.0	2.9	1.1
Tuvalu	0.01	400c	...	...	...	...	...	...	...
Vanuatu	0.2	1150	130	45	85	...	12.5	4.4	8.2
Wallis and Futuna Islands	0.014	1400	...	...	...	...	...	...	...
Western Samoa	0.2	1120	40	...	...	...	4.5	3.1	1.4
High-Performing Asian Economies									
Hong Kong	6.2	22990	748	144	604	...	4.3	1.9	2.4
Indonesia	193.3	980	12	4	8	3	1.5	0.7	0.8
Korea, Rep.	44.9	8260	390	160	230	161	5.4	1.8	3.6
Malaysia	20.14	3890	77	33	44	90d	3.0	1.3	1.7
Singapore	3.0	26730	547	316	231	406	3.5	1.1	2.4
Taipei, China	21.1	12790	515	268	246	...	4.9	2.6	2.3
Thailand	58.2	2740	73	17	59	22	5.3	1.4	3.9

MAIN SOURCES: World Bank, 1993a, 1996a, 1996c, 1997a; WHO, 1994a, 1995c, 1997b. (a) GDP per capita 1988; (b) GDP per capita 1991; (c) GDP per capita 1994; (d) social security contributions, 1993; (e) World Bank, 1992a; (f) WHO, 1996b.
*In some cases, the numbers do not add up because the data comes from different sources.
Note the following abbreviations: China - People's Republic of China; Korea, DPR - Democratic People's Republic of Korea (North Korea); Lao, PDR - People's Democratic Republic of Lao; Viet Nam - Socialist Republic of Viet Nam; Kyrgyz, Rep. - Republic of Kyrgyz; Micronesia, FS - Federated States of Micronesia; Korea, Rep. - Republic of Korea (South Korea); Taipei, China - Republic of China (Taiwan).

Overall, we see that expenditure data are limited, with only 14 of the 44 countries reporting information on all of the sources of the expenditures. The relative importance of the public and private sectors in health financing varies among countries. In India and Hong Kong, for instance, the private sector predominates, while the opposite is true for Mongolia, Tonga, and Uzbekistan.

As we stated in Chapter 1, there is no rule of thumb defining the optimal combination of private and public resources. Jamison (1996) suggests that, to resolve inequality problems and health market failures, the public sector in a developing country should spend on average the equivalent of 4 percent of the country's GDP. Although the 4-percent hypothesis can be taken as a reference, the optimal level of public expenditures depends in practice on the distribution of those expenditures among different uses, on the total national expenditure constraint, and on factors such as the level of education of the population and its access to health services (discussed above).

Table 2.8 shows that there is relatively good reporting on the broadly used indicators of health infrastructure and manpower—hospital beds, physicians, and nurses per 1,000 population—with 36, 38, and 34 countries reporting this information, respectively. It is also clear that there is no obvious relationship between hospitals or doctors and national health status. Countries such as Kazakhstan and Mongolia have a relatively high number of beds (11.6 and 11.5 beds per 1,000) and trained personnel (3.6 and 3.7 physicians per 1,000), yet their health statistics (presented in Table 2.10) show relatively high child mortality (35 and 74 deaths per 1,000 live births) and maternal mortality (53 and 240 maternal deaths per 1,000), respectively.

An Estimation of Individual and Provider Behavior. Data describing behaviors in quantitative terms are hard to generate. Although the changes in utilization of health services resulting from change in unit price can be measured as price elasticities in practice, no data describing these "preferences" have systematically been collected and synthesized for analytic consumption. Some data exist in the research literature or consulting reports, mostly related to how individuals and providers respond when faced with changes in price. We provide this type of information when we discuss financing health care in Chapter 4.

Other phenomena, such as the influence of cultural and social factors in the decision to follow medical advice, are difficult (if not impossible) to quantify. The traditional economic model of demand for health services, where "tastes" are treated as givens, has little or no application in this type of analysis. Indeed, when the services do not have a price (e.g., immunization campaigns), an economic model fails to explain why some individuals demand the services and others do not.

Despite all these difficulties, the role of social and cultural factors in health reform is critical, as we discuss in Chapter 6. An inadequate recognition of the nature of culture and social organizations and their involvement in health practices can drive any reform to failure. Indeed, we will argue that some behaviors can neutralize the effects of a given policy; therefore, not including them in the analysis might lead to misspent resources. Specifically, we look at qualitative data that describe common practices in different domains (e.g., work, nutrition, sanitation, family planning) that are intrinsic to some societies and to important stakeholders.

Table 2.8

Health Infrastructure and Manpower in 44 Asian Countries

Country	Distribution per 1000 Population		
	Hospital Beds	Physicians	Nurses
South Asia			
Afghanistan	0.2	0.1	0.1
Bangladesh	0.3	0.2	0.1
Bhutan	1.6	0.2	0.4
India	0.8	0.5	0.5
Maldives	0.8	0.4	1.13
Mauritius	2.9	...	...
Nepal	0.2	0.1	0.2
Pakistan	0.7	0.5	0.3
Seychelles	...	...	...
Sri Lanka	2.7	0.327	0.74
Southeast Asia			
Cambodia	2.1	0.1	0.3
Lao, PDR	2.5	0.2	1.4
Myanmar	0.6	0.289	0.22
Philippines	1.4	0.1	0.4
Viet Nam	3.8	0.4	1.7
East Asia			
China	2.4	1.6	0.7
Korea, DPR	13.5	2.97	...
Mongolia	11.5	2.7	3.7
Central Asian Republics			
Kazakhstan	11.6	3.6	12.4
Kyrgyz, Rep.	10.9	3.2	...
Uzbekistan	8.4	3.3	10.4
Pacific Islands			
Cook Islands	7.1	...	...
Fiji	0.5	0.6	2.2
Kiribati	4.3	0.2	2.0
Marshall Islands	2.3	0.4	2.3
Micronesia, FS	...	0.4	3.2
Nauru	...	...	...
New Caledonia	...	1.8	...
Niue	...	2.0	10.0
Papua New Guinea	4.0	0.1	0.6
Solomon Islands	2.8	0.2	2.3
Tokelau Island	...	1.0	8.0
Tonga	3.3	0.5	2.0
Tuvalu	...	...	...
Vanuatu	2.1	0.1	...
Wallis and Futuna Islands	...	...	...
Western Samoa	1.3	0.3	1.8
High-Performing Asian Economies			
Hong Kong	4.3	1.3	4.2
Indonesia	0.7	0.2	0.5
Korea, Rep.	4.1	1.2	0.7
Malaysia	2.0	0.4	1.4
Singapore	3.6	1.4	4.1
Taipei, China	4.9	1.3	0.5a
Thailand	1.7	0.2	1.1

MAIN SOURCES: World Bank, 1993a, 1996a, 1996b, 1997a; WHO, 1994a, 1996a, 1996b, 1997b. OTHER SOURCES: (a) Peabody, 1995.
Note the following abbreviations: China - People's Republic of China; Korea, DPR - Democratic People's Republic of Korea (North Korea); Lao, PDR - People's Democratic Republic of Lao; Viet Nam - Socialist Republic of Viet Nam; Kyrgyz, Rep. - Republic of Kyrgyz; Micronesia, FS - Federated States of Micronesia; Korea, Rep. - Republic of Korea (South Korea); Taipei, China - Republic of China (Taiwan).

An Assessment of Clinical Practice. There is an enormous amount of literature in medical journals (also summarized in textbooks) about the best tests, drugs, treatments, and surgical procedures for given diseases. This literature reports the results of studies that evaluate clinical practices.

The data often come from very carefully designed experiments that compare the health status of individuals who were subject to a given intervention with the health status of similar individuals who did not receive the intervention. These studies must be cautiously interpreted; they must be assessed to see if their results and conclusions are externally valid for the relevant population.

It is not possible to summarize this type of data in a few tables within this book. However, systematic reviews of clinical data are available through medical databases, journal publications, and academic books that practitioners around the world use and share. The Cochrane Collaboration is an excellent example of a database that can be used in developing countries.

We argue that the demographer, the economist, and the policy analyst must be able to have a basic facility with the medical literature. In an unregulated private market, each individual, given the available information, is free to evaluate what drugs and treatments he/she would like to get and what price he/she is willing to pay for them. However, when part of those services are financed by the government under a budgetary constraint, choices have to be made. A widely promoted criterion for making these choices is the cost-effectiveness of the interventions (i.e., the number of lives that can be saved for a fixed amount of resources by using the intervention).

A review of health care priorities and cost-effectiveness of alternative interventions is an arduous task. This task is broadly undertaken for Asia in Chapter 3, where we prioritize clinical interventions by objectives, burden of disease, cost-effectiveness, and the role of government. (See Tables 3.11a and b, 3.14, and 3.16a and b.)

An Assessment of the Political, Social, and Institutional Environment. Information on the political, social, and institutional environment certainly exists, but, like information on individual and provider behaviors, it has rarely been systematically collected. However, unlike with information on individual and provider behaviors, the bigger issue with political, social, and institutional sources is determining what kinds of information or factors are important to health care reform.

In terms of political information, policymakers want to understand the ideologies, electoral power, strength in legislative bodies, and position all relevant political parties have about the organization of the health sector.

In terms of institutional information, policymakers are more aware of the institutions that design policies for the health sector (at both central and lower levels). They should make researchers and analysts aware of the linkages of these institutions to executive power, their management and organization, and their degree of autonomy. Nevertheless, data about all public institutions that support health services—specifically their organization and management, mechanisms for budget design, sources of financing, the size of social organizations (e.g., unions of workers, physicians), the interests they pursue, and the privileges they have— are pieces of information that affect the policy process. One important area, often ignored, is private providers of health care—their size, organization, sources of

---

Box 2.2: Closing the Information Gap: The Cochrane Collaboration

To determine the effects of health interventions on health outcomes, medical researchers use RCTs to reliably distinguish between useful and useless medical treatments. Over 20 years ago, British epidemiologist Archie Cochrane drew attention to the existence of a large gap between published RCT data and their use in making informed decisions in clinical practice. That gap continues to this day. For example, a recent study showed that despite a 1988 article published in the *Lancet* on a pragmatic RCT that established the substantial benefits of using thrombolysis in treating acute myocardial infarction, five years later only around 30–50 percent of potentially benefited patients in England's Trent region had received the recommended thrombolysis treatment described in the 1988 article. (See Freemantle et al., 1995.)

The increased attention drawn to the health care information gap by Cochrane's criticism and by many other examples like the one above led to the establishment of an organization intent on closing it. The Cochrane Collaboration was established institutionally in 1992 as the UK Cochrane Center at Oxford. Its responsibilities include overseeing collaborative review groups and preparing and maintaining *The Cochrane Database of Systematic Reviews*. In 1993, a sibling organization, the National Health Service (NHS) Centre for Reviews and Dissemination, was set up at the University of York; its functions include overseeing and performing systematic reviews, disseminating the research results to facilitate effective decisionmaking, developing and maintaining review databases, and developing an information service. (See Sheldon and Chalmers, 1994.)

Since its establishment, the Cochrane Collaboration has grown considerably, consisting today of 8 international centers, 37 collaborative review groups, and 7 methods working groups from around the world. The review process is driven by members of the review groups. For example, the Cochrane Pregnancy and Childbirth Group, comprising 30 reviewers and 6 editors, is responsible for maintaining 600 systematic reviews of RCTs, as well as for dealing with between 200 and 300 new RCT reports per year. The group is composed of international reviewers from Africa, Australia, Europe, and North America. The reviews are incorporated in the main database and produced as a specialized database—the Cochrane Pregnancy and Childbirth Database. These databases are available on-line, on CD-ROM, and on diskette to all clinicians in Asia. (See Hayward et al., 1996.)

As the Cochrane Collaboration increases its reach throughout the world, including developing countries in Asia, it will have a two-way benefit: Health professionals in Asia will have greater access to current data on the best clinical practices, and the world will benefit from the inclusion of Asian research in Cochrane reviews. As the coverage widens, both in terms of content and worldwide experience, the information gap will close.

Those who would like to examine Cochrane Collaboration material may do so by paying for a subscription and obtaining the quarterly reports; by accessing the (limited) information that is available through the website (http://hiru.mcmaster.ca/cochrane/default.htm); or, if these are not affordable, by writing to the review authors directly and requesting material. The Cochrane Collaboration also has a special interest/working group that focuses on applications in developing countries.

---

political support or power, and their motivations for policy change (or likely resistance to it). This type of information comes from case studies and is necessarily country-specific.

In terms of social information, policymakers need to understand the key organizations that affect public policy; this includes understanding the social support, electoral power, goals, and position about the organization of the health sector of all relevant social organizations.

Drawing from the types of information needed and discussed above, Table 2.9 illustrates what such information looks like for two Asian countries—Kazakhstan and Viet Nam in 1996. While the data are not current, this table reflects the breadth and qualitative nature of political, social, and institutional knowledge but masks the depth and detail of this type of data. Typically, in-depth case studies and expert committees are needed to fully understand issues in these areas. To generate useful, policy-relevant guidance, both the breadth and depth of such information would ultimately need to be more extensive than what we see in Table 2.9.

Measures of Health Outcomes. Table 2.10 compiles aggregate versions of the most commonly used health outcome measures—life expectancy at birth, under-five mortality rate, IMR, and maternal mortality. Life expectancy is widely available (in 43 of the 44 countries). As we saw in Chapter 1, life expectancy begins to plateau as it approaches an undefined limit of human survival, which, in the aggregate, is still potentially over 80 years in Asia. The infant mortality rate is available for all 44 countries. We see that infant mortality rates tend to be a larger percentage of the child mortality rate as health outcomes improve in developing countries. The under-five mortality indicator is a more elaborate statistic than infant mortality, but it is unavailable for four of the Pacific Island countries.

An extremely valuable indicator, because of the effectiveness of clinical interventions in the area, is the maternal mortality rate. The definition of death during childbirth varies across countries, however, so the maternal mortality indicator is difficult to use in comparisons across countries. To make matters worse, many maternal deaths are not registered, particularly those in rural areas. Thus, countries with an important share of the total population living in rural areas tend to underestimate this indicator. With these caveats, we see that data are available for only 38 of the 44 countries. Tragically, maternal mortality rates are extremely high for many of the countries that report the indicator, and the three-digit mortality rates we see in some countries suggest that women's health must be a high priority.

The data on mortality rates show that even if the rates were cut by half in the last 15 years, they are still high compared with standards in countries with developed market economies. As is the case for other indicators we have analyzed, the situation is critical in countries such as Afghanistan, Bhutan, Lao, and Bangladesh. Differences in income and education partly explain the differences in mortality among countries, but, as we show in Chapter 1, different health policies also appear to be fundamental.

Better Data for Policymaking—The Long and Short of It

The Importance of Public Investment in Data Development. What can be done about the "data gap" problem? Developing countries, in general, have not been able to adequately invest in information systems to generate routinely collectable data. And in many cases, short-run urgencies make it impossible to consider the value and potential savings from conducting specially designed surveys and experiments, so a limited share of the public budget is allocated to these activities.

Table 2.9

Political, Social, and Institutional Factors: An Illustration Using
Kazakhstan and Viet Nam In 1996

Factors	Kazakhstan	Viet Nam
POLITICAL PARTIES • Status of main party and competitors	Main political force is People's Unity, led by Nazabaev Nursulatan, which has kept many old Soviet-era structures; no known succcessor to Nazarbaev Main opposition party is National Democratic Party of Kazakhstan and Jeltoqsan; activities scrutinized by authorities and access to media restricted	Vietnam Communist Party (VCP), led by President Le Duc Anh since September, 1992, is the only party and most important political force Social support of other political organizations (operating outside borders), such as the Viet Nam Quoc Dan Dang (VNQDD), is growing fast, but influence on public policy is still marginal
SOCIAL ORGANIZATIONS • Key organizations	Peasant's Union, led by Zhanatov Koshebaib, generally supports government policy Opposing group, Independent Trade Union and Business Association, led by Leonid Solomin, aims for more dynamic process of political and economic reform	The Free Vietnam Alliance (FVA) aims to democratize the political system; focus is on abolishing parts of constitution that endorse Marxism-Leninism and vest the party with absolute and total power, on separating party's apparatus from government, the public security forces, and the armed forces, and on abolishing all limits on basic rights
INSTITUTIONS THAT DESIGN POLICIES FOR HEALTH SECTOR • Management and organization • Level of centralization/ decentralization	Ministry of Health (MOH) highest level of management, headed by health minister and members of cabinet of ministers of republic Next level are oblast's (province's) departments and health departments of oblast's administration that execute policies Public health budget decentralized— MOH does not directly influence health budget for each region	Health services organized along 4-tiered pyramid: MOH, provincial/district health bureaus, and commune people's committee formulate/execute health policy; commune health centers at bottom of pyramid MOH operates at provincial level through provincial health services department funded by central government
PUBLIC INSTITUTIONS PROVIDING HEALTH SERVICES • Management and organization • Sources of financing • Size/nature of social organizations (unions of workers, physicians)	Structure of public health services varies, including new organization forms like family medical ambulance stations, centers of outpatient surgery, and daytime hospitals Services include 3,527 ambulatory polyclinic and 1,649 hospital establishments, funded by 8.78% of general budget Wages of medical workers low—MOH has proposed that wages be paid in accordance with quality/quantity of work	MOH manufactures/distributes pharmaceuticals, trains doctors, coordinates medical research, and provides all curative/preventative health services MOH assisted by specialty agencies: Institute for Protection of Mothers and New Born, Institute for Hygiene and Epidemiology, National Institute of Nutrition, and others responsible for research, training, and patient care in areas such as cancer and pediatrics 9,800 commune health centers provide primary health care
ORGANIZATIONS OF PRIVATE PROVIDERS • Size and type	Volume of fee-for-services represents 1-2% of total health expenditures; expected to increase to 8-10% Expansion of private market viewed as way of increasing medical workers' welfare	Private health services multiplying rapidly, with 1/3 of physicians in commune health services in private practice 2 to 2–1/2 hours per day Large number of full-time private physicians in both rural and urban areas, with daily number of patients examined over 5 times higher than in public sector

SOURCES: ADB, 1996b; World Bank, 1992a.

Table 2.10

Aggregate Version of the Most Commonly Used Health Outcome Measures in 44 Asian Countries

Country	Life Expectancy at Birth 1995	Under-5 Mortality Rate (per 1,000 live births) 1995	Infant Mortality Rate (per 1,000 live births) 1995	Maternal Mortality (per 100,000 population) 1990–1996
South Asia				
Afghanistan	45	237	159	1700
Bangladesh	58	115	78	450
Bhutan	52	97	70.7	380
India	62	95	74	420
Maldives	70.6	47	32	200
Mauritius	71	20	16	112
Nepal	56	118.3	78.5	539
Pakistan	63	127	91	340
Seychelles	72	19	15	...
Sri Lanka	73	19	17.7	40
Southeast Asia				
Cambodia	53	158	109	900
Lao, PDR	52	147	92	660
Myanmar	59	100.73	49.7	518
Philippines	66	53	40	280
Viet Nam	68	49	41	105
East Asia				
China	69	43	35	115
Korea, DPR	72.7	32	14.1	48
Mongolia	65	74	56	240
Central Asian Republics				
Kazakhstan	69	35	27	53
Kyrgyz, Rep.	68	42	30	80
Uzbekistan	70	48	30	43
Pacific Islands				
Cook Islands	69e	28	17.5a	189a
Fiji	72	25	21	90
Kiribati	58	75	56	225a
Marshall Islands	63	29	63a	2a*
Micronesia, FS	64	40	33	14a
Nauru	56e	...	26a	...
New Caledonia	73	19	16	16
Niue	...	...	10a	...
Papua New Guinea	57	95	65	930
Solomon Islands	62	52	41	30
Tokelau Island	m:65,f:70a	...	19a	...
Tonga	69	23	19	126
Tuvalu	67a	56	73.6a	434
Vanuatu	64	51	42	280
Wallis and Futuna Islands	68a	...	22a	...
Western Samoa	69	27	23	35
High-Performing Asian Economies				
Hong Kong	79	6	5	7
Indonesia	64	81	55	390
Korea, Rep.	72	14	10	30
Malaysia	71	14	12	34
Singapore	76	6	4	10
Taipei, China	76	7	6	...
Thailand	69	21.53	15.35	10.68

MAIN SOURCES: WHO, 1996a, 1997b; World Bank, 1996a, 1997a; ADB, 1996a; (a) WHO, 1995c. *Data are from 1985. m=male. f=female. Note: Figures adjusted on the basis of UNICEF, 1992 and DHS Reports, 1987–1994.
Note the following abbreviations: China - People's Republic of China; Korea, DPR - Democratic People's Republic of Korea (North Korea); Lao, PDR - People's Democratic Republic of Lao; Viet Nam - Socialist Republic of Viet Nam; Kyrgyz, Rep. - Republic of Kyrgyz; Micronesia, FS - Federated States of Micronesia; Korea, Rep. - Republic of Korea (South Korea); Taipei, China - Republic of China (Taiwan).

Data collection and research depend on public financing to support their development. Just as governments are responsible for setting policy, they are also responsible for much of the data gathering and research studies needed to guide policy. Information is a public good in the sense described earlier in Chapter 1:

One person's use does not reduce the amount another can consume. Indeed, better policy that results from better data generates savings that can be used for other public goods and services.

The problem, of course, is that data collection and research are often expensive, which leads to a temporal trade-off issue for governments: While better information may make better use of resources in the long run, gathering data and doing studies incur costs in the short run. In cash-strapped developing countries, affording data collection and research is an acute issue, even though the marginal payoff of better policies is potentially much higher for poorer countries.

One potential solution is to allow the richer developing countries in a region to do the research and transfer the information to the poorer countries. Thus, the wealthier countries would subsidize the poorer ones by doing the data collection and the research. Unfortunately, such data collection and research cannot always be left to wealthier countries. The epidemiologic transition, for example, is different in wealthier countries, because they have different burdens of disease. For instance, China is more worried about the unusual incidence of oropharyngeal carcinoma and, logically, less concerned about the high prevalence of malaria than poorer East Asian countries are. In short, countries often have different research agendas.

International organizations and NGOs are ideally positioned to assume the data-generation role. Already, they have stimulated and participated in the development of national surveys (e.g., LSMS under the aegis of the World Bank, and the DHS under the aegis of USAID and others) and experimental studies (e.g., the Maternal and Child Health—Family Planning (MCH-FP) programs in Matlab-Bangladesh). However, the number of countries covered in Asia is still limited (e.g., of the 58 DHS surveys, only 8 have been developed in Asia). This suggests that, just to meet basic data needs in Asia, the current resources invested in the generation of new household data alone would have to be doubled or tripled.

Another option, given the expense of data collection, is for analysts and policymakers to continue to explore the effectiveness of rapid-assessment methods to evaluate policy. These methods are cheaper and can be developed in shorter periods of time. Examples are mini-surveys, used for marketing and assessment of customer preferences (see Satia et al., 1994); cluster surveys (see Henderson and Sunderesan, 1982); lot quality assurance sampling, often used to look for the emergence of a disease (see Lanata et al., 1990); anthropological methods, useful for gaining insights on how to improve services and stay "close to the customer" (see Manderson and Aby, 1992); focus groups, helpful to estimate consumer behavior (see Dawson et al., 1993); sentinel sites, useful for monitoring trends and alerting public health officials of diseases such as HIV infection, when precise counts are not needed and clinical care is available or will be introduced if the disease appears (see Frerichs and Khin, 1989); and Delphi panel methods, useful for generating expert opinion. (See Oranga and Nordberg, 1993.) Each of these approaches is useful in investigating issues that cannot be studied using more-formal techniques. However, caution must be used whenever they are proposed in place of household or facility surveys. (See Sandiford et al., 1992.)

Ways to Improve Data Quality in the Short Term. Beyond the problem of not having data and the long-term solution of investing public money in data collection, there are also some problems with the existing data that can be addressed in the short term.

Below, we discuss four such problems that can be corrected without significant new investments in information gathering: (1) lack of frequent updates and efficient dissemination; (2) lack of disaggregation; (3) registration problems; and (4) uncertainty that comes from model estimation. To illustrate these problems, we refer as appropriate to Tables 2.2–2.10.

Lack of Frequent Updates and Effective Dissemination. Even if good-quality data are available in the areas policymakers need, the data themselves are not updated frequently enough, limiting their usefulness. Specifically, there is an important lag between the time the information is gathered and the time it is published. As one can see by simply looking at the tables above, post-1994 data are available for very few of the indicators. In some cases, the data delay is as much as 10 years (e.g., the income distribution data shown in Table 2.4). Having frequently updated data is a critical issue for Asia—it is a dynamic region where demographic and socioeconomic factors change rapidly. Improvements are rapid—yesterday's problem is today's solution and new problems emerge. The area of financing options for health care is an example where the health sector continues to change.

Even when data are available, disseminating them poses another problem. Such dissemination problems occur in the area of access to health care data (shown in Tables 2.5 and 2.6). Household surveys are the usual means to generate these indicators; however, despite the fact that the number of countries implementing household surveys has been increasing since the 1950s, the results have not been widely disseminated, so the indicators are hard to find.

Bottlenecks can occur in three phases of the data generation process—collection, analysis, or reporting. Correcting the reporting or dissemination bottlenecks may be the easiest to address because it is less costly than commissioning new studies or training better analysts. Fortunately, the ability to collect and analyze data has improved in remarkable ways since the late 1950s, when India was the first developing country to adopt household surveys to gather information on morbidity and utilization. (See Kroeger, 1983.) Today, collection and analysis can be expected to improve with better technology for survey field work, data entry, and programming. The ability to disseminate information with relative ease supports the notion that, more than ever before, there is an information revolution transforming the health sector.

A word of caution is in order. Cibulskis and Izard (1996) point out that computerization has not always been the panacea many had anticipated, because of a lack of staff skilled in programming, archiving, hardware maintenance, software utilization, and system upgrades. (See Cibulskis and Izard, 1996.) (The transfer of expertise from the developed world is a key concern in this area.) Nevertheless, computers are a powerful technology that provides tools and incentives for gathering and analyzing data. Developments in information technology through telephones, satellite communication, facsimile, and electronic mail are now used throughout Asia and offer equal promise for dissemination.

In addition, we believe that many more data exist than what are publicly available (i.e., published). This suggests that the "owners" of the data and funders of studies should improve their dissemination mechanisms.

Lack of Disaggregated Data. Of course, even if data are available in a timely manner, the data may still be too aggregated to be useful. Data's usefulness is often constrained because the data are not disaggregated by region, income, age, or sex. Ideally, for example, indicators of nutrition and access to education, water, sanitation, and health services (shown in Tables 2.5 and 2.6) should be available by sex, age, income group, and geographic region. Only then can interventions be targeted, thus concentrating resources on those population groups with limited access (as we discuss in more detail in Chapter 5).

In Table 2.5, for example, we see urban/rural splits for Cambodia in access to safe water and for the Solomon Islands and Vanuatu in access to sanitation, but we do not have the same information for the other countries. In Table 2.6, the access to prenatal care for China shows an urban/rural split and reveals a significant variation (98 percent urban versus 72 percent rural). But again, such splits are not available for the other countries in the table.

Indicators of access to health care (shown in Tables 2.5 and 2.6) should be disaggregated into inpatient and outpatient services. Doing so provides flexible allocation of resources by service types—a subject that is discussed in more detail in the next two chapters. Moreover, to have a real policy impact, these indicators should also be available by income group, region, sex, race, and age.

Another example of disaggregation problems occurs in the indicators used for infrastructure and manpower (as shown in Table 2.8). Such indicators are rarely available by region (urban/rural) or income groups (i.e., thousands of the population with less than a given level of income). Moreover, the indicators shown in Table 2.8—which are critically important to the planning and budgeting process—are far too crude to be operationally useful. To be truly useful, the data should be disaggregated to reveal more-specific information about medical equipment, drug supplies, electricity, and refrigeration.

Disaggregation problems are unavoidable in some measures such as DALYs, because they are meant to be aggregate measures. For the most part, however, data resulting from routinely collected information systems and surveys can readily be presented at different levels of disaggregation. "Owners" of the data should redesign the formats they use to collect and present the data. Similarly, the "source" of the data (e.g., hospital records) should be revised so researchers and analysts can collect data along the necessary disaggregated dimensions. These tasks can be enormously facilitated by means of the Internet and attached electronic files.

Data Registration Problems. Systems of routinely collected data, like discharge data and invoices in public hospitals or distribution of expenditures of the Ministry of Health, may suffer from poor quality, primarily because an efficient system of data registration (i.e., the entry of data) is not available. This problem can be corrected with routine computer entry and data programs that immediately screen for incorrect entries. Where computerization does not exist, other steps are possible. Efficiency can be improved by administrative oversight, incentives, and controls that are often absent.

Uncertainty Problems Created by Model Estimation. Despite the lack of high-quality data, health policies must still be designed and implemented. The process of reform cannot be delayed until a first-rate information system for each country is available. Thus, policy is often based on adjusting current data and using them to project, interpolate, and estimate related indicators through mathematical models. For example, it has been estimated that in Asia (excluding China and India) only 11 percent of deaths are registered; thus, the mortality estimates that are currently used must be based on models and adjustment algorithms. Another practice that has become frequent is making recommendations using data that were not specifically collected for the purpose (e.g., designing a basic plan of health services based on discharge and invoice data from a sample of public and private hospitals). Although this type of analysis is better than no analysis at all, policies designed this way should be carefully monitored.

In fact, most of the indicators currently available are the result of adjustments made by researchers, NGOs, and international organizations to the data collected by governmental agencies or to their own data. Because in most cases we cannot measure the accuracy of those adjustments, the indicators should, as a rule, be interpreted with circumspection. By extension, when key policy decisions are made using these numbers, policy must be followed exceptionally closely to ensure that these projections are not fatally flawed.

DISCONTINUITIES BETWEEN POLICYMAKERS AND RESEARCHERS

Beyond the lack of available data, there are more fundamental data-related issues that can cause problems for policymaking. To be effective in this era of change and complexity, policymakers need to understand the strengths and limitations of information. This requires a basic understanding of data quality and how data are reported. Recalling Figure 2.1 at the beginning of the chapter, we see that policymakers and researchers interact in two areas: Policymakers commission the studies researchers conduct, and they interpret the analyzed data researchers produce. In the absence of basic knowledge, policymaking can suffer from discontinuities. Here, we examine some that can affect policymaking.

Variations in Data Quality by Research Study Type

Given that policymakers commission studies for researchers, there is a mutual obligation for researchers to explain and policymakers to understand the range of studies possible, along with their advantages and disadvantages. For example, problems will occur if policymakers are allowed to assume that studies yield similar levels of data quality and plan health policy accordingly.

Table 2.11 breaks studies down into two broad categories—cross-sectional and longitudinal—and summarizes the advantages and disadvantages of the individual study types within the two categories. In the last column, we have ranked the quality of the data, from Class 1 (the highest quality) to Class 5, to indicate the strength of the conclusions that can be drawn from each type of study. At a quick glance, the table underscores the fact that longitudinal studies yield better-quality data than cross-sectional studies—longitudinal studies have a more rigorous study design.

References to the various types of studies and to the classifications of data quality show up in our discussions of the evidence throughout the remainder of the

Table 2.11

Advantages and Disadvantages of Different Types of Studies

Type of Study	Advantages	Disadvantages	Quality of Data
Longitudinal Studies			
• RCTs - Clinical or community trials - Blinded/double blinded - Crossover	• Experimental design • Eliminates differential bias • Establish causality • Strong internal validity	• Expensive • Difficult to implement in many settings • Ethical issues may prohibit implementation	Class 1
• Prospective Cohort or Incidence Studies (Prospective) - Experimental - Observational	• Establishes sequences of events • Avoids bias in measuring predictors • Avoids survival bias	• Often requires large sample sizes • Potential bias from self-selection • May be expensive	Class 2
• Case Control (Retrospective)	• Short duration • Relatively inexpensive	• Potential bias from sampling two self-selected populations • Does not establish sequence of events • Limited to one outcome variable • Potential survival bias • Does not yield prevalence/incidence	Class 3
Cross-Sectional Studies			
• Prevalence	• May study several different outcomes • Control over enrolling the subjects • Control over measurements • Relatively short duration • Lower costs	• Does not establish sequence of events or causality • Potential selection bias in measuring predictors • Potential survivor bias	Class 4
• Laboratory	• Control over measurements • Done with controls • Strictly define environment • Can easily be conducted as RCT	• Difficult to implement outside of bench-science environment	Class 2 or 5
• Case Reports or Series and Case Studies	• Some control over external environment • Stimulates formulation of hypotheses	• Many potential biases • May not reflect causality • No controls	Class 4 or 5

SOURCE: Adapted from Newman et al., 1988.

book. Here, we discuss each type in more detail to highlight their differences and uses.

Longitudinal Studies. Longitudinal studies look at changes over time. In such studies, the investigator tries to understand the key parameters and then changes one (or more) factor(s) under investigation while keeping the other important factors of the system constant. These interventions are followed over time, usually in a before-and-after design. If other factors are also accounted for in the study, it is possible to find cause-and-effect relationships.

Longitudinal studies can be divided into RCTs, prospective cohort or incidence studies (PCSs), which are generally prospective, and case control studies, which are generally retrospective. These are important divisions because of the varying scientific (and statistical) inferences that can be made from the studies. They are, thus, worth a more detailed look.

Randomized Controlled Trial. The most powerful type of experimental design is a longitudinal RCT (ranked 1 in terms of data quality), in which the subjects (patients usually, but they can also be communities or providers) are randomly divided into two (or even more) groups. The groups are simultaneously treated or influenced differently. For instance, in a study of individual behavior, one group might be told to stop smoking, while the other would be told but also enrolled in a smoking cessation program. The first group is typically referred to as the *control group* and does not participate in the intervention. Individuals should be unaware (referred to as masked or blinded) of which group they are randomly assigned to. Randomization ensures that both groups are alike with regard to all "other" variables besides the treatment. While randomization does not ensure that both groups will be identical, it does ensure that no systematic *bias* favoring one treatment or the other can operate. Table 2.12 discusses this and other common types of biases that occur in studies.

Table 2.12

Examples of Types of Study Biases

Type of Bias	Definition
Sampling Bias	
Selection bias	Two populations differ in their outcomes not because of the intervention but because of some fundamental difference that existed before the intervention was introduced
Differential bias	Unknown exogenous factors (i.e., factors outside the study design) affect one study group more than another
Survivor bias	Found in studies trying to evaluate the effectiveness of an intervention to reduce mortality when individuals with a given condition who died are excluded (e.g., exercise treatment to protect against cardiac ischemia, where those who died are inevitably excluded from the final analysis)
Measurement Errors	
Observer bias	Consistent distortion, whether conscious or unconscious, in the perception or reporting of the measurement by the observer
Subject bias	Consistent distortion of the measurement by the study subjects
Hawthorn effect	Involves a true alteration in the phenomena under study caused by the process of being studied
Recall bias (respondent bias)	When the differences in the responses are determined by differences due to respondent's recall compared with what actually happened
Competing risk/synergy	Under- or overestimating the impact of an intervention because other impacts (e.g., increased susceptibility for competing risks) are not taken into account
Instrument bias	Results from a faulty function of a mechanical instrument
Other Types of Bias	
Pilot-test bias	Successful results of small-scale trials cannot be generalized because the trial had factors that cannot be duplicated in everyday environment
Prevalence-incidence bias	Effects of a risk factor on disease duration are mistaken for effects on disease occurrence
Reporting bias	Studies of interventions or evaluations (e.g., diagnostic tests) that do not show promise go unreported in the literature

SOURCE: Adapted from Newman et al., 1988.

When patients are switched from the intervention group to the nonintervention group, they act as their own controls, and it is called a *crossover* trial. Randomized crossover trials that demonstrate the same effect on both treatment groups are particularly substantive and convincing. Nonrandomized studies can often lead to exaggerated claims about the efficacy of an intervention because *confounders* (factors other than the intervention) are not randomly allocated between those who are using the intervention (drug, vaccine, education program) and those who are not. Similarly, the researchers in RCTs should not know which group receives the treatment (sometimes referred to as a *double blinded* study), because they are likely to be biased toward the group getting the treatment and thus overestimate the benefits of the intervention. RCTs are typically used to determine whether such interventions as new medicines or alternative surgical procedures are more effective than existing or established ones.

Cohort or Incidence Study. Another effective design, although slightly less powerful, is the cohort study (ranked as Class 2). Here, two (or more) groups or communities called cohorts are matched for varying confounders (often referred to as *covariates*), such as age and income, and followed over time. Even if the researcher does take care, it is possible for the groups to be systematically biased by unobserved factors. If the researcher introduces a treatment, it is an *experimental* design; if the study just follows the natural history, it is *observational*. Cohort studies focus on factors that influence the development of a given condition (e.g., disease or death) or practice (e.g., number of patients seen) and then follow the groups over time. By comparing the cohort of individuals for weeks, months, or even years and by identifying those who develop the condition or change their behavior, it is possible to assess which factors may be causative. Cohort studies are typically used to determine if epidemiologic factors, such as breastfeeding and birth spacing, lead to better outcomes for infants and mothers. They can also be used to see if policies lead to changes in patient or provider behaviors.

Case Control Study. A less powerful type of study (ranked as Class 3) is a longitudinal case control study. Here, one group is identified that already has a particular attribute or outcome, such as self-referral to a cardiologist, and is compared to a second group, such as those who did not choose a specialist but who have other similar features, such as risk factors. The obvious weakness with this design is that it is not possible to identify every distinguishing feature, such as family history or serum cholesterol, that would distinguish those who ask for specialist care from those who do not.

Cross-Sectional Studies. In contrast to longitudinal studies, cross-sectional studies are usually one-time studies and describe the state of affairs at a particular moment, independent of the effects over time. Cross-sectional studies can only make associations. The investigator does not typically control the setting or influence the factors that are under investigation and thus is limited to observing changes in the variables at one point in time. Because all variables in the system of study are changing simultaneously, it is difficult to isolate individual effects of one variable on another. This means that it is difficult to make strong statements about cause and consequence. This is a common type of study, especially for complex social and behavioral issues, but it leaves the researchers to hypothesize about plausible causality relationships.

Prevalence and Laboratory Studies. Prevalence studies (ranked as Class 4), such as those done to determine cases of diarrhea in a community, are typically cross-sectional. Laboratory studies (ranked as Class 5 or 2), can observe phenomena, such as the presence of motile trophozoites in amebic dysentery, that are also cross-sectional (Class 5). Laboratory studies can also be set up as longitudinal controlled trials. For example, when a patient with pneumonia is admitted to the hospital, a doctor will want the pathogen identified and treated with the most suitable antibiotic. In this setting, the researcher has complete control over the environment and can study the sensitivity of the bacterial pathogen to the proposed antibiotic (Class 2).

Case Report or Case Series Studies. Less powerful data in terms of showing causality (ranked as Class 5) come from case reports or case series studies. Case series are investigations that summarize similar cases and describe their common features. As such, they are really no more than anecdotal information and should be viewed with great care. In health services research, they are the equivalent of descriptive studies and exploratory research in which no causality is being determined. This type of study is intended to be preliminary and stimulate further research.

Case studies are detailed exploratory or explanatory investigations. They ask "how" or "why" things occur (marked as Class 4) in a setting over which the investigator has no control. Such studies are most useful in describing complex phenomena and in retaining the holistic relationships of the actual events. (See Yin, 1994.) The explanatory power of this methodology is suited to investigating the impact of such things as cultural, political, and anthropological features. Qualitative case studies, for example, help explain how institutions work and are the source of much of the information needed to understand political, social, and institutional factors.

Other typical types of case study investigation focus on the incidence and prevalence of particular diseases, or on mortality rates and disability. The general strategy is to divide the population by geographic regions and other variables such as sex, age, race, and socioeconomic status and then evaluate the level of the outcome variable. These studies can be very useful in identifying high-risk groups (e.g., HIV in military recruits in Thailand) and in assessing the distribution of health resources among populations and geographic areas (e.g., health status of mountain dwellers in Viet Nam). The policy-oriented goals of these studies may be to identify health service (curative and preventive) priorities, to generate hypotheses that aid in setting health service research priorities, or to aid in identifying potentially disadvantaged groups and targeting health interventions.

It is important to mention how case study research should be conducted and analyzed. Resource constraints will dictate that only a handful of sites can be selected. Selection is based on general characteristics (e.g., management changes in hospitals that are turned over to the private sector). If management issues in privatization are of interest, the chosen facilities should represent a spectrum of factors so that their relationships can be explored (what researchers refer to as data variation). These studies should be conducted on site, over several weeks to months, and should include interviews with people, reviews of documents, and direct observations. Analyzing case study results is an iterative process requiring a lot of expertise and even more patience. (See Yin, 1994.) The hope is that patterns will be apparent after several studies are distilled to their core elements. The picture that emerges will at least be descriptive and provide policy leaders with a list of policy alternatives. It might also be explanatory, for instance, providing future analysts with a better framework to evaluate business decisions relative to changing economic cycles. The final results will be based on pattern matching, explanation building, and reproducibility. The unique capability of case study research is the strong internal validity that allows a coherent story to be told. This is a powerful weapon in policy advocacy: A story is easily understood and often repeated. (See Nelson, 1987.)

The Value of RCTs and PCSs to Help Evaluate Government Policies. The above discussion and Table 2.11 show why RCTs and PCSs are considered the "gold standard" and "silver standard" for determining efficacy of treatment or policy interventions. Longitudinal experimental studies in general provide researchers and policymakers with more-accurate information about therapeutic interventions and health services and have been very valuable in helping to transform medical practice into evidence-based care.

However, RCTs and PCSs have been grossly underutilized in developed or developing countries when there is a need to evaluate interventions to change behavior, provide access for the poor, and investigate new management studies. The result is that medical interventions are chosen with good information about their likely outcomes, while government policies are chosen based on very limited information. This is ironic—while it may be important to know what the best drug is to treat hypertension, that is a small problem compared to understanding whether social insurance will increase the number of women who have a supervised delivery, or whether user fees will drive the poor from government-run clinics.

In terms of the question of the effect of user fees on utilization, there has been, to date, only one large randomized social experiment to look at the effects of copayments on utilization. The RAND Health Insurance Experiment (reported in 1988) showed that decreases in user fees increased utilization but had no measurable impact on health outcomes. This landmark study cost over US $80 million and took seven years to complete, but it yielded many insights and had far-reaching policy impact. Despite its success, however, it still remains one of the only studies of its kind. Many similar social experiments would be useful to investigate the effects of pricing strategies on utilization and provider productivity.

Despite the advantages, there are many reasons that RCTs and PCSs are not always suitable. For example, they are typically expensive (although misguided treatment may be more costly) and technically difficult to plan and implement. Moreover, if the phenomenon of interest is rare or takes a long time to happen, such as the development of adenocarcinoma of the lung in smokers, it is difficult to obtain an adequate sample size. More important, there may be ethical problems of randomization in using RCTs. For instance, no one would conceive of asking one group to smoke and another to abstain to show cause and effect.

Interpreting Research Design and Research Data

Even when it is understood that the type of study determines the quality of the data and their usefulness for evidence-based policy, there is another common problem. The analyzed data cannot be used if policymakers cannot interpret how data are linked to policy and how they are commonly presented.

**Box 2.3: A Prospective Controlled District Study in Indonesia:
The Example of Health Plan III**

RCTs are widely used to evaluate clinical interventions. But when evaluating social behaviors or the impact of public policies, researchers are typically limited to using cross-sectional designs or simple, uncontrolled longitudinal analyses. The real question is, can RCTs be used to help governments choose policies? The example of a randomized district trial in Indonesia provides some answers.

In 1990, Indonesia introduced a five-year, $47 million project—Health Plan III—to improve health care in two provinces: one, a relatively wealthy oil and timber exporting province, and the other, a poor, agriculture-based province. To sustain these efforts, the government wanted to find alternative sources of revenue when the project was over and thus wished to explore the revenue potential of increased user fees. But user fees can be a complicated path to increased revenues. They can lead some who need care to choose not to use it, because of the increased cost. This problem may be particularly severe for the poor, who, faced with the same choices as others, are generally more price-responsive. In addition, if the price responses are too large, the increased fees can actually reduce revenues. Thus, the government needed to know how user fees would affect revenues and how fee increases would influence health outcomes, particularly among the poor.

The government proposed that these revenue and health outcome questions be considered as part of the Health Plan III project and commissioned a pilot study before fee increases were considered throughout the country. A team of researchers proposed a prospective controlled study: User fees would be increased in some districts within the two provinces (the treatment areas) at the beginning of the study, while the remaining districts (the control areas) were restrained from increasing fees until after the study.

The policy question required that the effects of the fee changes be measured independently of any other shocks. To do this, researchers first considered the local political processes, because these dictated the size of the area where user fees could be influenced. Fees could be implemented at the district level, but no lower. With only six districts in each province, randomized assignment to treatment and control areas would not be effective. Rather, districts were matched, based on their economic and health characteristics, and similar districts were split between treatment and control areas.

A population-based survey interviewed a representative sample of 6,000 households (and matched facilities) from both treatment and control areas, just before the experimental fee increases. The same households and facilities were then resurveyed two years after the baseline to evaluate the effects of the fee changes. Because the result of fee changes was critical to future policy in other parts of the country, the researchers carefully examined the trade-off between decreased access and increased revenue. What they found gave them valuable clues to how user fees could be introduced elsewhere.

For Indonesia, the pilot study clearly showed how its citizens, especially the poor, would respond to fee changes. For other developing countries, this study showed how a rigorous experimental design with case controls and longitudinally collected panel data could be used outside of the typical clinical setting to provide data on access to care while controlling for social and demographic factors. (See Gertler and Molyneaux, 1996a.)

Linking Study Design to Policy. Does understanding "how data are generated" lead to better interpretation and better policymaking? Jamison and Jardel provide a framework that addresses this question and describe what data are needed for the rational evaluation of policy. (See Jamison and Jardel, 1994.) But this work stops short of linking study design to data quality, which is also important. Throughout the rest of this book, we will present examples of data, the studies that generated those data, and the resulting analysis that informs policy. For example, if policymakers know that researchers use modeling strategies to generate burden-of-disease calculations (and, thus, that the data are imputed), they will learn not to read too much into changes in numerical values. Also, knowing that researchers use qualitative studies to investigate institutions and political constraints should tell users that information from this method is hard to generalize to another setting. Finally, to understand how service choices have to be made, researchers use financial information to prioritize interventions, but policymakers need to know that those costs are not *actual* costs—they are estimated from imputed costs.

A few common study designs are frequently used to inform various types of policy decisions. Cross-sectional and longitudinal facility surveys of hospitals and clinics are used to find out about such things as the quality of care, the cost or the charges for services, and the types of patients who use the facility. Facility surveys, however, are biased because they capture only those who seek care and do not include all those who need care or who get care elsewhere. Household studies are used to determine the demand for services and make estimates about the population, regardless of whether they receive care or not. If a new benefits package is under consideration by the legislature, policymakers might want to see if the new package decreased overall utilization or if it pushed consumers to the private sector; so they would use a household survey. In the analysis, using a technique called regression, they could isolate the impact of income and location on utilization. This allows analysts to say that the household data showed that the new benefits package increased (or decreased) access to primary care clinics, irrespective of where people lived.

Data Presentation. It seems clear that nearly everyone involved in the health sector and in policy reform will need, at some time, to understand statistical analyses and reasoning to make sense of data. (See Moses, 1992.) The real question is, can knowledge of a few simple statistical techniques help policymakers and policy analysts understand a majority of research in scientific publications? Just such a question was asked in a review of the *New England Journal of Medicine*. The results might surprise those who shy away from understanding statistical analysis. A reader who knew only descriptive statistics—percentages, means, and standard deviations—could understand 58 percent of the articles. Adding t-tests and contingency tables increased comprehension to 73 percent. (See Emerson and Colditz, 1992.) Below, we briefly discuss the key statistical terms policymakers should understand. Table 2.13 defines the most commonly used statistics in policymaking and explains their common uses.

Most policymakers are familiar with *means*, which are merely the average value (x) in a sample, and *standard deviation(s)*, which, in turn, are a measure of how a sample typically varies around the mean. *T-tests* provide confidence intervals that allow researchers to attach certainty (typically 95 percent or *p values* of <.05) to a sample, to differences in means between two samples, or to matched samples. *Chi-square* tests are used to test differences between observed and expected findings and to estimate if the overall deviation was by chance or because it is from a different population. *Power*, loosely defined, is the size of the sample that has to be taken to detect useful differences between two groups. *Sensitivity*

Table 2.13

Common Statistical Terms and Their Use in Health Policy

Statistic/Term	Definition	Common Use in Policy
Mean	Average value of random variable in the sample	Used to summarize measures of samples such as population, utilization, income, and costs
Standard deviation	Measures how a sample varies around the mean	Used to measure the precision of summary measures—for example, age, prevalence, and health status
T-tests	Provide confidence interval that allows researchers to attach certainty, typically 95%, to a sample mean, or to differences in means between two samples, or to matched samples	Found in tests that look at differences, e.g., hospital discharge status or disease incidence between men and women, or between rich and poor populations
Chi-square test	A hypothesis test based on the difference between observed and expected values of categorized variables	Commonly used to evaluate relationships, such as sex ratios at birth, and to test the dependence between two variables, such as education of parents and their children's health status
Power	The size of the sample that has to be taken to detect useful differences between two groups	Used in designs of population or health surveys to determine the needed sample size
Sensitivity analysis	Evaluates the changes in outcome when assumptions or inputs are changed	Often found in decision analysis to see whether the optimal choice will be sensitive to changes in assumptions; it can be used, for example, in the analysis of investment decisions on health projects
Cost-benefit analysis	Compares the monetary costs against the monetary benefit to see whether the benefit of a policy or project outweighs the costs	Widely employed in project appraisal and policy evaluation; it can be used when both costs and benefits are measured in monetary terms
Cost-effectiveness analysis	Compares the costs with measures of effectiveness of a project or a policy by putting nonmonetary items into monetary terms	Also used widely in project appraisal and policy evaluation; it can be used when the benefit, such as patients' satisfaction, cannot be measured directly in monetary terms
Regression analysis	Explores the causality relationship between two or more variables	Widely used to study the relationship between health status/outcome, health policies, and sociodemographic factors, or, for example, the relationship between health policies and development, national income and education

analysis evaluates how results change if the assumptions or input data are varied. Finally, *cost-benefit analysis* compares the monetary costs against the monetary benefits, while *cost-effectiveness* puts nonmonetary items such as patient satisfaction into monetary terms. In either case, various cost-benefit/effectiveness strategies are then compared to determine policy priorities.

It should not be surprising that regression, an analytical method, does not eliminate the biases found in cross-sectional design. However, *linear and multivariable regression*, used extensively in the social science literature, is an enormously powerful tool that obviates some of the problems in observational (and longitudinal) studies. Regression uses statistical relationships in cross-sectional studies to draw inferences about causality between two observed phenomena. If data are collected longitudinally, regression controls for other concurrent changes and isolates the impact of the intervention. In the simplest case of linear regression, the *dependent variable* (Y) changes as the *independent variable* (X) changes.

If, for example, we are interested in the effect of per capita public spending on under-five mortality, we would write the equation as {Child Mortality = a (per capita public spending on health) + b}. Changes in utilization correspond to the coefficient "a" (also the slope), multiplied by spending. A *coefficient* can be positive, as it is in this case, or negative. The value of Y is equal to b when X is zero and corresponds to the intercept on the Y axis.

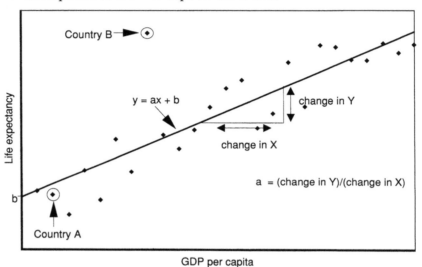

Figure 2.3—An Illustration of Linear Regression

Figure 2.3 (above) provides an illustration of linear regression that measures the relationship between longevity and income. The Y axis represents life expectancy, and the X axis represents GDP per capita. Each point in the graph is associated with a country. Thus, country A has a lower per capita GDP than country B, and it also has a lower life expectancy. In fact, for these data, as the per capita GDP increases (i.e., as we move to the right across the X axis), the life expectancy also increases. The straight line captures the positive relationship between the per capita GDP and life expectancy. The slope of the line (a) tells us by how much life expectancy would increase if we increase per capita GDP by one unit. Deviations from the line represent deviations from the estimated relationship between GDP and life expectancy. Thus, while country A does almost as well as estimated, but not quite, country B—an outlier—has a much higher then expected life expectancy for its amount of GDP.

These simple concepts can be extended for multiple variables so that analysts can simultaneously evaluate several independent effects on the dependent variable, such as education (also a positive coefficient), income (or consumption in developing countries), and sex (women typically use more health services than men). The power of regression allows researchers to "hold everything else constant" and thus isolate the effect of one factor, such as education or income, on the outcome of interest.

Each coefficient for each independent variable is associated with an *error term* that accounts for the degree of imprecise correlation. Error in this sense means "wandering" and corresponds to difficulties in measurement or inherent variability (such as country B in Figure 2.3) that occurs in behavior and biologic phenomena. The overall equation itself has a *correlation coefficient* (r) to test the ability of all the independent variables to explain the variation in the dependent variable. A key caveat is that these relationships depend on assumptions of independence, normal distribution, and noncorrelation in the error terms. Multivariable regression can be extended to include nonlinear effects such as income, which is usually a logarithmic function, and to discover discrete outcomes through a variety of well-established statistical and econometric methods.

Differing Perspectives

Beyond problems policymakers may have in understanding the issues of study data quality and interpreting analyzed data, differing perspectives can affect policymaking.

Sometimes, researchers' agendas and policymakers' expectations do not match. For example, the researcher, to validate conclusions, may be better served by ensuring that the results of a study are internally valid. In 1954, polio researchers compared a placebo with an attenuated virus in children between 6 and 9; as a result, the researchers narrowed the focus to this age group and were able to conclude that the virus worked for all *like* children. Policymakers, however, wanted to know if the researchers' conclusions were externally valid—i.e., true for older and younger children—a question the initial investigation could not answer.

Another difference centers on the different timeframes policymakers and researchers often operate in. Specifically, when they need to make choices, policymakers often have a limited time frame—a concern that is often antithetical to researchers, who are reluctant to finish ahead of schedule or to present partial results and data.

Finally, differences often center on the political dimensions discussed in Chapter 1. Researchers trying to provide data for policymakers may have to suffer with a poorly defined policy problem that does not consider both additional social or cultural factors and the political realities involved. In these instances, policy analysis is needed to frame the problem. For example, the problem may be conflicting values between different groups within the country, limited managerial skills, or inadequate and unsustainable funding.

POLICY IMPLICATIONS

What can we say about evidence-based policy when we look across these findings? First, regardless of whether a policy intervention is clinical, managerial, or financial, the quality of the evidence needs to be critically evaluated and there are limitations on how the data can be used. Adhering to these "data-use" principles should limit wasting valuable resources on interventions where the quality of the evidence is insufficiently convincing. Often, data quality can be

Box 2.4: Differing Perspectives of Policymakers and Scientists:
The Case of Vitamin A Supplementation Policy

In conducting studies to gain the high-quality data needed to make decisions about medical interventions, one of the major problems is that the perspectives of policymakers and the scientific community may differ—a difference that can have a significant impact on the timing and certainty of policy implementation. The example of Vitamin A supplementation is a case in point.

Xerophthalmia, a disease that results partly from a deficiency in Vitamin A, is considered one of the most common causes of blindness among children aged two to four in developing countries. In 1983, a group of researchers led by Sommer showed that the probability of dying altogether was also higher for children with Vitamin A deficiency than for those without it. (See Sommer et al., 1986.) Using a randomized controlled trial (RCT) of children living in Indonesian villages, researchers estimated that Vitamin A supplementation reduced the mortality rate for children by 34 percent.

Based on these results, policymakers in UNICEF and USAID planned to incorporate Vitamin A supplementation into the group of basic interventions given in the developing world. However, the scientific community had a different perspective: It questioned the validity of the results, arguing that since the original RCT was not double-blinded—i.e., the researchers knew which group was receiving the treatment—the results could be biased, thus overestimating the efficacy of the Vitamin A supplementation.

Confronted with these concerns, most policymakers suspended policy efforts to implement Vitamin A supplementation programs until more convincing evidence was available. During the mid-1980s, other scientific studies took place in countries like Brazil, Indonesia, India, Haiti, and Nepal, and by 1993, the results of almost all the trials confirmed that Vitamin A supplementation reduces childhood mortality, with a meta-analysis showing a nearly 23 percent reduction.

improved without significant costs—for example, by improving dissemination or by using better-disaggregated data. There is a tremendous need for high-quality evidence to evaluate management and financial interventions. This is important because such interventions not only have a much wider impact on health outcomes than clinical interventions have, they also entail using significantly more resources.

Second, while policy will continue to be made in the absence of solid evidence, policymakers should fund rigorously designed studies (such as RCTs and PCSs) that use control groups and employ before-and-after designs to get evidence. Pilot tests should be done when possible and then carefully scaled up to ensure effective resource allocation. As this chapter shows, good study designs can even be used to evaluate government's macro-policies.

Third, once policies are implemented, policymakers need to rigorously evaluate them to determine the benefits they yield, the harm they cause, and how cost-effective they are. This is imperative for policies implemented in the absence of any compelling data. As shown in Figure 2.1, there is a feedback loop from improved health outcomes back to studies. To do this, data users and leaders alike need to have basic literacy in study design and data presentation.

Fourth, governments and international public agencies must play the central role in funding data collection efforts for the public good. The unshakable corollary is that governments and international groups must also take a long-term view by investing in better routine data collection (both human and technologic capacity)

Although the data compellingly argued that improving Vitamin A intake for young children in populations where xerophthalmia exists should be a high priority, implementing Vitamin A supplementation policies was stalled again by the differing perspectives of policymakers and researchers. Specifically, debates emerged between scientists and international policymakers over the internal versus external validity of the studies. By the early 1990s, policymakers at UNICEF and WHO were supporting the introduction of Vitamin A supplements through existing immunization programs, reasoning that adding the relatively inexpensive supplement would be cost-effective and feasible to implement. Such reasoning assumes the Vitamin A supplementation results are externally valid across a broader range of ages—from several months to six years—and not just the two year interval demonstrated in the original studies. However, many scientists argued against the broader ranges, reasoning that the data showing the benefits of Vitamin A supplementation are only internally valid for older infants and young children.

Currently, this controversy has subsided—Vitamin A supplementation is widely recommended for children of all ages—but this controversy has given way to a new one on differences over how to give Vitamin A. Vitamin A intake can be increased either through supplements and food fortification or through changes in eating habits and agricultural practices. Not surprisingly, making a decision about how to give Vitamin A requires new studies and, once again, there are new controversies between policymakers and scientists. Changing behaviors such as eating habits requires doing research that is difficult, getting results that are more difficult to measure, and, if effective, implementing interventions that are slower to develop. This new research, besides being inherently uncertain and involving short-term costs, incurs another problem: The new approach to treating Vitamin A deficiency potentially makes it more difficult to sustain existing solutions, such as supplementation, which have already been shown to be effective. While scientists may argue that in the long run dietary sources are more effective, policymakers see supplementation as a program that works, and may want to turn their research attention and resources elsewhere.

and by supporting studies that answer unique policy questions. The focus, in the absence of baseline data collection, should be more on commissioning special surveys, such as household and facility surveys to evaluate a primary care intervention, and on local data collection and feedback, such as manual reporting at health facilities that do not have electronic or national systems.

Just as international agencies need to invest in data collection efforts for the public good, they need to fund disease-specific or developing-country-specific research and development (R&D) efforts. R&D funding should be aimed at "orphaned diseases"—diseases that affect the poor but are of little commercial interest. This includes both the diseases, such as malaria and post-partum hemorrhage, and enabling interventions, such as primary care health education strategies and community financing strategies.

CHAPTER 3: SUMMARY OF POLICY QUESTIONS, FINDINGS, AND IMPLICATIONS

ISSUES	EVIDENCE
• What is the burden of disease in Asia, both now and projected into the future?	• Asian countries simultaneously face an unfinished agenda of communicable diseases and a growing burden of noncommunicable ones.
• What are the best ways to measure the burden of disease given the data that are available?	• DALYs and similar measures combine morbidity and mortality and can be used to estimate disease burden, if their limitations are understood.
• What factors should be considered to match the disease priorities with health interventions?	• Costs, effectiveness, and other factors need to be considered to prioritize interventions.
• What is the best way for countries to reduce the burden of disease?	• Interventions can be prioritized into essential, desirable, and unnecessary packages.
• How effectively can Asian countries fund the necessary interventions?	• Funding high-priority interventions, although hard, is possible even for poorer countries and can significantly improve national health status.
• How can Asian countries get more efficiency out of their constrained resources when implementing the necessary interventions?	• Using traditional medicine, improving quality of care, and exploiting synergies can yield efficiencies.

POLICY IMPLICATIONS

- To prioritize interventions, policymakers need to rely on population-based measures of morbidity and mortality.
- Given that there is strong evidence, based on well-designed studies, that effective and affordable interventions exist, it is critical that policymakers consider medical efficacy when they prioritize interventions.
- Policymakers at the national and international level should ensure that present and future technologic developments from research and development are available and affordable even in the poorest of countries.
- Policymakers should pursue a broad policy that pursues the goal of universal availability of high-quality primary care.

PRIORITIZING MEDICAL INTERVENTIONS: DEFINING BURDEN OF DISEASE AND COST-EFFECTIVE INTERVENTIONS IN THE PURSUIT OF UNIVERSAL PRIMARY CARE

OVERVIEW

Prior to 1940, many people argued that medicine offered little to improve health or prolong life. However, since the discovery of sulfonamides in the mid-1930s, a panoply of medications, surgeries, and preventive measures have contributed enormously to human well-being, with new interventions and better therapies being developed every year. Just as important, there is a better understanding of the complex interactions between disease and the environment, between health and economics, and between social development and collective welfare.

Today, scientific investigations have shown that some therapies are effective, safe, and in many cases affordable to even the poorest of individuals. Other therapies are effective but are more expensive and, thus, require careful balancing of the costs and benefits, which vary with location, culture, and social structure. Still others are less efficacious but still are provided in place of more efficacious, better substantiated, and less-expensive interventions.

Choosing the right set of interventions is therefore an increasingly complex task of public policy. In some cases, the evidence for therapies is so overwhelming that all governments should try to make these interventions available as widely as possible; in other cases, the evidence is conflicting or, more commonly, incomplete. Thus, decisions are much harder to make and governments must be more cautious. In addition, whatever choices governments make are inevitably constrained by resources. And what makes choosing among interventions even more complex is that these choices have life-and-death consequences.

Prioritization is key, because, as discussed in Chapter 1, governments cannot—and should not—invest everywhere, nor can they afford to take an ad hoc approach to making decisions. They must take a more reasoned approach that is based on knowing what interventions work and how much they cost. How much interventions cost is about expenditures and about receiving value for expenditures. Thus, costs must be considered alongside medical efficacy. The information on efficacy comes from clinical data; therefore, the nature of the studies conducted to get those data is an important factor in making decisions about how much interventions cost.

In addition, the interventions should be prioritized in terms of their effectiveness. This includes the relative size of the burden of disease averted by the intervention, as well as its value in improving non-health outcomes (such as increases in education, income, and leisure time). So when should governments intervene?

From a public policy point of view, interventions should meet the following criteria: (1) They prevent or correct market failure, providing a necessary public good, and (2) they ensure equity, addressing disparities in health status among subgroups of the population.

Given these needs, we formulate six questions. Their answers form the basis for the rest of the chapter:

1.   What is the burden of disease in Asia, both now and projected into the future?
2.   What is the best way to measure the burden of disease given the data that are available?
3.   What factors should be considered to match the disease priorities with the health priorities?
4.   What is the best way for countries to reduce the burden of disease?
5.   How effectively can Asian countries fund the necessary interventions?
6.   How can Asian countries get more efficiency out of their constrained resources when implementing the necessary interventions?

As the last two questions show, this chapter necessarily touches on the areas of resource allocation and equity, both covered more extensively in Chapters 4 and 5, respectively. In terms of resource allocation, this chapter focuses on working *within* the existing resource constraints to fund interventions, while Chapter 4 focuses on how *additional* resources can be mobilized to pay for health interventions, as well as on how populations can be protected from market failures. In terms of equity, this chapter looks at improving equity using the most effective clinical interventions, whereas Chapter 5 specifically examines what approaches are available to governments to reduce gross disparities among vulnerable populations.

THE UNFINISHED AGENDA OF COMMUNICABLE DISEASES

Asia is undergoing a rapid demographic shift. Although the population growth rate (from 1985 to 1990) has slowed to 1.85 percent, this aggregation hides the variation between countries such as Pakistan (3.4 percent), Cambodia (3.1 percent), and Lao People's Democratic Republic (PDR) (2.8 percent) and the more affluent developing countries, such as Indonesia (1.8 percent) and Kazakstan (0.9 percent). (See ADB, 1994b, 1994c.) Such changes in growth reflect more than just changes in mortality from childhood deaths and communicable diseases. They are fundamentally influenced by changes in fertility. When the population base is continually expanding, the age structure is highly skewed toward the young; when the fertility starts to slow, as it has in Asia, the number of births each year no longer expands and the age structure changes from a broad-based pyramid to a rectangular-shaped column. In effect, this means that there is a rapidly growing adult population. The general decline in the fertility rate and concomitant aging of the population, both now and as projected into the future, are most dramatic in the wealthier, more-developed countries in the region.

This demographic transition is correlated closely with the epidemiologic change in disease patterns we are witnessing in Asia. As the population ages, diseases associated with insufficient nutrition and infection are giving way to degenerative disease. Driven by demographic change, many diseases are being influenced by concurrent changes in behaviors associated with increased personal (and national) wealth. For example, dietary choices lead to an increased percentage of caloric intake from cholesterol and saturated fats that, in turn, lead to an increased incidence of cardiovascular or cerebrovascular disease and death. Similarly, smoking, ubiquitous throughout Asia, and the chewing of tobacco in the betel quid, seen in South Asia and the Pacific, are behaviors that lead to lung and oral cancers, respectively. World Bank projections show that, compared to industrialized countries where mortality from vascular disease and malignancy will not change significantly, developing countries will have almost double the percentage of deaths over the next 30 years (from 26 percent to 49 percent) from these three diseases. (See Bulatao et al., 1990.)

Clearly, Asia represents a heterogeneous group of countries at different stages of economic, demographic, and epidemiologic transition. While large parts of Asia remain firmly in the grip of poverty, with relatively high mortality and morbidity largely from communicable diseases (e.g., South Asia), other areas are rapidly joining the ranks of more-developed countries with a very different epidemiologic profile that tends toward noncommunicable diseases (e.g., East Asia).

Throughout Asia, there are changes in living arrangements, urbanization, diet, lifestyle (smoking, alcohol), environmental pollution, occupational hazards, and demand for and use of health care services—all of which point toward the need to reevaluate the burden and distribution of ill health in Asia and its consequences for health-sector priorities and objectives. (See World Bank, 1993a; Feachem et al., 1993.)

Because of the heterogeneity within Asia in terms of socioeconomic development and its attendant health problems and priorities, this chapter (as does the book as a whole) concentrates mainly on developing economies in Asia, the two largest countries in Asia, India and China, and other countries—Bangladesh, Cambodia, Indonesia, Laos, Mongolia, Papua New Guinea, Pakistan, Philippines, Sri Lanka, Viet Nam, and the Central Asian Republics—where information is more plentiful. However, we will also draw on the experience of countries inside and outside of the region when appropriate. First, we will examine the current situation and then look at what the future holds.

Current Burden of Disease in Asia

Table 3.1 shows the burden of disease, as measured by DALYs, in China, India, and other Asian and Pacific Island countries (a heterogeneous group of 49 countries with Bangladesh and Nepal at one end of the economic development and epidemiologic transition spectrum, and Taiwan and Singapore at the other) in the context of the rest of the world. The data show that 50 percent of the total burden of disease is concentrated in Asia—670 million DALYs out of a total 1.3 billion DALYs.

Leaving aside China for the moment, when we look at "India" and "Other Asia and Islands," we see that about 50 percent of this burden is attributable to communicable diseases—diarrhea (9 percent), vaccine-preventable childhood infections (5 percent), respiratory infections (10 percent), and perinatal causes (8

Table 3.1

Burden of Disease by Cause and Demographic Region, 1990

Cause	World	India	China	Other Asian and Pacific Island Countries	Latin America and the Caribbean	Middle Eastern Crescent	Sub-Saharan Africa	Formerly Socialist Economies of Europe	Established Market Economies
Population (millions)	5267.0	850.0	1134.0	683.0	444.0	503.0	510.0	346.0	798.0
Communicable diseases (%)	45.8	50.5	25.3	48.5	42.2	51.0	71.3	8.6	9.7
Tuberculosis	3.4	3.7	2.9	5.1	2.5	2.8	4.7	0.6	0.2
STDs and HIV	3.8	2.7	1.7	1.5	6.6	0.7	8.8	1.2	3.4
Diarrhea	7.3	9.6	2.1	8.3	5.7	10.7	10.4	0.4	0.3
Vaccine-preventable*	5	6.7	0.9	4.5	1.6	6.0	9.6	0.1	0.1
Malaria	2.6	0.3	...	1.4	0.4	0.2	10.8	...	...
Intestinal nematode	1.8	0.9	3.4	3.4	2.5	0.4	1.8	...	...
Respiratory infections	9.0	10.9	6.4	11.1	6.2	11.5	10.8	2.6	2.6
Maternal causes	2.2	2.7	1.2	2.5	1.7	2.9	2.7	0.8	0.6
Perinatal causes	7.3	9.1	5.2	7.4	9.1	10.9	7.1	2.4	2.2
Other	3.5	4	1.4	3.3	5.8	4.9	4.6	0.6	0.5
Noncommunicable diseases (%)	42.2	40.4	58.0	40.1	42.8	36.0	19.4	74.8	78.4
Cancer	5.8	4.1	9.2	4.4	5.2	3.4	1.5	14.8	19.1
Nutritional deficiencies	3.9	6.2	3.3	4.6	4.6	3.7	2.8	1.4	1.7
Neuropsychiatric disease	6.8	6.1	8.0	7.0	8.0	5.6	3.3	11.1	15.0
Cerebrovascular disease	3.2	2.1	6.3	2.1	2.6	2.4	1.5	8.9	5.3
Ischemic heart disease	3.1	2.8	2.1	3.5	2.7	1.8	0.4	13.7	10.0
Pulmonary obstruction	1.3	0.6	5.5	0.5	0.7	0.5	0.2	1.6	1.7
Other	18.0	18.5	23.6	17.9	19.1	18.7	9.7	23.4	25.6
Other (%)	11.9	9.1	16.7	11.3	15	13	9.3	16.6	11.9
Motor vehicle	2.3	1.1	2.3	2.3	5.7	3.3	1.3	3.7	3.5
Intentional	3.7	1.2	5.1	3.2	4.3	5.2	4.2	4.8	4.0
Other	5.9	6.8	9.3	5.8	5.0	4.6	3.9	8.1	4.3
Total (%)	100.0	100.0	100.0	100.0	100.0	100.0	100.0	100.0	100.0
Total millions of DALYs	1362.0	292.0	201.0	177.0	103.0	144.0	293.0	58.0	94.0
Equivalent infant deaths (millions)	42.0	9.0	6.2	5.5	3.2	4.4	9.0	1.8	2.9
DALYs per 1,000 pop.	259.0	344.0	178.0	260.0	233.0	286.0	575.0	168.0	117.0

SOURCE: Murray and Lopez, 1994. *Childhood infections.

percent)—that could be prevented or reduced with better education and improvements in the household environment. Another 40 percent is from noncommunicable diseases, such as cancer (4 percent), cerebrovascular disease (2 percent), and schemic heart disease (around 3 percent), while the final 10 percent is from other causes, such as injuries.

Within this distribution—50 percent communicable, 40 percent noncommunicable, 10 percent other—we see that Asia is fairly evenly burdened by both the unfinished agenda of communicable diseases and the growing burden of noncommunicable diseases. Asia is struggling to control both ends of the demographic and epidemiologic transition simultaneously. This is a different story from what we find in the established market economies, which are driven by the burden of noncommunicable diseases, or sub-Saharan Africa, which is driven by the burden of communicable diseases.

The example of China—25.3 percent communicable, 58 percent noncommunicable, and 17 percent other—shows the epidemiologic transition in process from poorer Asian countries to those among the established market economies. For example, if we compare China with India (Table 3.2), we see that China, unlike India, has already completed its demographic transition and is currently at or near replacement fertility. Beyond China's rapid decline in fertility, its health profile is also driven by a successful health infrastructure. These two factors have combined to significantly reduce the risk of maternal death and the risk of communicable diseases.

Table 3.2

Comparison of Two Countries at Different Stages of the Demographic and Epidemiologic Transition

Characteristics	India	China
Demographics		
Population (millions, 1995)	936	1,221
GNP per capita ($US, 1995)	340	620
Life expectancy at birth (years, 1995)	62	69
Annual population growth rate (1991-2000)	1.8%	1.3%
Proportion of population 0-14 (1991)	35.8%	27%
Proportion of population 65+ (1991)	4.0%	6.6%
Proportion of population that is urban (1995)	26.8%	30.3%
Relative Burden of Disease (using DALYs) (1995)		
Communicable and maternal	50.5%	25.3%
Noncommunicable	40.4%	58.0%
Other (including injuries)	9.1%	16.7%

SOURCES: World Bank, 1993a, 1996a, 1997a; Murray and Lopez, 1994.

The other countries in Asia lie in between India and China, largely because the huge populations of Indonesia, Bangladesh, Viet Nam, Philippines, and Thailand represent about 80 percent of the total remaining population of this region; as a result, their epidemiologic profile dominates.

Finally, a notable point that is often overlooked is the substantial burden of injuries in Asia, particularly in China: While injuries have a variety of causes, many of them are preventable, and there needs to be a higher level of consciousness about this issue.

While the burden of disease in Asia differs from other regions of the world and within regions of Asia itself, it is only part of the story. The true heterogeneous nature of Asia shows up when we examine the burden of disease in cross-country comparisons. Table 3.3 examines, for selected countries, one of the causes of

Table 3.3

**AIDS and HIV Infections in Selected Asian
Countries, January 1995**

Country	Reported AIDS Cases	Estimated HIV Infections
Bangladesh	7	<20,000
Bhutan	0	<300
India	2,940	2 to 5,000,000 [a]
Indonesia	108	34,000
Lao PDR	17	550
Papua New Guinea	177	4,500
Philippines	273	18,000 [b]
Pakistan	64	40,000
Myanmar	1,349	150,000
Nepal	53	<5,000
Sri Lanka	68	<1,000
Thailand	44,471	750,000 [a]

MAIN SOURCES: WHO, 1997; WHO/SEARO, 1995b; OTHER
SOURCES: [a] Harvard School of Public Health and United
Nations Programme on HIV/AIDS (UNAIDS), 1996; [b] WHO,
1996c.

burden of disease in Asia—AIDS and human immunodeficiency virus (HIV) infections. As the table shows, the Asian epidemic is concentrated in India and Southeast Asia. In Thailand, 1 in 50 individuals is already infected. Also note the wide variation in reported AIDS cases and estimated HIV infections, from 0 and less than 300, respectively, in Bhutan, to 44,471 and 750,000, respectively, in Thailand. While some variation comes from underreporting, the range is still noteworthy.

Diarrhea, as mentioned above, has one of the heavier burdens of disease in Asia (around 9 percent). However, as Table 3.4 shows, the burden of this treatable disease varies widely in selected countries in Asia. The range in episodes per child less than five years old during a year is as low as 0.7 in Sri Lanka to as high as 3.9 in Bhutan.

As a final example, tuberculosis kills or debilitates more adults, age 15–59, than any other disease. It is responsible for about 2–4 percent of the burden of disease.

Table 3.4

Estimated Diarrheal Morbidity In Selected Asian Countries

Country	Estimated Total Diarrhea Episodes in Children Less Than 5 Years (in thousands)	Estimated Diarrhea Episodes per Child Less Than 5 Years per Year
Bangladesh	65,716	3.5
Bhutan	386	3.9
India	192,943	1.7
Indonesia	18,589	0.8
Myanmar	8,207	1.3
Nepal	11,171	3.3
Sri Lanka	1,261	0.7
Thailand	7,253	1.3

SOURCE: WHO/Southeast Asia Regional Office (SEARO), 1995a.

In developing countries, it accounts for an estimated 2 million deaths a year or about 5 percent of all deaths and 25 percent of preventable adult deaths. In India, for example, tuberculosis is the single leading cause of death. More women of childbearing age die of tuberculosis than from causes associated with pregnancy and childbirth.

The annual incidence of tuberculosis varies from 50 to 260 per 100,000 in the developing world, with more than half of these cases being infectious or sputum-smear positive. Table 3.5 shows the variations of reported cases for selected countries in Asia. For most forms of tuberculosis, 50–60 percent of those infected will die if untreated, with the case fatality being highest for smear positive cases—at an estimated 60–70 percent. (See Murray et al., 1993; Olakowski, 1973.)

Table 3.5

Reported Tuberculosis Cases and Percentage of Smear-Positive Cases in Selected Asian Countries

Country	Reported Tuberculosis Cases	Smear-Positive Cases (%)
Bangladesh	56,052	35
Bhutan	996	30
India	1,555,353	22
Indonesia	469,832	16
Kazakhstan	10,519	...
China	386,804	29
Lao PDR	1,135	66
Papua New Guinea	5,335	11
Pakistan	73,175	15
Fiji	996	27
Philippines	180,044	49
Myanmar	16,440	72
Nepal	8,893	47
Sri Lanka	6,174	54
Thailand	50,185	75

SOURCES: WHO/SEARO, 1995a; World Bank, 1996c; WHO, 1996c.

Future Burden of Disease in Asia

As mentioned earlier, Asia is going through a dramatic demographic and epidemiologic transition. Fertility rates are dropping, life expectancies are growing, and the population is aging. In the future, the burden of ill health will shift away from communicable diseases (which dominate the current environment) and toward noncommunicable ones.

Figure 3.1 compares the burden of disease in 1990 with the projected results in the year 2020 for China, India, and other Asian and Pacific countries. The information must be viewed cautiously because of the set of assumptions needed to perform a 30-year projection. Despite the data limitations, there is an important message: In Asia the burden of communicable disease is expected to be cut by half. Between 60 and 80 percent of the total burden of disease will be attributable to noncommunicable diseases.

However, in contrast to the classic epidemiologic transition that occurred in the West, the transition in Asia is somewhat different. First, the epidemiologic

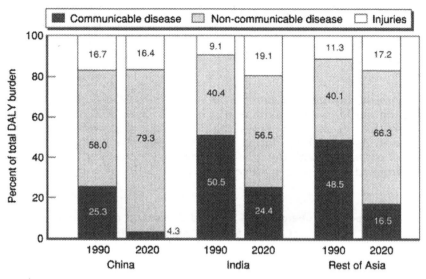

SOURCE: Adapted from WHO Ad Hoc Committee, 1996.

**Figure 3.1—Current and Projected Burden of Disease for
China, India, and Other Asian and Pacific Island Countries**

transition in the West was essentially reciprocal—communicable diseases went down and were replaced by a rising burden of noncommunicable diseases. In the developing countries of Asia, however, there is an overlapping transition, with countries having to face significant burdens of communicable disease and noncommunicable diseases simultaneously. In part, this overlap is fueled by fertility or birth rates that have not declined as far as they have in the West and by the decline in death rates (and, thus, the rise in life expectancies) that has not leveled off as fast as in the West. The combination leads to a much wider "gap" in Asia than in the West. This is demonstrated in Figure 3.2, which shows the demographic transition in England and Wales versus the transition in Sri Lanka.

Second, the transitions are happening much faster for the developing countries in Asia than they did for countries in the industrialized West, where rapid economic growth and improvements in health care infrastructure paralleled the shift in the causes of ill health. As Figure 3.1 showed, the shifts in China, India, and other Asian and Pacific countries are very rapid over the period of 1990 to 2020.

Beyond the differences in birth and death rates shown in Figure 3.2, the growth of AIDS throughout Asia will drive this residual burden of communicable diseases. Figure 3.3 (above) compares current HIV levels with other communicable diseases for selected countries in Asia. Table 3.6 shows the projected growth in AIDS in Asia and other regions of the world out to the year 2000.

Over 80 percent of the estimated 8.8 million people infected with HIV in 1990 lived in a developing country, where HIV is primarily a disease of heterosexual adults, with substantial perinatal infection of young children. Already 7,500 persons are being infected every day, and Asia is in the center of the explosive

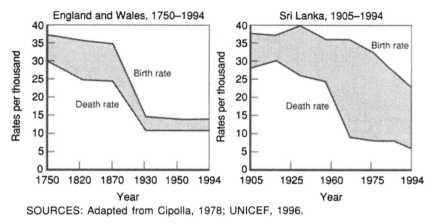

SOURCES: Adapted from Cipolla, 1978; UNICEF, 1996.

**Figure 3.2—The Demographic Transitions in the West and Asia:
Comparing England and Wales with Sri Lanka**

growth of HIV/AIDS projected worldwide over the next five years. As Table 3.6 shows, by the year 2000, 1.3 million people in Asia will be newly infected with HIV every year, HIV prevalence will have reached 9 million, and yearly AIDS deaths will total 600,000.

Thus, developing countries in Asia are facing a transition that has important consequences for the decisions that they have to make today about the types of

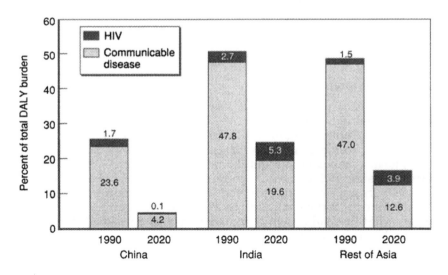

SOURCE: Based on Table 3.1.

**Figure 3.3—Current and Projected Burden of Disease from
Communicable Diseases and HIV**

Table 3.6

Evolution of the HIV-AIDS Epidemic

Region	HIV Incidence (millions/year)		HIV Prevalence (millions)		AIDS-Related Deaths (millions)	
	1990	2000	1990	2000	1990	2000
Demographically developing group	1.6	2.5	7.4	25	0.3	1.7
Sub-Saharan Africa	1.1	1.0	5.8	12	0.3	0.9
Asia (India, China, and other Asia and Pacific Island countries)	0.3	1.3	0.4	9	**	0.6
Established market economies and formerly Soviet economies of Europe	0.1	**	1.4	1	0.1	0.1
Total	1.7	2.5	8.8	26	0.4	1.8

SOURCE: World Bank, 1993a. **Less than 0.05 million.

investments in research and technologies. The challenge of the future for health planners in Asia, then, is how to deal with the rising tide of noncommunicable diseases, given relatively constrained financial and logistic resources, while simultaneously not neglecting the significant residual burden of communicable diseases.

DALYs AND SIMILAR MEASURES

To deal with the burden of ill health, both now and in the future, policymakers must be able to measure it effectively. Here, we examine some traditional measurements—morbidity and mortality—and then turn our attention to a more recent measurement scheme—Disability Adjusted Life Years, or DALYs. We then discuss some common data problems plaguing all classification schemes. Next, we show the results of comparing different diseases using different measurement schemes. Finally, we look at the results of using DALYs to measure the burden of ill health in Asia.

Morbidity and Mortality

Historically, health problems have been measured on two scales. The first scale, *morbidity*, describes the number of cases resulting for a particular disease entity/health problem. Morbidity is further stratified by distinguishing between *incidence*—the number of new cases in a given year for the particular disease/health problem in question—and *prevalence*—the number of cases currently existing (which includes both earlier cases that have not been cured and new cases). In practice, the distinction between incidence and prevalence is hard to make in most national statistics, and what is actually reported is the number of cases recorded in health facility registers in a given calendar year, regardless of when the health problem actually began.

The second scale, *mortality*, measures the number of deaths resulting from a particular disease entity/health problem. This scale includes measures such as infant and maternal mortality rate, but it can also include disease-specific causes of death. One problem often noted in the scientific literature is that, without an autopsy, the cause of death may be incorrectly assigned in over half the cases. Thus, even mortality figures should be interpreted carefully.

With regard to measuring ill-health burdens, both schemes have strengths and weaknesses. Morbidity calculations have the weakness of not being able to distinguish between levels of severity. Clearly, a case of dermatitis is not as severe a problem as a case of lower respiratory tract infection. And while mortality calculations provide a less unambiguous and relatively easily measured severity metric, mortality rankings of ill-health burdens omit the impact of conditions that produce a great deal of suffering but do not necessarily result in death (e.g., nutritional deficiencies, worm infestations, psychiatric conditions, and arthritis). Thus, most rankings of health problems by country/region have resorted to ranking health problems on both the number of deaths (mortality) and the number of reported cases (morbidity).

Disability Adjusted Life Years (DALYs)

In recent years, DALYs have been promoted as a new burden of ill-health classification scheme. (See Murray, 1996; World Bank, 1993a.) DALY classifications incorporate a number of features that distinguish them from conventional morbidity and mortality measures, including the following:

- *Measure of a joint burden of mortality and morbidity.* DALYs combine both morbidity and mortality into a unitary scale;

- *Measure of morbidity from handicaps, pain, or other disabilities.* DALYs combine morbidity from acute nonfatal diseases with long-term disability and other sequellae of illness;

- *Measure of potential years of life lost.* DALYs weight the death or disability of a prime-age adult more than that of an infant or an elderly person. This explicitly values economic productivity rather than giving equal weight to the death of infants, laborers or professionals, and the elderly;

- *Weight of disease and death as a function of time.* In the DALY scheme, years of life gained or lost in the future are discounted over time so that the near future is valued more than the distant future.

Healthy Life Years (HeaLYs)

The approach of using healthy life years (HeaLYs) to measure burden of disease was developed by the Ghana Ministry of Health Planning. It is a composite indicator that combines morbidity and mortality to provide quantitative measures of life loss from particular diseases and gains from particular interventions. (See Morrow and Bryant, 1995.)

The health status of a population is determined by the amount of healthy life its people achieve as a proportion of the total potential amount that they could enjoy under optimal health conditions. The total disease burden of a population is computed by adding together the years of healthy life lost per 1000 population from disability and premature death attributable to all diseases with onset in a given time period. Similarly, the benefits to be derived from a health program can be expressed as years of healthy life gained per 1,000 per year.

The main difference between HeaLYs and DALYs is that the latter directly integrate social preference values with the amount of healthy life.

Caveats to Using DALYs. The attraction of DALYs lies in their synthesis of conventional morbidity and mortality classification schemes into one unitary metric. However, their use and implementation involve a number of factors that need to be carefully weighed. (See World Bank, 1993a; Anand and Hanson, 1995; Hammer, 1997a.) First, calculating DALYs requires accurate information on age of death and cause of death, as well as the incidence and duration of morbid conditions. Accurate data on all these dimensions (especially the latter) are hard to come by in developing countries. Thus, model-based estimates and projections are used, which are difficult to validate. Moreover, this modeling makes cross-country and cross-cultural comparisons even more limited.

Second, the total number of DALYs depends on age structure. Since mortality and morbidity in children and young adults are weighted more heavily than similar conditions in older adults, countries with younger populations end up with a larger DALY burden. Because different weights are given to years lost at different ages, there is an emphasis on economic productivity in assessing ill health. Thus, a year lost to morbidity from tuberculosis for a 24-year-old adult yields more DALYs than a year lost to morbidity from tuberculosis in any other age group.

Third, the discounting of future years of life lost implies that lives saved in the future count less than lives saved today.

Fourth, the actual disability "weights" depend on the assessments of "experts." For example, how does one compare morbidity from uterine prolapse to morbidity from a lost limb, or from depression? To further complicate matters, disability is also determined by social and cultural factors that vary depending on who assigns the weights.

Finally, normalizing disability weights to 1 means that the impact of a disease is weighted less for disabled people than for people without any disability. (See Anand and Hanson, 1995; Prost and Jancloes, 1993.)

Data Problems with All Classification Schemes

Regardless of what ill-health classification scheme one uses, there is a generic issue about the utility and representativeness of nationally reported health statistics. Most developing countries have relatively poor recording systems, so what gets reported is information about those who make it to some kind of officially sanctioned health care facility. Because individuals have different propensities to seek treatment, using hospital data may lead to a number of biases. For example, if only severe cases that end up in the hospital get reported, the incidence/prevalence of each category would be underreported. In addition, because the threshold of health care facility use may vary greatly by disease category, recording will be much more complete for some types of disease entities than for others. For example, in Viet Nam, there are specific vertical programs focused on identifying cases of tuberculosis and malaria. Thus, more of these cases may be recorded than cases of diarrhea and acute respiratory infection, which might lead to artifacts in the rank order of different morbidities. Moreover, hospital and clinic reporting may be much more complete in some regions than others, leading to spurious regional differences. Finally, because of access barriers, poor, rural individuals may be less likely to go to health facilities than rich, urban individuals, which would lead to overestimating diseases that affect rich, urban individuals.

Some of these artifacts in the rank order of different morbidities and mortalities can be seen in the reported data. For example, when we look at trends in the five leading causes of morbidity and mortality for selected countries in Asia as reported by WHO, there appears to be significant volatility in the rankings—volatility that is unlikely to represent real changes in disease prevalence or fatalities and is probably the result of classification biases. For the period 1988–1990, circulatory system diseases in India were shown as the second leading cause of mortality; however, three years later in the 1991–1993 period, there is no mention of circulatory system diseases in the top five causes of mortality. Similarly, in Sri Lanka, while injury/poisoning was the leading cause of mortality in the period 1983–1985, it completely disappeared from the top five rankings in 1988–1990, then reappeared as the third leading cause of mortality in the 1991–1993 period.

The information required for a more accurate listing of disease or health burdens involves getting data from a random sample of the population. As described in Chapter 2, this sort of information is hard to come by and exists only in the few developing countries that have good surveillance systems. However, even with good surveillance systems, attributing causes of deaths, especially for adults, is a tricky business and involves a lot of ad hoc judgments. For example, time-series data from the Matlab (Bangladesh) surveillance system on causes of death show some unexplained but significant variation in certain types of causes. Specifically, cardiovascular mortality ranged from 10–20 percent of all deaths within the relatively short 1987–1991 time period. Again, this is most likely a classification bias rather than any real change in the pattern of disease.

The bottom line is that regardless of which classification scheme is used, national health statistics in developing countries should be viewed cautiously. This is particularly a problem with the DALY and HeaLY calculations, since they integrate information not only about deaths (which are hard enough to classify) but also about incident cases, their duration, and severity. Clearly, better microlevel data are needed to accurately gauge the magnitude and distribution of ill health in the population.

The Results of Measuring the Burden of Ill Health with Different Classification Schemes

In the absence of high-quality population-level information on morbidity and mortality, it seems prudent to use more than one burden of disease rankings (e.g., mortality and morbidity statistics and DALY calculations) and view the rankings as rough guidelines. Instead of trying to distinguish between entities close to each other in rankings, it makes sense to consider entities as a cluster (e.g., 1st through 5th versus 5th through 10th).

A comparison of mortality statistics with DALYs for the demographically developing countries is instructive. Tables 3.7 and 3.8 show that with respect to

Table 3.7

Comparison of DALYs Versus Deaths in Demographically Developing Countries by Categories of Disease

Category of Disease	DALYs (%)	Deaths (%)
Communicable maternal, and perinatal diseases	47.6	39.98
Noncommunicable diseases	43.4	52.02
Injuries	10.0	8.0

SOURCE: World Bank, 1993a.

death classifications, DALY classification schemes give more weight to diseases that predominantly affect children and young adults and diseases that cause disability but not death.

Communicable problems that mostly affect young children (such as acute respiratory tract infections, perinatal problems, diarrheal diseases, and childhood-immunizable problems) get more weight in the DALY than in a standard death classification. In addition, conditions such as HIV and helminth (intestinal parasite) infections, which cause a lot of disability but relatively few deaths, also end up with increased weights in the DALY classification. Since many noncommunicable diseases (such as cardiovascular diseases, malignant neoplasms, chronic respiratory problems, digestive problems) occur later in life, they are down-weighted in the DALY classification relative to the death classification. Two broad classes of problems that not only have been underrecognized but that also cause a lot of long-standing disability and relatively fewer deaths—nutritional deficiency-related problems and psychiatric problems—get significantly more weight in the DALY classification than in the mortality

Table 3.8

Comparison of DALYs Versus Deaths in the Demographically Developing Countries, Males

	DALYs			Deaths	
Rank	Disease	% of Total Burden	Rank	Disease	% of Total Burden
1	Acute respiratory tract infections	9.50	1	Cardiovascular	21.58
2	Cardiovascular	8.74	2	Malignancies	10.39
3	Perinatal	8.47	3	Acute respiratory tract infections	9.56
4	Diarrhea	7.95	4	Diarrhea	6.97
5	Neuropsychiatric	6.15	5	Perinatal	6.49
6	Child cluster (immunizable diseases)	5.54	6	Chronic respiratory disease	5.99
7	Malignancies	4.69	7	Tuberculosis	5.85
8	Tuberculosis	4.15	8	Child cluster (immunizable diseases)	4.97
9	Nutritional deficiencies	3.99	9	Digestive	3.96
10	Chronic respiratory disease	3.46	10	Motor vehicle accidents	2.33

SOURCE: World Bank, 1993a.

classification. Finally, with respect to injuries, there is not much difference between the two types of classification schemes.

Although the two schemes yield differing rankings and differing proportions of cause-specific ill-health burdens, the reality is that 8 out of the top 10 health burdens for males of all ages are the same for both schemes (this is also true for females).

The Impact of Using DALYs to Measure Burden of Ill Health in Asia

For the developing countries in Asia, which tend to have a bigger burden of communicable diseases and diseases that affect children, the correspondence between the two schemes is likely to be high. Roughly two-thirds of the DALYs currently lost in Asia's developing countries are from premature death. Thus, in the absence of DALY calculations, countries can use mortality classification schemes supplemented by morbidity classifications as a first approximation to gauge the societal burden of ill health, without fearing that they will be overlooking important areas of concern.

In summary, DALYs mostly confirm our existing understanding of health-sector priorities in Asia based on mortality rankings, but in addition highlight the contribution of specific nonfatal disease conditions. Thus, DALYs can be used, as long as the limitations noted above are taken into consideration.

COSTS, EFFECTIVENESS, AND OTHER PRIORITIZING FACTORS

Having established the burden of ill health in Asia and ways to measure it, governments must sift through the range of potential interventions for addressing that burden and prioritize them. Clearly, the cost-effectiveness of the interventions is central to determining which interventions to choose, but cost factors alone are not sufficient; other noncost factors should be included in considerations. Below, we discuss a series of factors to be used in prioritization, starting with cost-effectiveness.

Cost-Effectiveness in Prioritizing Health Interventions

Given there is always a limit on resources, governments intervening in the health sector have a responsibility to get the maximum benefit for society at the minimum cost. First, governments must determine costs and effectiveness. Second, they must allocate funds for interventions according to some measure of cost-effectiveness—defined here as the net gain in health (compared to doing nothing) divided by the cost of the intervention.

Caveats to Measuring Cost-Effectiveness. Estimating the costs or the effectiveness of health interventions is not without challenges. A number of factors affect such calculations, both for the same disease and across diseases. (See Prost and Jancloes, 1993.) Thus, one cannot really talk about a specific cost-effectiveness ratio for an intervention regardless of setting. A range of values is more likely. If cost-effectiveness is done properly, it can take local factors into account. However, in developing countries this may not always be possible given data constraints.

Poor-Quality Cost Data. Good empirical evidence on costs of interventions is generally not available in most developing countries, and Asia is no exception. This is true for both the health-system and household costs. In the case of health-system costs, budgets typically are disaggregated by inputs, not by programs/interventions. As a result, reported costs-per-consultations or costs-per-bed-days aggregate across many interventions and are thus not useful in determining intervention-specific costs. For household costs, there are even fewer empirical data. For instance, very little household survey data exist to gauge opportunity and travel costs of seeking care. (See Jamison, 1993.)

Not Treating Effectiveness and Costs as Separate Parameters. Many health providers and analysts view effectiveness and costs as independent parameters. The problem is that people equate effectiveness in an individual patient with effectiveness in a population. So while many health providers would reject a 50-percent effective intervention in favor of a 100-percent effective intervention on an individual level, on a population level, it might make perfect sense to consider such an intervention, especially if the 50-percent effective intervention is much cheaper. Cost-effectiveness analysis, if properly done, can take this into account. Thus, from a public-health perspective, one should consider the total number of individuals in the population who are better off given a set amount of resources.

A case in point is the use of streptokinase versus tissue plasminogen activator (TPA) as anti-clotting agents to treat evolving coronary artery blockages. On an individual basis, streptokinase is slightly less effective than TPA as an anti-clotting agent; however, TPA is much more expensive. Thus, given a fixed set of resources, it makes much more sense to advocate using streptokinase instead of TPA because many more patients would be helped.

Analytic Importance of Marginal Costs. Marginal costs—the costs incurred from the incremental expansion of the program/intervention—are critically important for evaluating the costs of health interventions. (See Mooney and Creese, 1993.) In most situations, health planners are primarily concerned with the costs of expanding the scope of operations. But the relevant issue is how much more it would cost to treat an additional case of a disease, not the average cost of treating those with the disease.

Allocation of Joint or Shared Costs. A big challenge in calculating accurate marginal costs of a particular intervention is deciding what proportion of joint costs shared by the health system should be attributed to the intervention. For example, when estimating the costs of short-course chemotherapy for tuberculosis, we can easily attribute the costs of anti-tuberculosis drugs, chest X-rays, and other modalities for diagnosis intervention, so we can calculate the additional cost by case treated. But how do we estimate the costs of personnel and infrastructure? What proportion of the salaries of hospital/clinic staff should be attributed to the TB intervention?

The Probability of Dying as a Result of the Disease. The case fatality rate matters in cost-effectiveness determinations if the metric of effectiveness weights death more than disability (e.g., cost/per death averted versus cost per DALY). Thus, immunizing against measles is more cost-effective than treating a child with oral rehydration solution (ORS), because immunizing against measles is more likely to prevent death than treating a child with ORS.

Disease Transmission Rates. Transmission rates of diseases matter because interventions that prevent transmission are more cost-effective than interventions that affect single individuals. Thus, because of their higher population impact (social benefit), interventions against communicable diseases are generally more cost-effective than those against noncommunicable ones.

Furthermore, if rates of transmission are high rather than low, cost-effectiveness is increased. This is why treating core groups in STDs/HIV and vector control are cost-effective in localized highly endemic areas, but not cost-effective when these same interventions are applied to the population at large.

Competing Risks and Synergy. The issue of competitive risk and synergy is very important. Naive calculations of effectiveness give the impression that a case cured is cured forever and that the patient will not be at risk for other diseases. This is the claim typically made for ORS, which temporarily averts the risk of watery diarrhea. However, counting up the cases of watery diarrhea averted underestimates the overall mortality/morbidity impact of ORS, precisely because these children are now at risk of getting other diarrheal diseases—most important, dysentery. Of course, this is not to say that children with diarrhea should not be rehydrated—only that ORS will not completely restore them to their original health. (See Hammer, 1997a; Martines et al., 1993.) By contrast, measles immunization is effective not only because it permanently protects the immunized child against measles but also because it raises general immunity and thus prevents the development of other conditions, such as acute respiratory tract infections.

Social Costs for Vulnerable Groups. One of the biggest potential deficiencies in reported cost-effectiveness estimates is that in most cases the costs are calculated only from the perspective of the health care system. Other costs borne by the patients are not included. Thus, the total social cost of a successful outcome for an intervention may vary by treatment, by gender (treatment of women may cost more), age (treatment of children may be more expensive because of the travel and opportunity cost of the accompanying adults), income (because of labor market inflexibility and the absence of paid sick leave, the poor may incur considerably higher costs for successful treatment), and region (higher travel costs in some regions).

Generalizability of Cost Estimates. Cost estimates of interventions typically represent the experience of vertical programs or randomized controlled trials that use information from a relatively small sample size. This raises the issue of the generalizability of those cost estimates, which depends on a number of factors. For example, a well-run pilot program or a controlled trial may have significantly lower costs than implementation on a larger scale, where there is more room for inefficiency and poor supervision.

Discount Rate. The discount rate used in estimating the present value of future payoffs also has a large impact on cost-effectiveness. Interventions where most of the payoffs are in the future (such as Hepatitis B immunization and investments in water and sanitation) become much less cost-effective than interventions that lead to immediate payoffs (such as the treatment of pneumonia or surgery for appendicitis). (See Hammer, 1997a; Jamison, 1993.)

All of these factors can be addressed if cost-effectiveness is calculated properly and the necessary data are available. In highlighting these methodologic challenges, we draw two conclusions: First, defining social benefits requires that judgments, based on unique values, be made. Second, given that data drive the analyses, if results confound common sense, the supporting information should be reexamined.

Table 3.9

Summary of the Cost-Effectiveness of Major Public Health Interventions

Condition	Intervention Strategy	Cost-Effectiveness per DALY Averted
Acute respiratory infections	• Screening and referral	• $20 to $70 per DALY with variable efficacy
	• Behavior change	• Approximately $50 per DALY with multiple benefits, including averted infant mortality
	• Immunization	• Approximately $70 per DALY for ages less than 18 months. Moderate efficacy in children over two years
Diarrheal diseases	• Immunization	• $10 to $75 per DALY, depending on realized efficacy of vaccine
	• Environmental control	• Cost-effectiveness unknown, but estimated to reduce diarrhea morbidity and mortality by about 30 percent
	• Behavior change	• Approximately $170 per DALY, depending on case-facility reductions, incidence rates, and wage levels
Measles	• Immunization	• $2 to $15 per DALY depending on case-fatality rates and cost of measles portion of immunization program
Protein-energy malnutrition	• Targeted mass chemoprophylaxis	• $70 per DALY, depending on target population
	• Food supplementation	• $25 per DALY, can affect birth weights significantly depending on target population
Tuberculosis	• Immunization	• $7 per DALY, but cost-effectiveness drops substantially when annual risk of infection is less than 1 percent
	• Targeted chemoprophylaxis	• Suspected to be reasonable though not on large scale

SOURCE: Jamison, 1993.

Estimates of Cost-Effectiveness in Developing Countries. Estimates of cost per DALY have been published by the World Bank for the 50 interventions that are the most relevant for developing countries. (See Jamison, 1993.) In Table 3.9 (above), we summarize the main public health interventions and their cost-effectiveness. As the table shows, targeted screening and immunizations are among the most cost-effective interventions. Indeed, the cost of averting one DALY ranges between $0.5 and $75. Interventions focusing on behavior change, although relatively more expensive (ranging between $30 and $170 per DALY), are still low-cost interventions when compared with interventions such as spraying of chemical insecticide for Aedes mosquito ($2,200 per DALY).

The information presented in the table can be viewed as generally valid for the developing world, since no data have been systematically compiled at the country level. However, we should not assume that this information substitutes for specific country studies. Still, given the lack of data and bearing in mind the cost-effectiveness caveats discussed above, the estimates do represent average values under realistic representative conditions in developing countries today. As such, they are a potentially useful guide for priority-setting by policymakers.

Setting Priorities at the National Level

What can be done to prioritize at the national level when so many technical challenges exist? First, the medical efficacy of interventions and the quality of the data should be determined. Second in importance is the relative size of the burden of disease those interventions avert. In addition, the nonhealth benefits of interventions (i.e., their ability to improve conditions other than health per se) need to be considered. Finally, and perhaps most important, interventions need to be prioritized in terms of whether they address issues of market failure and equity. These additional considerations are discussed below.

The Medical Efficacy of Health Interventions. Regardless of how the burden of disease is measured, getting reliable population-level data on the medical efficacy of health interventions, although difficult, should be attempted. As mentioned in Chapter 2, the gold standard is evidence from RCTs, an expensive, logistically complex, and often lengthy process. Because of these constraints, data from RCTs or even PCSs are not available for many interventions. This means relying on the other, less-rigorous evaluation techniques discussed in Chapter 2, such as case-control studies, retrospective cohort studies, and in some cases, anecdotal reports. In the absence of RCT evidence, however, evidence of medical efficacy must be interpreted cautiously.

There are a number of problems associated with relying on non-RCT studies for evaluating the cost-effectiveness of interventions, which we discussed in Chapter 2. The most important of these include deceptive claims about the population efficacy of the intervention in question because of nonrandom allocation of confounders (factors other than the intervention) between those using and not using the intervention (drug, vaccine, education program); recall bias in nonprospective studies (see the definition in Table 2.12); and small sample sizes, leading to statistical imprecision. (See Prost and Jancloes, 1993.)

In the next section, we recommend a set of interventions—selected from a much larger list—in an effort to eliminate those therapies and procedures where the data and studies are not reliable enough to demonstrate medical efficacy. In some cases, where interventions looked promising, they are included; in all cases, the text includes a discussion of the state of the data supporting medical efficacy.

Burden of Disease Averted. When applying cost-effectiveness criteria in selecting interventions, it is not always the case that resources should be put first into the lowest cost per death or DALY intervention. The total burden of disease averted

> **Box 3.1: How One Country Prioritizes Health Interventions: Information Needs in Viet Nam**
>
> How can governments trying to prioritize their investments in health interventions combine many factors into a single set of coherent policies? They must consider the burden of disease, effectiveness of clinical interventions, information about cost-effectiveness, the relative size of disease burdens addressed by interventions, the viability of private alternatives, the presence of nonhealth welfare outcomes, and the need to address equity concerns. According to mostly anecdotal data, government expenditures in most developing countries are skewed toward prescriptive and hospital care. Relatively few empirical data break down public health expenditure by the nature of health interventions—prescriptive or curative versus preventive or promotive. The situation is even worse for household expenditures. Cross-national case studies indicate that financial decisions are often separate from health policy needs. Information for prioritization is needed so that governments know where their resources are going and what the private sector (households and individuals) is spending. Private spending is particularly important, since it gives us a guide to the sorts of services there is demand for and for which private individuals are willing to pay out of pocket.
>
> What is needed is a set of national health accounts (NHAs) that would allow analysts and policymakers to track both government and household health expenditures. However, these exist for only a very few developing countries. One such country is Viet Nam.
>
> Viet Nam national health accounts suggest that public-sector financing is a relatively small part of total health care sector financing (16 percent), with the bulk of health-sector financing coming from private or household sources. In addition, the vast bulk of public-sector financing (by some estimates, almost 90 percent) goes for curative care in hospitals. Only a small amount—about 3 percent—is reportedly spent on preventive health care, and an even smaller proportion (about 2 percent) is spent on the lowest level primary-care centers—the "commune" health centers. Moreover, the majority of household health care expenditure is for the purchase of drugs. Finally, while spending on preventive services is meager, almost all comes from the public sector.
>
> The few empirical data from Viet Nam show that government health expenditures are skewed toward relatively sophisticated curative services that serve urban/peri-urban areas and, thus, have little impact on the population at large. This pattern is probably repeated in other countries. And NHAs show that despite the curative bias of government health expenditures, the primary source of funding for curative care and drugs come from out-of-pocket spending.

should also be taken into account, and priority should be given to those health conditions that are both cost-effective *and* avert large disease burdens. That is, the population prevalence and incidence of diseases matter. The rarer the disease, the more expensive it is to get a desired reduction in the societal burden of disease from a fixed unit of intervention. For example, screening for cancers only makes sense for those conditions like cervical or breast cancer that have a moderately high prevalence. Otherwise, the lower the prevalence, the more people are likely to have a falsely positive test and less likely to have the disease. With regard to incidence, BCG immunization, for example, becomes less and less cost effective as incidence of tuberculosis falls, because more and more children have to be immunized to protect those children who would contract tuberculosis in the absence of immunization. This is in contrast to medical treatment or secondary case prevention using anti-tuberculosis drugs, which focuses on those who already have been diagnosed or exposed to tuberculosis.

The criteria for burden of disease averted is met differentially in different age groups. Most of the health interventions considered below for those under the age of five are both cost-effective and avert large disease burdens. This situation is also true for women age 15–44. As the population ages, its health problems generally become more expensive to treat, and the disease burdens averted by available interventions tend to be much smaller.

Nonhealth Benefits Produced. Another major consideration is that a cost per DALY approach limits government to evaluation based only on health outcomes. As we mentioned briefly in Chapter 1, the objective of health planning is not only to improve the population's health status but also to protect the population from the adverse economic consequences of ill health.

What if a health intervention provides other aspects of individual welfare (e.g., increases in income, education, and leisure time) in addition to health? For example, by allowing households to limit family size, family planning interventions not only provide health gains for children and mothers but also have important implications for future household income and welfare. Not only do water and sanitation investments reduce the burden of water-borne diseases, they also produce large time-savings that can be used for other activities, including income generation. And while hospital care may not be very cost-effective based solely on health gains, if the desire is to provide some kind of catastrophic health insurance, governments may legitimately want to subsidize some kinds of hospitalizations. (This type of trade-off is discussed more fully in Chapter 4.)

Whether the Intervention Averts a Market Failure. In Chapter 1, we discussed two roles governments must play in the health sector, one of which was stepping in to prevent market failures (where insufficient resources are being spent on effective health interventions). It is difficult to capture these benefits in cost-effectiveness analyses. But if an intervention exists for which there is insufficient private demand (i.e., households are unwilling to use their own resources to seek treatment) and the benefits accrue to the general population, then the government should invest in it. (Chapter 4 has more discussion on how governments can intervene to overcome market failures.)

Where the Intervention Addresses an Equity Consideration. The second role described in Chapter 1 is to improve equity. In such situations, governments may want to deviate from the general principle of cost-effectiveness to address disparities in health among population subgroups. Poor women and other vulnerable groups such as children and the elderly may not have the money to pay for care or may be forced to make unacceptable choices between paying for care and paying for other basic needs such as clothing. (Chapter 5 has more discussion on how governments can intervene to improve equity.)

Prioritizing by Types of Care

In addition to prioritization schemes that are based on estimates of effectiveness and costs, health providers and policymakers recognize that some types of interventions can be packaged together. Inputs, such as hospital facilities or medical staff, are one way to aggregate health care services. Outputs or services, such as prevention or curative care, are an even more useful way. Aggregation by outputs creates economies of scale. Counseling patients about avoiding diseases or dispensing drugs to treat or prevent a variety of complications are examples. Another advantage is that services with similar outputs can be provided in facilities that require different capital outlays, and then, under these general groupings, be prioritized.

Primary care, secondary or district-level care, and tertiary or referral care are common aggregations of types of care. Primary care—care that includes fundamental public health and appropriate treatment against common disease—is further characterized as being coordinated, continuous, and comprehensive. Table 3.10 provides a list of objectives and aims that build on a typology used by Jamison (1993).

What types of care, if optimally delivered, are most effective at improving national health? Some preventive strategies, but certainly not all, fulfill this criterion, particularly if the diseases are communicable. Promotive strategies, such as breastfeeding, exercising, and hand washing, can also improve health in the aggregate. Many curative and rehabilitative services do not, in fact, improve national health, although they alleviate individual suffering, reduce pain, and occasionally save individual lives. We argue, therefore, that the best type of care to pursue is universal access to high-quality *primary* care, because it provides preventive, promotive, and basic curative care.

ESSENTIAL, DESIRABLE, AND UNDESIRABLE PACKAGES

Taking into account the above issues, what is a reasonable strategy for Asian governments to use in prioritizing health-sector investments? We recommend the following approach. (See Hammer, 1997a; Jamison, 1993; Mooney and Creese, 1993.)

1. Governments should invest only in those health interventions the private sector either cannot or does not adequately provide to the nation's population.
2. Using the available data, these interventions should be ranked according to cost-effectiveness.
3. The most cost-effective investments should then be prioritized by interventions that avert high disease burdens.
4. Governments should separately consider financing or providing interventions that improve other aspects of individual or social welfare.
5. Thus, governments will need to take into account the need to prevent or correct market failure and to improve equity (e.g., for the poor, women, populations in remote regions), even though interventions to do this may not be the most cost-effective ones.

Based on this strategy, we prioritize health interventions into those that:

1. Should be pursued by all developing-country governments in Asia;
2. Require a higher national income for developing-country governments in Asia to consider pursuing;
3. Have *limited* effectiveness in reducing population health burdens and thus should be deemphasized by developing-country governments in Asia.

Table 3.10

Objectives of Health Care Interventions

Objective	Aim	Examples
Primary prevention	Reduce incidence of condition by lowering level of risk factors	• Immunizations • Control of the environment (water and sanitation improvements) • Changes in sexual behavior • Adoption of contraception • Smoking cessation • Screening for hypoglycemia and prophylactic treatment for exposure to tuberculosis
Promotion of health	Encourage behaviors that lead to better health and hygiene and the avoidance of disease	• Breastfeeding • Proper balanced diet • Sexual abstinence • Boiling of drinking water • Hand washing • Wearing seatbelts • Daily exercise
Secondary prevention	Reduce severity or duration of condition or physiologic risk factor to prevent progression to more adverse consequences	• Distribution of ORS • Anti-helminthic therapy • Food supplementation • Screening/referral for treatment of cancers
Cure of condition	Remove the proximate cause and restore function to preexisting status quo	• Most clinic-oriented interventions, such as medical treatment for acute respiratory tract infections, tuberculosis, malaria, leprosy, STDs
Rehabilitation	Partially or completely restore physical, psychological, or social functioning to levels prior to condition being treated	• Physiotherapy and psychological therapy for disabilities from accidents, strokes, polio, leprosy
Palliation	Reduce pain and suffering for condition with no means of cure or rehabilitation	• Pain therapy for cancer • Medical treatment of AIDS

SOURCE: Adapted from Jamison, 1993.

For the first two priority areas, we summarize our results in a table and then discuss the interventions and the evidence supporting their medical efficacy in more detail. For the final area, we simply provide a summary table.

Health Interventions That Should Be Pursued by All Developing-Country Governments in Asia

The minimum package of required health interventions in all countries is shown in Tables 3.11a and 3.11b. They show that the major focus of health interventions in developing countries in Asia should remain on reducing childhood morbidity and mortality from infectious diseases and malnutrition and on improving maternal health through interventions such as immunizations, micronutrient provision, and the promotion of breastfeeding and appropriate weaning. Not surprisingly, these conclusions are in keeping with other assessments by most national governments, WHO, UNICEF, and other multilateral bodies.

At the same time, however, the recommendations for the essential and desirable packages (Tables 3.11a and b, and 3.14) also reflect a significant extension of the existing focus on children and mothers in two important directions: (1) they accommodate the increasing significance of specific noncommunicable diseases, such as cardiovascular diseases, cancers, and cataracts, that have accompanied the ongoing demographic transition and the rise in national income in Asia; and (2) they account for the resurgence of old communicable diseases, such as tuberculosis and STDs, and the emergence of new communicable diseases, such as AIDS.

A common thread running through all the recommended interventions is that government intervention is *required*—either for reasons of market failure, equity, or both—since the private sector is unlikely to provide adequate levels of services. Many of the benefits accrue to those who do not pay or receive the services. In addition, while most of the recommended interventions are preventive in nature, not all preventive interventions are worth pursuing (e.g., food supplementation), and some simple curative interventions (e.g., treatment of tuberculosis, treatment of STDs, etc.) are highly recommended. In general, the vast majority of clinical interventions can be performed in a primary-care setting at facilities lower than district-level facilities.

Finally, some interventions, such as assessing the universal access to obstetric services, although not justifiable on purely health benefits criteria, are recommended because of other welfare benefits and equity concerns (e.g., maternal mortality has huge negative impacts on women and children, historically disadvantaged groups in most societies).

We discuss each of the interventions in Tables 3.11a and b in detail.

Immunization. In the past 25 years, developing-country governments, urged on by WHO and other multilateral agencies, have raised the proportion of children immunized from less than 5 percent in 1977 to roughly 80 percent in 1990. In addition, about 35 percent of pregnant women have been immunized against tetanus. This increased rate of immunization has resulted in a remarkable 23 percent reduction of the total global burden of disease among children under five.

Despite these impressive gains, significant gaps remain. Even with the major strides in immunization coverage and even at the current levels of immunization (80 percent), roughly 10 percent of the total burden of disease for children under five—which could be prevented—is not being prevented. (See World Bank, 1993a.) More specifically, in selected Asian countries there are still significant gaps in the percentage of children immunized, as shown by the EPI numbers presented in Table 3.12.

It is also likely that the figures in Table 3.12 overestimate coverage. For example, DHS statistics in Thailand report coverage for diphtheria-tetanus-pertussis (DTP) at 66 percent (versus 85 percent); polio, 66 percent (versus 84 percent); and measles, 45 percent (versus 74.3 percent). In Sri Lanka, there was better correlation

Box 3.2: Preventing and Treating Measles in Developing Countries: Public Health Interventions That Clearly Work

In many cases, we have good evidence that interventions are effective, but it is rare when we have interventions that have been shown to have an unequivocal and significant impact on improving survival at the population level. The measles vaccination is one such intervention. Studies from the Matlab surveillance area in rural Bangladesh clearly demonstrate that children under the age of three who are vaccinated against measles have significantly lower risks of death—as much as 46 percent lower—than their peers without measles vaccination. (See Koenig, et al., 1990.) This conclusion is based on a large RCT— in which over 16,000 children were randomly assigned to receive or not receive measles vaccination and were then subsequently followed for a period of up to three years to assess survival.

What made this study particularly noteworthy is that it accounted for two important issues that are known to complicate attempts to assess the population impacts of health interventions. First, it accounted for the potential selection bias introduced by intrinsically healthy individuals receiving the health intervention in question. And second, it accounted for the issue of competitive risk and synergy, where an intervention is examined in light of whether it not only does what it is supposed to do but also lowers the risk of getting other diseases. The study showed that children who were vaccinated against measles enjoyed markedly improved survival throughout early childhood, compared to their peers who were not. Measles immunization, therefore, both protected the child against measles and raised the general immunity, thereby preventing the development of other conditions, such as acute respiratory tract infections.

The message from this study is that the measles vaccination should be given a much more prominent role within the EPI. Furthermore, in settings where infrastructural weaknesses make it impossible to deliver the complete package of EPI, at least measles vaccination should be ensured.

Unfortunately, despite its unequivocal success in protecting children, the measles vaccination is not nearly as widespread as it should be in Asia. For example, in 1994–1995, Pakistan, Lao PDR, and Myanmar had measles immunization rates below 70 percent. (See WHO, 1996d.) Because the vaccination rates are low in many places, measles still kill nearly 2 million children annually.

Interestingly, treating children with Vitamin A seems as promising for treating measles as vaccine is on the prevention side. Based on another RCT (this one of 189 children in South Africa), even if children were not immunized but contracted measles, Vitamin A was shown to be very effective in treating conditions associated with severe cases, such as pneumonia, diarrhea, or croup. Compared with the control group, the Vitamin A group recovered more rapidly from pneumonia and diarrhea, had less croup, and spent fewer days in the hospital. And of the 12 children who died, 10 were from the control group.

As was true on the prevention side, such unequivocal results lead to obvious recommendations on the treatment side: Give all children with severe measles Vitamin A supplements, regardless of whether they are thought to have a nutritional deficiency.

between DHS and EPI numbers. For example, DTP coverage in DHS was 91 percent versus 89 percent in EPI, although measles immunization was 67 percent compared to 82 percent.[1]

---

[1]These figures probably vary because of the way the data are collected: EPI uses "card" (medical record) information and imputes missing values from the "card note," while DHS uses maternal recall along with card information.

Table 3.11a

Health Interventions That Should Be Pursued by All Developing-Country Governments in Asia

Intervention	Prioritization Factors				
	Type/ Objective of Intervention	Cost per DALY Averted	Evidence of Medical Efficacy	Burden of Disease	Corrects Market Failure/ Improves Equity
Immunization (measles, diphtheria-pertussis-tetanus, polio, hepatitis B, tuberculosis)	P.Prevent	$12, $17; or $25-$30 if middle-income country	4+, RCT data very good	High	Yes/yes
Micronutrient fortification/ supplementation (iodization of salt, fortification of sugar with Vitamin A, semi-annual dose of Vitamin A)	S.Prevent	$1-$25	3+, some prospective data; 4+ RCT data for Vitamin A	High	Yes/yes
Targeted mass anti-helminthics	S.Prevent	$15-$30	3+, data limited	High	Yes/yes
Oral rehydration distribution in community	S.Prevent	$25-$75; up to $350 if complicated	4+, RCT data convincing		No/yes
Family planning promotion (contraception, birth spacing)	Promo/ Prevent	$15-$75 up to $250 for community distribution	3+, some-what limited study design, albeit good evidence	High	Yes/no
Breastfeeding and appropriate weaning practices	Promo/ P.Prevent	$25-$30	4+, good prospective design	High	Yes/no
AIDS/STD prevention education	Promo/ P.Prevent	$25 (condoms)	3+, data inconclusive in every case, good design	High	Yes/no
Antibiotic treatment of STDs in targeted risk groups	Cure/ Promo	$40	4+, clinical efficacy certain	High	Yes/yes
Programs to reduce smoking, alcohol, and other drug use	Promo	$25	2+, data not conclusive; social experimental design needed	High	Yes/no
Anti-tuberculosis chemotherapy	Cure/ S.Prevent	$3-$25	4+, clinical efficacy certain	High	Yes/yes

SOURCE: Adapted from Jamison et al., 1993.
NOTES: P.Prevent = Primary prevention; Promo = Promotion of health; S.Prevent = Secondary prevention; Cure = Cure of a condition.
Evidence: 4+ = Good prospective, randomized studies with convincing results; 3+ = Some prospective well-designed studies; 2+ = Cohort cross-sectional data; 1+ = Case study or common practice only.

The result of such coverage gaps is increases in the burden of disease. For example, half of all the new cases of polio in the world are in India. At least 25 million Indians have been severely disabled in the past 25 years. Of the 100,000 polio cases reported each year, 80 percent come from India, Bangladesh,

Table 3.11b

Health Interventions That Should Be Pursued by All Developing-Country Governments in Asia (continued)

Intervention	Type/ Objective of Intervention	Cost /per DALY Averted	Evidence of Medical Efficacy	Burden of Disease	Corrects Market Failure/ Improves Equity
		Prioritization Factors			
Antibiotic treatment of STDs in targeted risk groups	Cure/ promo	$40	4+, clinical efficacy certain	High	Yes/yes
Clinic services for pregnancy and delivery care	Promo/ cure	$30–$250	3+, prenatal care effective, elements of care	High	Yes/yes
Medical treatment of acute respiratory tract infections	Cure	$20–$50	4+, uncertain 4+ clinical efficacy very good	High	No/yes
Cataract removal	Cure	$20–$40	3+, clinically effective but efficacy in population depends on use/avail- ability of post-op connective lenses	High	No/yes
Cancer pain palliation	Pallia	$150	4+, for pain relief	Moderate/ high	No/yes
Rehab from injuries, leprosy, and polio	Rehab	$200–$225	3+, variable, depending on condition	High	No/yes
Treatment of injuries and minor trauma	Cure/rehab	$25–$250	3+, clinical efficacy excellent depending on type of injury	High	No/yes

SOURCE: Adapted from Jamison et al., 1993.
NOTES: Promo = Promotion of health; S.Prevent = Secondary prevention;
Cure = Cure of a condition; Rehab = Rehabilitation; Pallia = Palliation.
Evidence: 4+ = Good prospective, randomized studies with convincing results; 3+ = Some prospective well- designed studies; 2+ = Cohort cross-sectional data; 1+ = Case study or common practice only.

Myanmar, Nepal, Pakistan, Sri Lanka, and Thailand. The actual number of cases in India may be 10 times higher, according to WHO estimates. (See WHO, 1996d.)

Two expansions of the current EPI program are needed. First, coverage should be extended to 95 percent of all children. Second, the EPI package should be expanded to include hepatitis B, polyvalent pneumacoccal vaccines and, when it is generally available, a retrovirus vaccine.

In terms of medical efficacy, immunization to prevent the cluster of childhood diseases—measles, diphtheria, pertussis, tetanus, and polio—has been one of the

Table 3.12

Variations in Immunization Coverage in Selected Asian Countries, 1994

Country	Diphtheria-Pertussis-Tetanus (% infants immunized)	Polio (% infants immunized)	Measles (% infants immunized)	Tuberculosis (% infants immunized)	Hepatitis B (% infants immunized)	Tetanus Toxoid for Pregnant Women (% live births)
Bangladesh	74	74	62	95	...	61.8
Bhutan	83	82	69	92	...	27.0
India	90.3	90.8	85.8	96.5	...	79.4
Indonesia	99.2	94.8	90.3	96.2	34.88	63.9
Nepal	71.	72	66	83	...	26.8
Myanmar	73.2	73.1	71	80	...	72
Sri Lanka	89.8	89.5	82.9	88.5	...	85.3
Thailand	84.9	84.2	74.3	100	15.4	73.2

SOURCE: WHO, 1995a.

major advances of the past 50 years. A variety of well-controlled randomized cohort and case control studies have substantiated these benefits. (See Foster et al., 1993; Steinglass et al., 1993.) Immunizations are the quintessential public good, because the benefits accrue to more than those paying for the services. Because the private market will not provide adequate amounts of immunization, publicly funded and provided immunization coverage remains the alternative of choice.

Furthermore, immunizations are one of the most cost-effective health interventions available. The cost per DALY gained varies between $12 and $17 in low-income countries (those with high fertility and mortality and an average per capita income of $350) to $25–$30 in middle-income countries (those with low mortality and fertility and average per-capita incomes of $2,500). (See World Bank, 1993a.)

Micronutrient Fortification/Supplementation. People in developing countries frequently suffer from three major micronutrient deficiencies: iron, iodine, and Vitamin A. (See Levin et al., 1993.) Iron deficiency is the most common and produces a range of clinical problems, including reducing physical productivity and hampering children's capacity to learn in school. It may also diminish children's future growth by reducing appetite. Women are particularly vulnerable, because menstruation and pregnancy raise their needs for iron. If iron is not available in the diet, iron deficiency anemia results, which increases the risk of death from hemorrhage in childbirth. The problem is particularly severe in South Asia: In India, for example, it is estimated that 88 percent of pregnant women are anemic. For the rest of Asia, the figure approaches 60 percent, except for China, where it is no more than 40 percent. This contrasts with 15 percent of pregnant women in developed countries.

Iodine deficiency—which can cause severe and mild mental retardation; delayed motor development; stunting; impaired reproduction; and neuromuscular, speech, and hearing disorders—is estimated to be the leading preventable cause of intellectual underdevelopment in the world.

Vitamin A, an organic substance the body cannot produce, is essential for normal vision, growth, and immune function. Vitamin A deficiency can cause various degrees of vision loss and is the primary cause of acquired blindness in children. About 42 million children under the age of six are estimated to have mild or moderate xerophthalmia. (See Sommer et al., 1986.) Deficiencies in Vitamin A also affect the severity and survival chances of children with measles and diarrhea.

Micronutrients can be provided either by fortifying daily foods or by providing separate supplementations. Fortifying daily foods is a very effective means of raising micronutrient levels, since it does not involve a change in eating habits, which is much harder to implement. Many experimental programs have shown the value of fortification. For example, fortification of monosodium glutamate with Vitamin A in Indonesia is estimated to have cut mortality by as much as 30 percent. In Chile, the addition of iron to powdered milk and soybean-based infant formula decreased anemia substantially.

In terms of iodized salt fortification, a case-controlled, cross-sectional study in the Guizhou province of China examined the effects of iodized salt on the hearing of otherwise normal 7–11-year-old children, one, two, and three years after prophylaxis. The study found a significant positive effect of the intervention. (See Wang and Yang, 1985.) The study of another salt iodization program in one Chinese village showed that the program improved the intellectual capacity of the village residents and raised their productivity. The average income per capita increased from 41 yuan in 1981 to 223 in 1982 to 414 in 1984. (See Levin, 1987.) And Brazil's national salt iodization program, which began in 1978, greatly reduced endemic goiter in areas of iodine deficiency. (See World Bank, 1993a.)

Supplementation is more difficult than fortification, since it often requires regular, frequent contact with the target population. Still, there are many well-designed, randomized controlled studies that show Vitamin A supplementation to be effective. A study by Schroeder et al. (1995) concluded that food supplementation interventions decrease infant mortality rates 23 to 64 percent on their own and 25 to 77 percent in combination with other health care interventions. Another study in Ghana showed that Vitamin A supplementation significantly reduced the overall incidence of severe illnesses, clinic attendance, hospital admissions, and mortality. (See Ross et al., 1995.) A meta-analysis done on eight field trials of Vitamin A supplementation in children age six months to five years indicated that population mortality rates in children under five were reduced by nearly 23 percent in those with some clinical signs of Vitamin A deficiency. (See Beaton and Ghassemi, 1982.) Finally, if provided in the form of capsules at intervals of one week to six months, Vitamin A substantially reduces the risk of blindness.

Similarly, studies show that oral doses of iodized oil protect for two to four years against iodine deficiency. Supplements for women of reproductive ages prevent mental retardation in their children and reduce the risk of infant mortality.

Iron supplements are the least effective of the three micronutrients, since iron tablets need to be taken every day and often cause side effects (mostly gastrointestinal ones). Because of this, iron supplementation should be reserved for specific target groups, such as pregnant women or children in high-risk areas after deworming (e.g., South Asia).

Targeted Mass Anti-Helminthics. Worm infestations (roundworms, hook-worms, whip worms, and schistosomiasis) affect more than one-third of the world's population, including 100 to 400 million school-age children worldwide. Certain types of helminthic infestations, such as schistosomiasis, are among the top 10 primary infectious diseases in Asia, Africa, and Latin America as defined by prevalence, morbidity, and mortality.

Helminthic infections have significant consequences, especially for children. The consequences include failure to thrive, mental retardation, iron deficiency, anemia, impaired cognition, and an increase in morbidity and mortality. These consequences, combined with high prevalence of most helminthic infection, suggest the importance of intervention and control from the standpoint of both economic productivity and general welfare.

Worm infestations can be treated by low-cost, single-dose oral therapy. Well-controlled studies of single-dose oral therapy in India, Kenya, and the West Indies have shown significant spurts in growth and development and cognitive improvement at costs per DALY of $15–$30. (See Bundy et al., 1989; Jamison and Leslie, 1990; Warren et al., 1993.)

A major problem in endemic areas is the risk of reinfection. Within 12 months of treatment, children in such areas get reinfected with roundworm and whipworm (for hookworm, within 24 months of treatment). The key to addressing this issue is to lower the overall level of contamination of the environment from the infective stages of the worms. Treatment of school-age children (the most heavily infected group) reduces both individual infection and the risk of infection in the community.

There are three different strategies for controlling helminthic infections in a population—mass treatment, targeted mass treatment of a portion of the population, and screening. Mass treatment (e.g., mass chemotherapy) involves treating a total population, regardless of whether it is infected. Another type of mass treatment involves targeting a certain segment of the population (e.g., a specific age group such as children). The alternative strategy is screening: treating only affected members of the population whose infection is demonstrated by standard diagnostic procedures. These strategies have different implications in terms of cost and effectiveness.

A simulation study of the costs and effectiveness of chemotherapy based on representative data from the three approaches shows that, if only effectiveness is considered, mass chemotherapy is the best option, because it can effectively treat 90 percent of heavily infected cases; targeted mass chemotherapy ranked second, with 80 percent of cases treated effectively; and screening proved to be the least-effective option, with only 60 percent of cases treated effectively. If budget constraints are introduced, the screening option is still the least cost-effective strategy. The higher the budget level, the more effective and less costly the mass treatment is relative to targeted mass treatment. The mass treatment strategy is justifiable when the prevalence of the infection is sufficiently high. The screening option is more cost-effective only if drug costs are high relative to screening costs. (See Jamison, 1993.)

Oral Rehydration Solution Distribution in Community. The development of oral rehydration therapy (ORT) in the late 1960s has been hailed as one of the major medical advances of the twentieth century. It involves using oral rehydration solution (ORS), which combines electrolytes and glucose, sucrose, or rice powder, for treating watery diarrhea. Clinical studies have shown that ORS can successfully rehydrate 90–95 percent of cases of acute watery diarrhea, thus substantially reducing the requirements for intravenous rehydration. Not only is ORS as effective as intravenous rehydration in most cases, it is also less hazardous, especially in settings where the risk of infection is high.

While clinical studies in hospital settings uniformly show very high effectiveness for oral rehydration therapy, field trials show more variability in its effects to combat watery diarrhea. (See Levine et al., 1986; Tekce, 1982.) This is probably because of the complexity of preparing home-based rehydration solutions and because of the difficulties of administration. Nevertheless, the overall findings tend to be positive. A variety of studies in India and Egypt show a sharp reduction in diarrheal mortality for children under five associated with the use of oral rehydration. (See Kielman and McCord, 1977; el-Rafie et al., 1990.)

Until recently, ORT has been the mainstay of international and national programs in the field of diarrhea control. It has been claimed that since diarrhea accounts for 20–40 percent of all child deaths and since ORT can greatly reduce mortality from watery diarrhea, it would have a very significant impact on overall child mortality rates.

However, the past decade of experience with vigorous ORT programs in the developing world has not fulfilled the heightened expectations about sharp reductions in child mortality from diarrheal disease, despite relatively high ORS access rates. (The access rate is defined as the proportion of children less than five years old with reasonable access—i.e., living within one hour travel time—to a trained provider of ORS who receives an adequate supply of ORS.)

Table 3.13 shows the estimated ORS access and use rates for selected countries in Asia. While the access rates are fairly high, the use rate—defined as the proportion of all cases of diarrhea in children less than five years of age treated with ORS or recommended home fluid (RHF)—is significantly lower for most of the countries. (See McDivitt et al., 1994.)

A more careful examination of the complexity of diarrhea diagnosis and treatment—one that accounts for the nonapplicability of ORT in dysentery or in complex and persistent cases of diarrhea, the substantial prevalence of ineffectively provided ORT, and the presence of competitive risks—shows that at most only 40 percent of life-threatening diarrhea episodes can be potentially averted by the use of ORT. Because of these considerations, costs per DALY average $25–$75, but they may be as much as $350 for clinical interventions. (See Jamison, 1993; Lerman et. al, 1985; Shepard et al., 1986.)

The policy implication is that much more emphasis must be placed on primary prevention and on more-comprehensive case management of life-threatening diarrhea; this would include ORT but would go beyond it to embrace the correct use of antibiotics follow-up. (See Martines et al., 1993.)

Table 3.13

Estimated ORS Access and Use Rates
in Selected Asian Countries

Country	ORS Access Rate (%)	ORS Use Rate (%)
Bangladesh	75	26
Bhutan	85	85
India	77	37
Indonesia	92	78
Myanmar	57	37
Nepal	80	14
Sri Lanka	100	76
Thailand	90	65

SOURCE: WHO/SEARO, 1995a.

Family Planning Promotion. Fertility patterns affect both maternal and child health in a variety of ways. For example, births to young and old mothers, to those mothers with high parity, and closely spaced births pose significant risks to mother and child. Mothers who give birth before age 18 are three times as likely to die in childbirth as those who give birth between ages 20 and 29. Women over 35 face maternal mortality rates five times as high as their peers 20–24. Maternal mortality also rises with parity above three and with maternal age above 30. (See Cochrane and Sai, 1993; Peabody, 1995.)

With regard to children, evidence from Indonesia suggests that babies born to mothers age 18 and under are 50 percent more likely to die than those born to mothers age 20–24. Research from Kenya shows that infants born within 18 months of the birth of the previous child are more than twice as likely to die as those born after 24 months. (See Hobcraft et al., 1985.)

Promoting family planning is one of the most effective means of reducing the burden of ill health for women and children. Options to be considered include providing information on the health effects of fertility reduction and regulation, teaching couples about effective methods of contraception, removing restrictions on marketing contraceptives, and, in specific situations, distributing contraceptives in communities and households. (See Bongaarts, 1987, 1988; Trussell and Pebley, 1984.)

Family planning services provided through community-based distributions are a highly cost-effective way of improving maternal and child health. (This is discussed in more detail in Chapter 6.) This is particularly true of countries where both fertility and mortality are high, as is the case in most of the developing countries in Asia. Community health workers serve a dual purpose of both spreading information about family planning and providing contraceptives, including pills, condoms, and foaming tablets. In many parts of Asia (especially South Asia) where social restrictions make it difficult for women to go to relatively faraway clinics, community distribution of contraceptives has been the key to fertility decline and birth spacing. For example, as we discussed earlier in Chapter 2, controlled trials suggest that the dramatic decline of fertility in Bangladesh—from a total fertility rate of 7 per cent in 1975 to 3.4 in 1995—is largely a result of the community distribution of contraceptives. (See Cleland et al., 1994.)

Even with this evidence, the effectiveness and the costs per DALY for family planning promotion services clearly depend on a host of factors, including the level of program sophistication, the use of community distribution of contraceptives, and the prevailing levels of mortality and fertility. When limited to education efforts to increase the use of condoms and other contraceptives, costs per DALY vary between $15–$75. Community distribution of contraceptives is, of course, quite a bit more expensive but also more effective. While exact costs are unknown, they are likely to be as high as $250 per DALY. (See Cochrane and Sai, 1993.)

Promotion of Breastfeeding and Appropriate Weaning Practices. Probably the most valuable component of nutrition education is the promotion of breast-feeding. Longitudinal cohort studies from Brazil show that infants who have been exclusively breastfed for the first four to six months of life are 18 times less likely to die from diarrhea and three times less likely to die from respiratory diseases. This increased protection results from a higher volume of calories and from increased resistance to disease because of the transfer of maternal antibodies to infants. Not only do infants benefit from breastfeeding, so do their mothers. Breastfeeding helps to preserve maternal iron stores by suppressing menstruation (lactation amenorrhoea). In addition, it helps mothers by spacing out births, decreasing the risk of breast or ovarian cancer, and possibly by reducing the amount of postpartum bleeding. (See Martines et al., 1993; Briend et al., 1988.)

Breastfeeding promotion projects have been shown to be effective in increasing both the number of mothers initiating breastfeeding and the duration of exclusive and partial breastfeeding. Research estimates suggest that the promotion of breastfeeding can reduce diarrhea morbidity by 8–20 percent in the first six months of life and 1–4 percent for children under five. Mortality rates can be reduced by 24–27 percent in the first six months and by 8–9 percent for children under five. (See Feachem and Koblinsky, 1984.) Recent research using longitudinal, population-based studies from Bangladesh suggests that these estimates may in fact be conservative and that breastfeeding may provide protection against diarrheal deaths and severe diarrhea up to the third year of life. (See Clemens et al., 1986.)

Such programs of breastfeeding promotion need to educate both mothers and health professionals who often encourage milk substitutes. In addition, they must take into account the heavy time burden associated with breastfeeding. To be really effective, promotion of breastfeeding may require changes in work schedules of women. Results from the few adequately designed breastfeeding promotion programs show that they are consistently effective in increasing rates of breastfeeding. (See Huffman and Combest, 1988.)

In addition to breastfeeding, improved weaning practices can potentially have a significant impact on reducing malnutrition-associated diarrheal morbidity and mortality in children under five. Data from a number of developing countries—including Bangladesh, India, and Nigeria—support this finding. (See Chen et al., 1980; Bhan et al., 1986; Tomkins, 1981.) While lack of parental access to proper foods is a part of poor weaning practices, food taboos and lack of knowledge about appropriate nutrition contribute significantly. The few weaning educational programs that have been properly evaluated suggest that weaning education can halve the proportion of children at less than 75 percent weight for age who die from diarrhea. (See Ashworth and Feachem, 1985.)

With regard to cost-effectiveness, Jamison et al. (1993) estimate a cost of approximately $25–$30 per DALY for breastfeeding promotion by various methods, including changes in hospital routine and mass-media education. This cost assumes a reduction in nonbreastfeeding of 40 percent for children less than 2 months, 30 percent for children between 3 and 5 months, and 10 percent for children between 6 and 11 months. In the case of weaning, Jamison et al. (1993) estimate a similar cost-effectiveness of $25–$30 per DALY in children between six months and five years who are less than 75 percent weight for age.

AIDS/STD Prevention Education. Unknown before 1981, AIDS now is perhaps the most significant new public health challenge that developing countries in Asia face. (See Over and Piot, 1993.) The causative agent of AIDS, HIV, is transmitted through sexual intercourse and, like other STDs, can be spread by contact with contaminated blood (notably blood transfusions) and from mother to child during the perinatal period. Casual transmission from person to person has not been shown to occur.

Despite the absence of a vaccine or a cure, there is still a significant potential for reducing the spread of HIV/AIDS. The primary health intervention is prevention through two major components: providing education and encouraging condom use. Education should focus on reducing the number of sexual partners, on the importance of using condoms, on refraining from certain high-risk sexual acts (such as anal sex), on avoiding high-risk individuals (such as sex workers as sexual partners), on avoiding contact with contaminated blood, and on seeking prompt treatment for STDs.

The key to cost-effective intervention is to focus on changing sexual behavior and reducing transmission in core affected groups, such as sex workers and their clients, rural-to-urban migrants, members of the military, truck drivers, and intravenous drug users. (The subject of changing behavior is discussed in more detail in Chapter 6.) As the infection spreads beyond high-risk core groups to the population at large, it becomes more and more difficult to control.

Community trials show that condom use can slow the spread of both HIV and STDs but it needs to be vigorously encouraged. In Zimbabwe, a community intervention estimated to cost $85,000 successfully reached 1 million individuals, distributed 5.7 million condoms, and reduced STDs in the general population by 6–50 percent in different areas. The program was also successful in changing behavior among sex workers: The proportion using condoms rose from 18 percent before the intervention to 72 percent afterwards. (See World Bank, 1993a.)

Thailand, which is facing a historically unprecedented AIDS/HIV epidemic with 1 in 50 adults infected, has made AIDS prevention its highest priority. It has established the world's most comprehensive national HIV surveillance system, which reports twice a year on HIV prevalence in all risk groups in all provinces in the country. Acknowledging the difficulty in eradicating commercial sex, which is widespread in the country (as it is in many other Asian countries), the government has mandated a policy of 100 percent condom use by commercial sex workers and has aggressively supported treatment of STDs, particularly among high-risk groups. Preliminary evidence shows very high rates of condom use, with demand increasing from 10 million a year to 120 million a year, and some reductions in the incidence of STDs. (See World Bank, 1993a.)

Despite Thailand's positive experience with mandating condom use among commercial sex workers, it is worth noting that in most countries mandatory programs are unlikely to be very effective given the clandestine nature of commercial sex interactions and the privacy of sexual activities. As Over and Piot (1993) point out, influencing behavior change in commercial sex workers is difficult and works best when peer training programs use trusted fellow prostitutes as the source of the persuasive message. A program following this approach in Cameroon increased the reported use of condoms (at least half the time) from 28 percent to 72 percent over a 12-month period. (See Monny-Lobe et al., 1989.)

Given the prohibitive cost and low effectiveness of medical treatment of AIDS (e.g., a year of zidovudine costs more than $3,000), treatment options for AIDS patients in developing countries should be limited to alleviating pain and managing opportunistic infections, such as tuberculosis, diarrhea, and candidiasis, using outpatient treatment and home-based palliation wherever possible.

For most developing countries in Asia and elsewhere in the foreseeable future, the major focus should be on prevention through education and improved access to condoms. Cost-effectiveness calculations, while still preliminary, suggest that the use of condoms to prevent STDs and HIV can be carried out for as little as $25 per DALY.

Antibiotic Treatment of STDs in Targeted Risk Groups. One of the key factors that has led to the undervaluation of STD control in developing countries is the failure to account for the benefits of preventing secondary and subsequent cases—preventing or curing one case of an STD often prevents many other cases. WHO estimates that there are approximately 250 million new cases of STDs each year worldwide, with women bearing roughly 80 percent of the total DALYs lost to STDs (excluding HIV). Women are particularly vulnerable because of the greater efficiency of male-to-female transmission for most STD pathogens; because of the lower likelihood that women will seek treatment given the largely asymptomatic nature of the conditions and the social stigma attached to being infected; and because of the lack of female control over means of prevention (the use of condoms). (See Piot and Holmes, 1989; Wasserheit, 1989.)

Although effective treatment, based on excellent clinical data, exists for many STDs, the lack of inexpensive and rapid field diagnostic procedures has limited the use of appropriate antibiotics. Thus, in the context of limited resources, interventions should be targeted to especially high-risk groups, such as pregnant women and their infants (e.g., the use of single-dose ophthalmic antibiotic ointment at birth to prevent gonococcal ophthalmic neonatorum). In these groups, case management of syphilis, chlamydia, and gonorrhea can be both cheap and effective.

In Zambia, for example, a demonstration syphilis treatment project for pregnant women achieved a two-thirds reduction in stillbirths, low birthweights, and neonatal deaths associated with syphilis, at a cost of only $40 per DALY. (See Hira and Hira, 1987; Laga et al., 1989.)

Programs to Reduce Smoking, Alcohol, and Other Drug Use. Prolonged cigarette smoking is one of the leading causes of morbidity and mortality in the developed world and is increasing in importance in the developing world, particularly in Asia. Tobacco is already responsible for about 30 percent of all cancer deaths in developed countries and affects a variety of organs, including the lungs, oral cavity, larynx, esophagus, bladder, pancreas, and kidneys. A relatively underappreciated fact is that even more people die of tobacco-related "noncancer" diseases, such as stroke, myocardial infarction, congestive heart failure, aortic aneurysm, and peptic ulcer. Aside from the direct effects on the smoker's health, smoking also has significant health effects on nonsmokers. Passive smoking increases the risk of lung cancer and decreases the birth weight of babies born to mothers who smoke.

While per-capita cigarette consumption is either decreasing or remaining constant in the developed world, it is expected to increase quite dramatically in the developing world—by about 12 percent between 1990 and 2000. In China alone, it rose from 500 billion cigarettes in 1978 to 1,700 billion in 1992, and if present smoking patterns continue, it could lead to about 2 million deaths a year from tobacco. In India, more than one-sixth of all deaths in males over the age of fifteen are estimated to be attributed to tobacco. (See Gupta, 1988.) Similar trends are prevalent in several other countries in Asia. (See Stanley, 1993.)

An additional problem in Asia is the rise in women who smoke. Originally a small percentage of the total Asian smoking population, women are an ever-growing proportion. (See WHO, 1996e; World Bank, 1993a.)

A variety of government policies can be used to discourage smoking. These include, first and foremost, educating the public about the dangers of smoking, with special attention to school-age children. Second, governments can regulate the promotion of cigarettes by restricting or banning direct and indirect cigarette advertising. Finally, tax policies on tobacco have been shown to reduce cigarette consumption. (See WHO, 1996e; WHO, 1983.)

Singapore has been a leader in the battle to reduce the consumption of tobacco in Asia. It has prohibited advertising since 1971, issued strong warnings on health effects, and created smoke-free zones. Tobacco consumption per adult seems to have fallen between 1975 and 1990. Perhaps the best example of the impact of public education about the dangers of smoking comes from the United States, where adult consumption of cigarettes has fallen dramatically, from 40 percent in 1965 to 29 percent in 1987. (See U.S. Department of Health and Human Services (USDHHS), 1989a, 1989b.)

Taxing tobacco has also been shown to have substantial effects in reducing consumption. In India, a longitudinal study showed that cigarette sales declined by 15 percent after the excise tax on popular cigarette brands was more than doubled in 1986. (See Stanley, 1993.)

Interventions against smoking are some of the most cost-effective options available to improve societal health and cost about $25 per DALY.

Box 3.3: Smoking in Asia: Cause for Alarm

Smoking takes a huge toll on human life throughout the world. Estimates show that one person dies every 10 seconds as a result of tobacco use. And this toll will soar in the future. Whereas tobacco products were estimated to have caused around 3 million deaths a year in the early 1990s, that figure is expected to rise to 10 million deaths per year by the 2020s or early 2030s. What's more, the toll will be heaviest in the developing world. Predictions are that 70 percent of those deaths will occur in developing countries, where tobacco consumption has risen steadily over the past 20 years. From 1970–1972 to 1990–1992, smoking consumption in developing countries rose by 2.5 percent, while smoking consumption in the established market economies has dropped by 0.6 percent. (See World Bank, 1993a; WHO, 1996e.)

And within the developing world, Asia bears the lion's share of the consumption: Eight Asian nations—China, India, Indonesia, Pakistan, the Republic of Korea, Philippines, Thailand, and the Democratic People's Republic of Korea—which represent 31 percent of the world's population, consume 55 percent of the world's tobacco crop. Seven out of the top twelve nations with the highest smoking prevalence are in Asia. Number one is the Republic of Korea, where an incredible 68.2 percent of the male population 15 or older smoke. In Fiji, which ranks number nine out of twelve, 59.3 percent of men and 30.6 percent of women smoke. (See WHO, 1996e.) Chinese men represent 10 percent of all the adults in the world yet smoke nearly 30 percent of the world's cigarettes. (See Pelto et al., 1996.) And, as the case of Fiji makes clear, the smoking prevalence among Asian women is rising rapidly, the direct result of tobacco company efforts to address the female market with western advertisements. (See WHO, 1996e; Pelto, 1996.)

Because Asia represents such an overwhelmingly large proportion of the world's smokers, the health burden from smoking will be particularly high in Asian nations. Tobacco use has both direct and indirect health costs. Approximately half of all regular cigarette smokers die from the habit, and China alone is projected to account for 2 million of the 10 million projected future deaths. In addition to the health cost of early mortality, smokers in the United States also take 50 percent more sick leave and are 50 percent more likely to be hospitalized. Smokers are also twice as likely to die during their working years; have twice as many on-the-job accidents; waste 2 to 6 percent of working time smoking; require corporations to increase cleaning, repair, and maintenance costs; and increase the irritation, discomfort, and health risk of their nonsmoking co-workers. Cigarette smoking also has indirect costs, such as lost income and nonmedical costs (including accidental fires and the loss of wood that is used for curing tobacco). Finally, there is the direct economic cost of cigarette smoking: The average cost of a pack of cigarettes in developing countries is US $1.00. (See Stanley, 1993.) These costs may differ somewhat across Asian nations, but it is clear that the increased prevalence in smoking will undoubtedly take a heavy toll on the health and economy of those nations.

Given the limited resources of many of the Asian nations, each of these factors represents a significant burden. In South Korea, the per-capita consumption of cigarettes per adult over 15 years of age is 1,505 per year. While the cost associated with this level of consumption in Korea is only 0.9 percent of per-capita income, the cost of consuming only 395 cigarettes per year in Viet Nam represents 10 percent of per-capita income. (See WHO, 1996e.)

The growing problem of tobacco use in Asia must be controlled by the appropriate health and economic policy adjustments. If left alone, smoking in Asia is likely to result in a health crisis of epidemic proportions throughout the region.

While alcohol and illegal drugs are a second-order problem relative to cigarettes, they also contribute substantially to disease and disability. As with cigarettes, the damage from alcohol and drugs is not limited to the users themselves; others also suffer indirectly because of drunk driving and drug-related crime and violence.

Anti-Tuberculosis Chemotherapy. Based on prospective randomized trials, there are two effective approaches to treating tuberculosis: (1) short-course chemotherapy, which uses three to five drugs over six to eight months; and (2) the "standard" course of two to three drugs taken over twelve to eighteen months. Short-course treatment is preferred because it has much higher patient compliance (60 percent of patients complete treatment versus 30 percent for the standard course); because it involves a smaller number of resistant organisms; and because it has a lower overall cost ($3 per DALY). Short-course chemotherapy is likely to remain cost-effective in most settings because there is less need for retreatment from noncompliance. (See DeJonghe et al., 1994; WHO, 1995b.) Standard-course treatment is more expensive, costing approximately $25 per DALY.

The emergence of HIV/AIDS has added a new dimension to the problem of tuberculosis. Persons with a history of usually subclinical infection by tubercle bacilli and HIV infection are at higher risk of developing active tuberculosis. In Southeast Asia, where 40 percent of the population is estimated to have latent/dormant tubercular infection, increasing HIV prevalence will lead to a significant increase in tuberculosis associated with HIV. Between 60 and 80 percent of AIDS cases in India, Myanmar, Nepal, and Thailand, for example, have developed tuberculosis. This is a particularly worrying development, because HIV-associated tuberculosis has a high risk of resistance to two main drugs—rifampicin and isoniazid; nearly one-fifth of these cases will develop multidrug resistance. (See WHO, 1995b.)

Clinical Services for Pregnancy and Delivery Care. A shocking 1 in 50 women in developing countries dies as a consequence of pregnancy and childbirth compared to only 1 in 2,700 in developed countries. Maternal mortality has huge consequences for the health of their children; for example, the chance of dying for children under five increases by about 50 percent when the mother dies. (See Walsh et al., 1993.)

Of all maternal deaths, 75 percent can be attributed to one of three causes—hemorrhage, sepsis, or eclampsia (convulsions resulting from hypertension during pregnancy). The statistics are somewhat obscured by the fact that death from the hemorrhage and sepsis that can follow abortion is not coded as a separate category. It is estimated that about 30 percent of pregnancies worldwide end in abortion. This is a total of approximately 55 million induced abortions in the world each year. Between 60,000 and 200,000 women die of abortion-related complications, with a substantial fraction of those in Asia. (See Reich, 1987.) The remaining 25 percent of maternal deaths include complications of illness that existed prior to pregnancy, such as hypertension, diabetes, and heart disease.

Effective family planning by reducing unwanted births, spacing out births, delaying first birth, reducing higher-parity births, and providing access to safe abortions can have a major impact on reducing the numbers of women at risk for maternal mortality. (See Fortney, 1987; Maine, 1981.) The bulk of maternal mortality occurs in demographically low-risk women, who do not have access to adequate prenatal and obstetric care. (See Maine et al., 1987; Trussell and Pebley, 1984.)

Some estimates suggest that extending prenatal, delivery, and postpartum care to 80 percent of women would reduce the burden of disease associated with unsafe pregnancy/childbirth by about 40 percent. (See Fauveau et al., 1991; Herz and Measham, 1987.) A reasonable program of pregnancy-related care would include three components: (1) information, education, and communications to create demand for prenatal care; (2) community-based obstetrics with trained birth attendants to provide prenatal care, obstetric first-aid, and effective early referral for complicated pregnancies and anticipated complications; and (3) district hospital facilities to provide essential obstetric services for preeclampsia, prolonged labor, and postpartum infections and hemorrhage. (See Lettenmier et al., 1988.) Clearly, while such programs are intuitively appealing, they should first be introduced on a controlled pilot basis and evaluated for unintended outcomes.

Given these three components, program emphasis will depend on local conditions. In rural areas with little infrastructure, the emphasis should be on good prenatal care (aimed mainly at correcting micronutrient deficiencies, STDs, and malaria) and access to emergency transportation to district health facilities for complicated cases. In urban areas with overcrowded hospitals, the emphasis should be on improving the quality of hospital care and the ability to deal with normal births. Depending on the clinical condition, costs per DALY range from $30 to $250.

Medical Treatment of Acute Respiratory Tract Infections. Acute respiratory tract infections (ARIs) account for 25–30 percent of the estimated 15 million deaths occurring each year among children under five. ARI is the leading cause of death for this age group in Bangladesh, Bhutan, Korea Democratic People's Republic of Korea, North Korea (DPR), India, Indonesia, Maldives, Mongolia, Myanmar, Nepal, Sri Lanka, and Thailand. Four countries in particular—Bangladesh, India, Indonesia, and Nepal—are estimated to contribute about 40 percent of the global ARI mortality.

Besides the high case fatality from ARI, these infections in young children are also a leading cause of morbidity, often the highest contributor to workloads in outpatient departments of health centers and hospitals. Effective case management could help reduce this burden significantly. (See Stansfield and Shepard, 1993; WHO, 1984, 1995b.) A recent review of several studies in developing countries (mostly in Asia) that used auxiliary health workers to apply a set algorithm for case management found strong evidence of effective case management, despite design flaws and confounding from the simultaneous introduction of other interventions. ARI-specific mortality declined by an average of 41.6 percent (ranging from 8 percent to 65 percent), whereas overall mortality was reduced by an average of 22.3 percent (ranging from 11.5 percent to 40 percent). (See WHO/ARI, 1988.) In particular, a controlled trial that used community health workers in Nepal to detect and treat pneumonia led to a 62-percent reduction in ARI-specific mortality and a 40-percent decline in overall mortality. (See WHO/ARI, 1991.) Similarly impressive results have been demonstrated in Pakistan and Indonesia.

The use of appropriate antibiotics in treating ARIs has been shown in a variety of situations to reduce mortality risk considerably, at a cost of about $20–$50 per DALY.

It is probable that more than 50 percent of ARI deaths can be averted by using the already available technologies of immunization (primarily measles), antibiotics, and improved case management. Breastfeeding promotion and malnutrition reduction are other supplementary interventions that act synergistically to reduce ARI mortality.

The effective implementation of ARI control programs is not without challenges. Three factors need to be given special attention: (1) reducing inappropriate use of antibiotics through a mix of education and regulation, (2) investing adequate laboratory resources to monitor antibiotic resistance, and (3) overcoming physician resistance to using auxiliary health workers to diagnose and treat ARI. (See Chapter 6 for a discussion of WHO guidelines for ARI case management.)

Cataract Removal. Cataracts, which lead to painless, progressive loss of vision resulting in blindness, are the most common cause of blindness today. For example, in China alone there are 5.4 million cases of cataract blindness. The analogous figure for India is 1.41 million, and for Indonesia, 1.28 million. Because of an increasing life span and a growing elderly population in the developing world, the prevalence of blinding cataracts is expected to double by the year 2010. (See Javitt, 1993; WHO, 1987.)

Blindness from cataract is associated with significant disability, increased need for support from family members, loss of social status, and frequently early death. Fortunately, unlike many other causes of blindness, cataract blindness is generally entirely reversible upon removal of the opacified lens. In fact, surgery is the only known treatment. Cataract extraction is highly successful, even with the limited resources, lower standards of sterility, and older instruments common in the developing world. Costs per DALY range from $20–$40. (See Venkataswamy, 1993.)

The long-term health benefits of cataract extraction are harder to quantify. Because an aphakic eye (one that has no lens after undergoing cataract extraction) is left with an extreme refractive error, corrective spectacles, contact lenses, or intra-ocular lens implants are required. Most commonly, aphakic spectacles are used in developing countries, because they cost less compared to contact lenses and intra-ocular implants. Aphakic spectacles are notably thick and uncomfortable to wear and cause considerable distortion of peripheral vision. This discomfort often means patients do not use the corrective spectacles. One study reported that as many as half of those in the developing world who received aphakic spectacles following cataract surgery did not wear them and, consequently, suffered extremely limited postoperative vision. (See Ellwein et al., 1991.)

Cancer Pain Palliation. Most cancers are not detected until a relatively late stage, at a point where adequate treatment of pain is perhaps the only reasonable treatment option. (See Barnum and Greenberg, 1993.) WHO estimates that 50–70 percent of cancer patients experience pain. About a third experience very severe pain and another 50 percent experience moderate to severe pain. As a result, WHO recommends a three-stage pain control program, extending from non-opioids (e.g., aspirin and paracetemol) for mild pain, through weak opioids (e.g., codeine plus paracetemol) for moderate pain, to strong opioids (e.g., morphine) for intense pain. It is estimated that appropriate pain management can provide relief to about 90 percent of cancer patients with pain for about $150 per DALY. (See Jamison, 1993; WHO, 1986a.)

Cancer pain management is currently inadequate because of a lack of knowledge/training about pain management, a lack of effective pain control agents, and the irrational fear of addiction to opiates. Better education of health professionals, legislative reform, and improved pharmaceutical treatment can help substantially alleviate the sufferings of a significant majority of cancer patients. (See Barnum and Greenberg, 1993.)

Rehabilitation from Injuries, Leprosy, and Polio. Although very few data on disabilities are available for developing countries in Asia, such disabilities are estimated to be a major emerging health problem (See Figure 3.1 above), with significant socioeconomic importance. A study conducted in the Varanasi district in India revealed that the disability rate among 5,329 school children was 101.88 per 1,000 children. (See WHO, 1995b.) In 1994, the Bangladesh DHS survey reported crude disability rates of 11 per 1,000 population. Because of differences in levels of aggregation, different systems of categorizations, and incomplete data, however, it is still difficult to draw definitive conclusions about disability levels.

Rehabilitation, especially from injuries, leprosy, and polio, might be an extremely cost-effective intervention to which little attention has been given so far. Even less is known about how to provide services on a population level. Currently, rehabilitation programs in Asia are primarily still orthopedic services, without strong linkages to rehabilitation services in leprosy, blindness, or deafness, or to social services and other special programs. At the moment, such rehabilitation programs range from $200 to $225 per DALY.

The Treatment of Injuries and Minor Trauma. Approximately 10–25 percent of individuals in developing countries suffer a disabling injury each year, and WHO estimates that 2 percent of the world's population is currently disabled as a result of an injury. The most significant causes of fatal injury in the developing world are motor vehicle collisions, burns, poisonings, drownings, and falls. The main causes of nonfatal injuries include laceration by cutting and piercing instruments, interaction with animals, minor motor vehicle collisions, and falls. (See Stansfield and Shepard, 1993.)

Injury control includes reducing the frequency, severity, and consequences of injuries. Reducing the risk of injury (e.g., by using regulations/education to reduce alcohol use, unsafe behaviors, and poor product design) should be a major preventive focus of developing-country governments. Once injuries occur, however, basic case management can have a significant impact in alleviating the severity and adverse consequences of injuries in developing countries. Two of the most important strategies in case management are improvements in the quality of care and improvements in the emergency transport system.

With regard to quality of care, there are various low-cost, viable options. At the community level, appropriate first aid (e.g., controlling hemorrhage, cleansing of wounds, stabilizing fractures) can have a major impact in reducing the severity of injuries. One study in India demonstrated the effectiveness of cooling burns with cold water. (See Mohan and Varghese, 1990.) At the primary-care clinic level, simple low-cost strategies can be used to provide adequate management of minor trauma, including minor fractures, open wounds, and burns. Simple removal of toxins and the use of appropriate emetics can sharply reduce the adverse consequences of poison ingestion. Furthermore, appropriate and immediate stabilization of complicated fractures, such as neck injuries prior to transport to more-specialized facilities, can prevent subsequent severe disability and paralysis.

With regard to emergency transport, there are many logistic and financial constraints on poorer countries in developing sophisticated rapid response systems. However, basic notions of triage, if implemented systematically, could make a big difference.

In general, injury control has not been a major priority for developing countries so far, despite the significant ill-health burden of injuries. Increased emphasis in this area with modest expenditures and administrative and educational changes is likely to have a significant beneficial impact. Costs per DALY for treatment of injuries and minor trauma range from $25 to $250.

Health Interventions That Require a Higher National Income for Developing-Country Governments in Asia to Consider Pursuing

Table 3.14 lists 11 interventions, which—though ranked lower than those in Tables 3.11 on all the prioritization factors—are reasonable to pursue, assuming that the preceding interventions are funded and additional national income is available. Below, The majority of these interventions and some of the most relevant research studies are described in detail below.

Screening for Easily Treatable/Preventable Cancers.

Mass screening of asymptomatic individuals to identify early disease only makes sense for health conditions that are highly prevalent, have long latency periods, and are amenable to cure by early treatment. An important example is cervical cancer, which is the leading cause of cancer death for women in developing countries, accounting for 150,000 deaths each year. WHO recommends screening for cervical (and endometrial cancers) with Papanicolaou (Pap) smears beginning with women over 35 and continuing every 5 years to age 55, as resources allow. Inexpensive outpatient treatment (such as freezing abnormal cells) makes it possible to diagnose, treat and often cure precancerous conditions. (See Barnum and Greenberg, 1993; Kristein et al., 1977.) Screening for easily treatable/preventable cancers ranges from $50 to $100 depending on the test.

Improvements in Household Sanitation, Water Supply, and Ventilation.

The household environment has a huge impact on the health of individuals, particularly the poor. It is estimated that diseases associated with poor household environments account for nearly 30 percent of the total burden of disease. Efforts to improve the domestic environment (water and sanitation, garbage disposal, crowding, indoor air pollution, vector control, etc.) could avert almost a quarter of this burden. (See Martines et al., 1993.)

Table 3.15, which estimates the burden of disease from the household environment and its potential reduction from improved services in demographically developing countries, shows that significant gains in reducing the burden of disease are possible. For instance, let us examine the lack of access to clean water

Table 3.14

Health Interventions That Developing-Country Governments in Asia Should Pursue but That Require a Higher National Income

Intervention	Type/ Objective of Intervention	Cost/per DALY Averted	Evidence of Medical Efficacy	Burden of Disease	Corrects Market Failure/ Improves Equity
			Prioritization Factors		
Screening for easily treatable/preventable cancers	S.Prevent	$50–$100	3+, some prospective data; if discovered, treatment moderately effective	Moderate	No/no
Investments in water supply and sanitation and household ventilation	P.Prevent and Promo	Unknown but likely to be high	2+, inferred from survey data	High	Yes/yes
Regulation of environmental pollution, traffic accidents, and occupational safety	Promo	Unknown but likely to be high	2+, limited data in many cases	High	Yes/yes
Vector control with chemical pesticides (malaria, dengue, onchocerciasis)	P.Prevent and Promo	$25–$250	2+, time series data; effectiveness likely	Moderate	Yes/yes
Health education on reduction of cardiovascular risk factors	Promo and S.Prevent	$75–$250	3+, limited prospective design	Moderate to high	Yes/no
Medical treatment of leprosy	Cure	$25–$75	4+, clinical data	Moderate to low	No/yes
Medical treatment of malaria with passive case finding	Cure and S.Prevent	$2–$250	4+, clinical data conclusive	Moderate to high	Yes/yes
Blood screening for HIV	S.Prevent	$25–$1000	4+, good data; effective if HIV prevalent	Moderate	No/no
Medical treatment of schizophrenia and manic depressive illness	Cure and Rehab	$250–$350	4+, good data; effective therapy	Moderate	No/no
Management of stable angina	Rehab and S.Prevent	$25–$250	4+, good clinical data; moderate effectiveness	Moderate to low	No/no
Medical management of diabetes	Cure, Rehab, and S.Prevent	$25–$250	3+, prospective RCT; efficacy difficult to attain	Moderate to low	No/no

SOURCE: Adapted from Jamison et al., 1993.
NOTES: P.Prevent = Primary prevention; Promo = Promotion of health; S.Prevent = Secondary prevention; Cure = Cure of a condition; Rehab = Rehabilitation.
Evidence: 4+ = Good prospective, randomized studies with convincing results; 3+ = Some prospective well-designed studies; 2+ = Cohort cross-sectional data; 1+ = Case study or common practice only.

and adequate sanitation, which is an endemic problem in the developing world and particularly in Asia (as shown earlier in Table 2.6). For South Asia as a whole, 70 percent lack access to adequate sanitation and 20 percent to clean water. In India alone, 71 percent of the population (approximately 665 million people) lack access to adequate sanitation, while 37 percent (approximately 346 million people)

Table 3.15

Potential for Reducing Burden of Disease Caused by Household Environment in Demographically Developing Countries

Principal Diseases Related to Household Environment	Relevant Environmental Problem	Burden of Disease (millions of DALYs per year)	Reduction Achievable by Feasible Intervention (%)
Tuberculosis	Crowding	46	10
Diarrhea	Sanitation, water supply, hygiene	99	40
Trachoma	Water supply, hygiene	3	30
Tropical cluster	Sanitation, garbage disposal, vector breeding around the home	8	30
Intestinal worms	Sanitation, water supply, hygiene	18	40
Respiratory infections	Indoor air pollution, crowding	119	15
Chronic respiratory disease	Indoor air pollution	41	15
Respiratory tract cancers	Indoor air pollution	4	10

SOURCE: World Bank, 1993a.
NOTE: These figures are from a different source, and thus do not exactly match Table 3.1.

lack access to clean water. In East and Southeast Asia, 64 percent lack access to adequate sanitation and 34 percent to clean water. The lack of clean water and adequate sanitation is the primary reason why diseases transmitted by feces—diarrhea, intestinal worms, schistosomiasis, guinea worms—are so prevalent in developing countries.

A review, which evaluated well-designed research studies that looked at the impact of water supply and sanitation on diarrhea, found that there was a median reduction of 27 percent in diarrhea morbidity and 30 percent in diarrhea mortality. Improvements in water quality appear to be less important than increased water availability and improved excreta disposal. (See Esrey, 1996.) From six randomized community trials, researchers estimated that a combined strategy of increased water supply, better excreta disposal, and hygiene education (particularly hand washing) could achieve reductions of 35–50 percent in diarrheal morbidity. By and large, the effects of these interventions are estimated to be greater on diarrheal mortality than on morbidity. (See Martines et al., 1993; Victora et al., 1988.)

Another environmental problem—indoor air pollution—contributes to ARIs in children, chronic lung disease, and cancer in adults, and possibly adverse pregnancy consequences for women. Data from Nepal and a variety of other countries suggest that sharply reducing indoor air pollution could lead to a 50 percent reduction in the incidence of childhood pneumonia. Studies from China, Nepal, and India suggest that up to half of adult women (relatively few of whom smoke) suffer from chronic lung and heart disease. Comprehensive improvements in indoor air quality could significantly reduce the burden of acute and chronic respiratory infections (by about 15 percent) and respiratory cancers (by about 10 percent). (See WHO, 1995b.)

Even though these problems may result from market failures (as shown in Table 3.14), public investments in improvements in household environments and sanitation are generally not cost-effective in terms of cost per DALY because of huge initial capital costs, logistical complexity, and bureaucratic inefficiency. Moreover, there is significant private demand and willingness to pay for household improvements, particularly in the urban sector. Thus, the most important determinants of improvements in household environment are likely to remain rising incomes and education levels. Governments have a supplementary role in setting and enforcing environmental standards and regulations and in disseminating information on hygiene practices and on the deleterious effects of exposure to smoke. But the biggest contribution of governments is in the realm of improving market mechanisms for providing water supply and sanitation services.

Recalling our earlier discussion of nonhealth benefits, investing in improving household environments yields substantial nonhealth benefits (e.g., savings in fuel used to boil polluted water and savings in time and energy for women who have to collect water from distant sources), leading to a possible rationale for government subsidies. (See Briscoe, 1984; Okun, 1988.)

Vector Control with Chemical Pesticides. Because of the localized nature of insect-borne diseases, the cost-effectiveness of this intervention drops sharply as one moves out of highly endemic areas. Thus, the intervention will have to be evaluated on a case-by-case basis, depending on the incidence rates and the geographical distribution of the human and insect vector population. The one factor that favors its promotion by governments is that vector control, like immunizations, is a classic public good with benefits that accrue to many others besides those paying for the services. Thus, it is an activity the private market will not provide. (See Shepard and Halstead, 1993; Najera et al., 1993.) Costs per DALY for vector control using chemical pesticides ranges from $25 to $250.

Medical Treatment of Leprosy. Leprosy is an infectious disease caused by Mycobacterium Leprae. The clinical spectrum of leprosy varies from a single benign hypopigmented skin patch that may heal spontaneously to widespread damage to nerves, bones, eyes, muscle, and kidneys. Persistent disease may cause severe mutilation of the face and extremities, and the associated psychological trauma is probably just as important as the physical deformities. Before the development of modern chemotherapy, leprosy was a lifelong affliction. In recent years, however, the use of multiple drugs (including dapsone, rifampin, and clofazimine) has drastically shortened the duration of illness, with chemotherapy presently taking between six months to three and a half years to cure a patient, depending on the level of the severity of the disease. (See Htoon et al., 1993.)

Because of low case-fatality rates, leprosy has tended to get low priority in terms of health interventions. However, the disability, social, and psychological problems and the economic loss associated with leprosy make it a significant health problem, particularly in Asia. Nine countries in particular—Bangladesh, Bhutan, India, Indonesia, Maldives, Myanmar, Nepal, Sri Lanka, and Thailand—account for approximately 66 percent of the estimated cases and 70 percent of the registered leprosy cases in the world. There has been a steady decrease in leprosy since about 1990, falling from a high of 4.3 million estimated cases to about 1.6

million cases in 1993. This substantial decline is largely the result of implementing vigorous early case detection and multidrug therapy programs. (See WHO, 1995b.)

Cost-effectiveness studies show that medical treatment of leprosy in primary-care clinics involving multiple drugs, monthly visits to the health center, and daily oral medication costs about $25–$75 per DALY. (See Ghana Health Assessment Project Team, 1981.) Clearly, drug resistance and compliance with medications are issues that need to be factored in and may raise costs considerably.

Medical Treatment of Malaria with Passive Case Finding. Despite vector control and other preventive measures (e.g., impregnated bednets), chemotherapy for malaria is likely to remain a mainstay of efforts to reduce the morbidity and mortality from this disease.

While the use of chloroquine has been a remarkably effective and cheap method of treating malaria, its indiscriminate use in many developing countries to treat minimally suspicious fever cases without smear confirmation has led to the rise of chloroquine resistance. Not only do the new drugs cost more, they also require more professional supervision, and some of them run into more serious problems of compliance with drug regimens. (See Najera et al., 1993.)

Costs per DALY can vary between $2 and $250 and are tied to the level of endemicity and the case-fatality rates. (See Kaewsonthi and Harding, 1986.) In endemic areas, priority should be given to extending coverage by the health care system and training health providers to recognize and test for new strains of malaria parasites.

Blood Screening of HIV. Although blood transfusions account for less than 5 percent of HIV transmissions worldwide, the use of infected blood almost invariably leads to infection. Thus, the first priority should be to reduce the need for transfusions (by reducing the level of anemia through programs of helminth control, malaria control, iron supplementation, and prenatal care) and to eliminate high-risk donors (by getting rid of incentive payments for giving blood). Only if blood transfusion is unavoidable should it be used, and only in those cases is there a need for screening.

The cost-effectiveness of blood screening varies dramatically—from $25 per DALY to over $1,000 per DALY—depending on the prevalence of HIV and the presence of preexisting screening infrastructure, such as blood banks. While this is clearly not a first priority, it is something that countries may consider if they have the requisite resources and if it will help maintain the population's faith in the medical community. (See Over and Piot, 1993; World Bank, 1993a.)

Medical Treatment of Schizophrenia, Manic-Depression, and Depression. Schizophrenia and manic-depressive illness affect 2 percent of the world's population during life's most productive years and have a profound effect not only on the patients but on their family members. Broadly defined, schizophrenia includes both brief and chronic forms of illness. Manic-depressive illness can occur in mild or severe forms. The diagnosis of both conditions relies on objective criteria that can be used by trained health professionals. (See Cowley and Wyatt, 1993.)

Recent WHO studies suggest that the incidence of schizophrenia in the developing world is between 7 and 14 per 100,000 in those age 15 and above. (See Jablensky et al., 1992.) Such individuals usually show at least intermittent symptoms (e.g., delusions of control, feelings of someone inserting thoughts, or auditory hallucinations) for the rest of their lives. Studies from Asia suggest an incidence between 2 and 11 per 100,000 in those age 15 and above, with China reporting an incidence of schizophrenia of about 11 per 100,000. (See Yucun et al., 1981; Wig, 1982.) For manic-depressive illness, estimates from Northern Europe suggest an annual incidence of between 11 and 21 per 100,000 for persons age 15 and older who seek treatment. (See Goodwin and Jamison, 1990.) Prevalence is suspected of being lower in the developing world, but no real epidemiologic evidence exists.

Very effective medications for both schizophrenia and manic-depressive illness exist. In the case of schizophrenia, antipsychotic medications such as fluphenazine, haloperidol, and chlorpromazine reduce the length of the psychotic episodes and can prevent relapse. In well-controlled double-blind clinical studies, antipsychotic medication has been reported to cause a 50–60 percent decrease in the severity of illness for both acute and chronic psychotic patients, as rated by standard clinical rating scales. (See Baldessarini et al., 1990.)

Approximately 80–90 percent of manic-depressive patients on lithium, evaluated in well-designed clinical trials, respond favorably, resulting in a 60–80 percent reduction in relapses. Lithium also sharply reduces the suicidal tendency of manic-depressive patients. (See Goodwin and Jamison, 1990.)

The cost per DALY is about $250–$350 for either the schizophrenic or manic-depressive treatment programs and depends highly on the clinical/societal perception of the disability. As in all chronic diseases having the need for regular medication, compliance issues can substantially raise costs. (See Cowley and Wyatt, 1993.) These, in turn, constrain the effectiveness of medical treatment of schizophrenia and manic-depressive illness. Despite these constraints, given the lack of consciousness about mental health and the very low rates of appropriate diagnosis and treatment in Asia, vigorous efforts to identify and treat these two conditions can potentially lead to substantial declines in the societal health burden.

Depression is even more common than schizophrenia or manic-depression. Varying methodologies and cross-cultural variations have made it difficult to estimate the population prevalence of depression until recently. However, in a 1996 cross-national study, researchers used population-based data and found that the lifetime prevalence rates for major depression only varied from 1.5 per thousand in Taiwan to 11.6 in New Zealand. Women are more affected than men, and the average age of onset is between 25 and 35 years of age, with insomnia and lack of energy being features seen across countries and cultures. Comorbid conditions such as substance abuse and anxiety are seen and individuals are more likely to be separated or divorced. (See Weissman et al., 1996.)

As with schizophrenia and manic-depressive illness, treatment is often lifelong and medication can be enormously effective. The estimated cost per DALY is $250–$350. Newer drugs such as the serotonin reuptake inhibitors present the dilemma of more-effective therapeutic options but at a cost that is prohibitive in developing countries.

Medical Treatment of Stable Angina and Diabetes. Because of the variable presentation, the need for self-referral, and the needs for regular medication and monitoring, these interventions can vary significantly in cost-effectiveness, from $25 to $250. In the case of diabetes, outpatient provision of oral hypoglycemics for about $25 per patient per year can be marginally effective in forestalling complications, including insulin-dependent diabetes. (See Pearson et al., 1993; Vaughan et al., 1993.)

Health Interventions That Have Limited Effectiveness and Should Be Deemphasized by Developing-Country Governments in Asia

The hallmark of the 23 interventions listed in Tables 3.16a and 3.16b is that they are often expensive, largely focused on individual case management in higher-level facilities, and have little impact in reducing societal ill-health burdens. A good example is medical management of unstable angina or acute myocardial infarction. Treating these complications of coronary artery disease not only requires a very advanced hospital and staff but also has a cost per DALY that may exceed $30,000. (See Jamison, 1993.)

An exception to the general rule of highly expensive interventions being of limited effectiveness is the issue of food supplementation to children and pregnant women, which, despite its modest expense and some notable successes in reducing malnutrition with high levels of supervision and careful targeting (e.g., Tamil Nadu), is generally very hard to implement effectively. Inadequate targeting, replacement of food from normal diet, and/or lack of attention to other causes of malnutrition often mean that the food is wasted. (See World Bank, 1993a; Pinstrup-Anderson et al., 1993.)

In a meta-analysis of the issue, about 200 food distribution and supplementary feeding programs for young children in developing countries were reviewed. (See Beaton and Ghassemi, 1982.) About half the reviewed studies provided quantitative or qualitative information about particular food programs. Even so, many of the quantitative data were drawn from research or pilot projects rather than ongoing programs. Most of the studies reviewed in the meta-analysis used cross-sectional data and not all programs had appropriate controls, although there were a few cases of longitudinally designed studies. In general, the studies showed that food supplementation programs may have some benefit, measured in anthropometric terms, but the outcomes were significantly influenced by the management quality of programs, extent of nutritional deprivation, ration size, and the food leakage problem. Given this, governments implementing food supplementation programs should evaluate the impact before and after the program, using a longitudinal cohort design. In addition, these programs are likely to be costly and their benefits, as measured by outcomes, need to be closely observed.

As developing countries go through the epidemiologic transition, the incidence and prevalence of noncommunicable diseases such as cancer and cardiovascular problems will increase. This will predictably happen first among urban elites, who can be expected, in turn, to put pressure on governments to allocate resources for the medical/surgical treatment of these conditions, most of which is expensive and of limited value in reducing societal health burdens. The challenge for developing countries is and will be to avoid the trap of spending scarce public resources on these highly cost-ineffective therapies.

FUNDING HIGH-PRIORITY INTERVENTIONS

Tables 3.11a and 3.11b presented the list of the 16 interventions recommended for all countries in Asia to pursue, and Table 3.14 presented 11 interventions recommended for those countries with the additional national income to afford them. The next question is: how easily can Asian countries afford these interventions and how should they allocate their resources to pay for them? Estimates from the World Bank indicate that for low-income countries[2] (14 of the 44 countries shown in Table 2.4), a minimum package of recommendations similar to those shown in Tables 3.11a and 3.11b involves a total per capita expenditure of $12. The $12 is divided between $4 for public health services and $8 for essential clinic/curative services. The same package of services would cost about $22 for middle-income countries (3 of the 44 countries shown in Table 2.4), with $7 for public health services and $15 for essential clinic/curative services. By efficiently targeting services to the poor, countries could create a broader and more generous package than the minimum prescribed here—funding, for example, some of the interventions shown in Table 3.14.

It is currently estimated that governments in developing countries as a whole spend approximately $21 per capita on health care services. Of this $21, only about $1 is spent for cost-effective public health services such as breastfeeding and family planning counseling. Another $4 to $6 goes for what are termed as primary health care services (i.e., those preventive, promotive, and basic curative services that are supplied by the primary-care facilities). In addition to the recommended essential curative services such as treatment of minor trauma and ARIs provided in primary-care facilities, a variety of non-cost-effective services such as endoscopy and many radiologic procedures are included. To make matters worse, these non-cost-effective services often go to the relatively better-off parts of the population. Finally, about $13 to $15 goes for completely discretionary services with very low cost-effectiveness such as treatment of cancer, cardiovascular diseases, and other chronic conditions.

Thus, implementing the minimum package shown in Tables 3.11a and 3.11b will require a significant reallocation of resources for middle-income developing countries. For the poorer developing countries it means generating substantially more health resources. In the case of the lower-income developing countries, implementing the recommended interventions would require a doubling of the total current health-sector allocations from approximately $6 to $12. Even if allnon-cost-effective health care interventions were eliminated and the funds were prioritized first to preventive services (for an allocation of $4), it would leave only $2 for essential curative care services, with a shortfall of about $6 per capita. For the poorer countries, such as Bangladesh (which has a GNP per capita of only $220), the shortfall would be even greater.

---

[2]The World Bank defines low-income countries as those with a per capita GNP less than or equal to $725 and middle-income countries as those with a per capita income of $726 to $8,955.

Table 3.16a

Health Interventions That Have Limited Effectiveness in Reducing Population Health Burdens and Should Be Deemphasized in Asia

Intervention	Type/ Objective of Intervention	Cost per DALY Averted	Evidence of Medical Efficacy	Burden of Disease	Corrects Market Failure/ Improve Equity
Food supplements to children and pregnant women	S.Prevent and Promo	$25–$75	3+, data reasonable	Variable	No/yes
Vector control for dengue using drainage and land management	P.Prevent	>$1000	Difficult to slow benefit	Low to moderate	Yes/yes
Fetal ultrasound	S.Prevent	Unknown but likely high	3+, limited prospective data show no impact on outcome	Not applicable	No/no
X-rays for low back pain	Cure	Unknown but likely high	4+, good clinical data show ineffective without other risk factors	Low	No/no
Angiography	S.Prevent	>$1000	4+, clinical data shown effective in subset of patients	Low	No/no
Surgery for cancers	S. Prevent and Cure	>$1000	4+, data show clinical staging is critical	Low	No/no
Surgery for coronary artery disease and rheumatic heart disease	S.Prevent, Cure, and Rehab	>$1000	4+, effective in limited number of patients	Low to moderate	No/no
Surgery for chronic obstructive pulmonary disease	Rehab	>$1000	2+, very limited role for surgery	Low	No/no
Surgery for leprosy complications	S.Prevent, Cure, and Pallia	$75–$250	2+, appears effective	Low	No/no
Medical treatment of tetanus	Cure	$75–$250	3+, clinical intervention can be effective	Low	No/no
Antibiotic prophylaxis of children with history of rheumatic fever	S.Prevent	$75–$250	3+, effective	Low	No/no

SOURCE: Adapted from Jamison et al., 1993.
NOTES: P.Prevent = Primary prevention; Promo = Promotion of health; S.Prevent = Secondary prevention; Cure = Cure of a condition; Rehab = Rehabilitation; Pallia = Palliation.
Evidence: 4+ = Good prospective, randomized studies with convincing results; 3+ = Some prospective well-designed studies; 2+ = Cohort cross-sectional data; 1+ = Case study or common practice only.

However, one should also consider that evidence from NHAs or similar projections (albeit crude) suggest that even in poor countries like Bangladesh, private (i.e., nongovernment) expenditure on health services is already about $4

Table 3.16b

Health Interventions That Have Limited Effectiveness in Reducing Population Health Burdens and Should Be Deemphasized in Asia (continued)

Intervention	Type/ Objective of Intervention	Cost per DALY Averted	Evidence of Medical Efficacy	Burden of Disease	Corrects Market Failure/ Improve Equity
		Prioritization Factors			
Management of MI and unstable angina	S.Prevent	>$1000	3+, data on outcomes show some efficacy	Low	No/no
Management of moderate hypertension	S.Prevent	>$1000	4+, good data for low-cost drugs	Moderate	No/no
Medical treatment of cancers	Cure and Pallia	>$1000	3+, many diseases to consider	Low to moderate	No/no
Medical treatment of chronic obstructive pulmonary disease	Rehab and Pallia	>$1000	1+, good data on clinical intervention but outcome data limited	Low to moderate	No/no
Medical treatment of hyper-cholesterolemia	S.Prevent	>$1000	2+, good data on effectiveness but not on outcomes	Low to moderate	No/no
Medical treatment for leprosy complications	Rehab and Pallia	>$75–$250	1+, limited data	Low	No/no
Medical management of dengue	Cure	>$250–$1000	2+, supportive care may be effective	Low	No/no
Hospital bed rest for premature labor	S.Prevent	Unknown but likely to be high	3+, clinical data show questionable efficacy	Low	No/no
Anti-secretory drugs for gastrointestinal disease	S.Prevent and Cure	$75–$250	1+, very effective to treat symptoms but sub-populations and/or long-term benefits undefined	Low	No/no
Non-steroidal anti-inflammatory treatment for arthritis	Rehab and Pallia	$250–$1000	2+, some effect for analgesia, but evidence showing long-term efficacy absent	Low	No/no
Routine use of newer-generation antibiotics	Cure and S.Prevent	>$1000	1+, increase in antibiotic resistance, limited studies on long-term benefits	Low	No/no

SOURCE: Adapted from Jamison et al., 1993.
NOTES: P.Prevent = Primary prevention; Promo = Promotion of health; S.Prevent = Secondary prevention; Cure = Cure of a condition; Rehab = Rehabilitation; Pallia = Palliation.
Evidence: 4+ = Good prospective, randomized studies with convincing results; 3+ = Some prospective well-designed studies; 2+ = Cohort cross-sectional data; 1+ = Case study or common practice only.

to $6 per capita. There is thus the potential for substantial expenditures from the private sector, especially if one is able to target services effectively to the poor and charge the nonpoor for services they are currently using. (The issue of financing and raising revenues is considered in detail in Chapter 4.)

If these new funds could be found through a judicious mixture of reallocation and fund recovery, the gain in health would be substantial. According to the *1993 World Development Report* (World Bank, 1993a), an expenditure of $15 per capita for developing countries as a whole would reduce the disease burden by about 25 percent. However, this gain would vary from country to country, depending on the distribution of the burden of disease/ill health. Estimates from the World Bank suggest that for low-income countries (such as Bangladesh and India), an expenditure of $12 per capita would result in reducing the disease burden by 30 percent. In China, the same expenditure would only result in reducing the disease burden by about 15 percent, but only because China has substantially dealt with diseases that affect children (the major focus of the set of recommended interventions) and already has a high burden of noncommunicable disease.

USING TRADITIONAL MEDICINE AND IMPROVING QUALITY OF CARE

In attempts to pay for the recommended package of interventions, governments can reallocate their resources more efficiently, as described above. Nevertheless, regardless of how efficiently governments allocate their resources, the practical reality is that government resources for health will not increase until economic growth occurs. Thus, a major goal of health policy in all countries—especially developing countries—is to produce better health outcomes using the same amount of resources. Here we explore two ways that government can do that: (1) exploiting traditional medicine; and (2) improving quality of care.

Traditional Medicine

The interventions discussed previously in this chapter are Western medical interventions. However, many developing countries in Asia have large numbers of traditional medicine providers. As countries grapple with limited resource allocation, an important policy question is: Can traditional medical interventions provide more-effective care at less cost? In Chapter 6, we explore another traditional medicine issue—integrating traditional medicine into a unified health care system as a way to improve access, alleviate health provider manpower shortages, decrease cost, and preserve the cultural suitability of health care delivery. Here, however, we focus on the therapies themselves and examine whether such therapies and approaches are effective enough to produce reductions in cost.

What do we mean by traditional medicine? Historically, the distinction between traditional medicine and alternative medicine has often been unclear. Whereas Western medicine emphasizes drug therapy and surgery, traditional medicine focuses on dietary and lifestyle changes, meditation, yoga or other forms of physical exercise, natural plant and herbal treatments, psychological support, religious practices, and various physical treatments to the body. Alternative medicine is another medical approach. It is a modern Western product that borrows heavily from older systems of traditional medicine.

Critics often tout scientific validation as a critical difference between traditional medicine and Western medicine. But this distinction is more apparent than real. As we discussed in Chapter 2, surprisingly few Western medicine treatments themselves are well supported by rigorous scientific validation, such as

---

Box 3.4: Traditional Medicine in Asia: How It Works

Oriental medicine, which originated in China more than 5,000 years ago, and Ayurveda, which originated in India at about the same time, are two ancient systems of traditional medicine. Despite their independent development, these systems have remarkable similarities and have provided the underpinnings of almost all traditional medicine practiced today in Asia.

How exactly do they work? Two related principles—balance and maintaining energy flow within the mind and body—underlie their approaches to maintaining health. Ayurveda views balance in terms of the three primal qualities—vata, pitta, and kapha—while Oriental medicine describes these three qualities as qi (or chi), yang, and yin.

When vata, pitta, and kapha (or qi, yang, and yin) are in balance and our bodies are in harmony, we exist in a state of health and vitality. When the balance is broken, the disharmony is expressed as pain or states of disease. Such a framework has one theoretical advantage: It lends itself to using techniques to restore optimal health even if no specific disease state has been diagnosed, for in traditional medicine good health is a state of balance and high energy rather than simply the absence of disease.

In both traditional medicine systems, pain is caused by the blockage of the flow of energy, an example of which is the development of muscular tenderness in areas of overuse. Over time, these blockages can lead to pain, discomfort, or dysfunction of bodily organs. Causes of imbalance include practically every pathogen we can think of in Western medicine terms, such as stress, toxins, drugs, and physical and emotional injuries.

Balance is restored by using herbs, and the flow of energy is restored by stimulating acupuncture points along the affected channels or by removing bodily impurities. To restore balance, hundreds of herbs have been developed over thousands of years—most of which are relatively free of side effects. The study of herbs affecting the immune system is an interesting topic of modern pharmacological research. For example, two herbs—echinacea and the Chinese astragalus root Astragalus membranaceus—have been found to have effects on the immune system. An interesting difference between Western medicine and traditional medicine is that the use of herbs in the latter is based not on their chemical composition but on their physical characteristics in terms of vata/pitta/kapha or yin/yang.

Compared to modern Western medicine, traditional medicine is relatively weak in terms of diagnostic and laboratory tools, but it makes up for this deficiency with an elaborate system of physical and pulse diagnosis. Traditional medicine techniques are most frequently used to provide symptomatic relief and a sense of well-being in treating chronic diseases for which Western medicine has no cure. Although clinical proof of the efficacy of such techniques is often lacking, traditional medicine provides a level of patient satisfaction and acceptance comparable to Western medicine treatments and is highly valued in many Asian cultures.

---

statistically significant findings from RCTs. (See Brook and Appel, 1973.) Instead, most Western medicine practices, like most traditional medicine treatments, are based on prevailing community standards. Moreover, substantial regional variations in Western medical and surgical treatments argue that Western medicine is not a consistently applied science. (See Wennberg and Gittleson, 1982.) The bottom line is that the clinical basis for many Western *and* traditional medicine therapies is observational and empirical and without strong scientific support. Thus, both types of medicine need to be subjected to more scientific scrutiny, and there may be no compelling reason in many situations to favor one style of treatment over another. This point has implications for policy in developing countries, where traditional and alternative medicine treatments are often less expensive and more available than Western medicine treatments.

The question is: What is the scientific evidence about the efficacy of traditional medicine? Although the origin of most indigenous traditional medical practices is observational and empirically determined by centuries of trial and error, the most widespread forms of traditional medicine, such as Oriental medicine and Ayurveda, are supported by substantial amounts of scientific research. There are also studies, many of them prospectively designed, that provide good scientific evidence, although the number is still limited compared to the clinical literature on Western medicine.

Much of the evidence is relevant to the primary-care setting, and that is where efficiencies can be gained. Ayurvedic health promotion has been shown to improve quality of life in outcome studies. (See Riegel et al., 1998.) Yoga and breathing exercises in Tai Qi, for example, have demonstrated beneficial effects in patients with arthritis and asthma, respectively, while aromatherapy has been shown to improve immune function and decrease depression and insomnia. (See Garfinkel et al., 1994; Komori et al., 1995.) Chiropractic treatment of acute low back pain has been shown to have similar efficacy to conventional treatment, while studies on massage have shown improved weight gain in premature babies and decreased incidence of atherosclerosis in animals, presumably because the release of neurochemicals from the skin following massage has autonomic nervous system effects. (See Meade et al., 1990; Field, 1995.) Meditation and relaxation techniques have been shown to benefit patients with a variety of medical conditions, including hypertension, chronic pain, irritable bowel disease, anxiety, insomnia, and infertility. (See Seer and Raeburn, 1980; and National Institutes of Health Technology Assessment Panel, 1996.) Stress management and relaxation training have benefited patients with coronary artery disease, presumably because they reduce psychosocial risk factors. (See Allison, 1996.) However, there is some controversy over how much impact behavioral medicine has on illness. Specifically, a meta-analysis of cognitive behavioral therapies in hypertension concluded that while they are superior to no therapy, they are similar in efficacy to credible sham techniques. (See Eisenberg et al., 1993a.)

In the area of prevention, nutrition plays a prominent role in both traditional and Western medicine. Diets lower in animal fats and higher in natural fruit and vegetable sources of antioxidants and fiber play a clear role in reducing hypertension, obesity, serum cholesterol, heart disease, cancer, and stroke. (See White and Frank, 1994; Gillman et al., 1995.) However, although many of the herbs traditional medicine providers use are generally considered safe even when they are not particularly effective, the literature reveals numerous examples of toxicity from herbs, giving reason for caution. (See Anderson et al., 1996.)

Acupuncture, used in both inpatient and outpatient settings, has been shown to be effective in a variety of illnesses, including chronic pain, anxiety, asthma, infertility, and musculoskeletal and inflammatory disorders. Acupuncture has also been demonstrated to have astounding utility in anesthesia. (See Zang, 1990; Chi, 1994.). By contrast, there is little scientific support for homeopathy. (See Kleijnen et al., 1991.) In more-advanced curative care, such as cancer treatment, a few studies have shown that alternative medicine therapies yield benefits, including increased survival in patients with breast cancer or malignant melanoma who received adjunctive psychological treatment (See Spiegel et al., 1989; Fawzy et al., 1993.) But there is controversy in this area; when researchers reexamined an earlier study by Spiegel, they discovered that the positive effect of psychosocial support on survival in breast cancer resulted from selection bias and was not a real effect. (See Morgenstern et al., 1984.) Unfortunately, this type of methodological problem is often seen in observational studies, which are typically used for traditional or alternative medicine therapies.

How does traditional medicine compare to Western medicine in terms of primary care? For many elements of primary care such as prevention, health promotion, and psychosocial support, the evidence suggests traditional medicine is comparable and sometimes superior. For curative care of acute illnesses, Western medicine is superior in many areas but the traditional practice could be substantially enhanced by training traditional medicine providers in the appropriate use of antibiotics. In terms of curative care of chronic conditions, traditional medicine and Western medicine use very different approaches; while Western medicine is more effective in many areas, it costs substantially more. If such traditional therapies are more cost-effective, implementing them typically requires integrating them into a unified health care system for most Asian countries. This issue is addressed in Chapter 6. Patients may ultimately need to decide based on their own assessments of costs and effectiveness. In most Asian countries, the two systems are poorly integrated. To take advantage of the often lower costs of effective traditional medicine, the two systems could be integrated at the primary-care level. Before this can happen, Western and traditional care must be integrated into a unified care-delivery system. This involves both government and providers. For the latter, the use of algorithms and clinical practice guidelines to standardize health care could certainly enhance this process. Policy change will also be required so that the benefits of traditional practices are promoted and the practices regulated. Ultimately, integration will require professional collaboration on policy.

In conclusion, many traditional medical therapies seem to be as effective as their Western counterparts, and some may even be more effective. They are often less expensive. But before substituting appropriate traditional medical therapies for Western ones, much more rigorous studies of their efficacy are needed.

Improving Quality of Care

Efforts to improve quality are an essential feature of national health care policy, both now and in the future. Of course, this presupposes we have a useful definition of "quality." Many definitions of quality have been proposed, reflecting the difficulty of arriving at a single simple definition. The definitions struggle with the problem of defining the multiple dimensions of quality and evaluating what better quality is supposed to accomplish operationally. Of these definitions, the one from the 1990 Institute of Medicine (U.S.) is perhaps the most useful for policymakers: "Quality of care is the degree to which health services for individuals and populations increase the likelihood of desired outcomes and are consistent with professional knowledge." (Institute of Medicine, 1990, pp. 20–21.)

Given that we can agree on a useful definition of quality (such as the one above), why do we care about improving quality of care? While there are a seemingly unlimited number of existing problems with current health care delivery systems that need attention, *measuring, improving, and monitoring the quality of care will lead to more-efficient use of resources and directly result in better health outcomes for developing countries.* The savings come either when care is provided more efficiently or when existing resources to fund interventions are allocated differently (e.g., to a district hospital and away from a tertiary-care facility). Here, we focus on improving the efficiency of how care is provided; in Chapter 4, we focus on reallocating existing resources.

When we talk about improving the efficiency of how care is provided, we are primarily talking about improving structure and process. Table 3.17 shows the linkages of structure, process, and outcome and the associated measures for prenatal care. Structural measures are such inputs as facilities, staffing, and drugs or other supplies used in implementing the interventions. This involves all the things needed to provide care and includes such measures as how many doctors, nurses, and midwives are in the clinic, city, or province. We are interested in how many facilities have running water and refrigeration and whether there is an adequate supply of medicines and basic equipment to treat common diseases. Structure is also concerned with the organization of care, such as how referrals are requested and how long it takes to get to a doctor.

Process measures are the practices of medicine—how doctors implement interventions. They can be divided into prevention, promotion, and prescription. These measures always describe the provision of services, such as immunization rates and prenatal visits. They can also include whether the right procedure was done, such as checking the blood pressure to screen for preeclampsia, or screening the urine for glucose and protein to identify high-risk pregnancies.

There are only a handful of studies that evaluate the quality of care in developing countries. Nevertheless, these studies consistently reveal that quality is wanting and that there are many opportunities to improve it. On the process side, for example, evidence from developing and developed countries has shown that medical practices vary, often extraordinarily, from country to country. For example, we find that polypharmacy (or "shotgun" prescriptions)—mixing many drugs (some of which may be inert) in one prescription to cover all possible types of therapy that might be needed—is quite common in Viet Nam; in addition, steroids are inappropriately used as standard therapy for common bacterial infections (41 percent of cases) such as pneumonia. (See Peabody, 1996b.)

A prospective study in Bangladesh showed that records were not maintained in half the cases of neonatal tetanus; this was associated with a case fatality rate of 64 percent. (See Begum and Salahuddin, 1991.) Peabody and Gertler (1996) found that better process-of-care measures were associated with higher birthweights in Jamaica. Interestingly, the same study showed that structural deficiencies were not related to differences in birthweight.

Polio is a good example of the importance of structural measures. As we pointed out earlier in this chapter, studies have shown that polio is still a significant problem in Asia. Part of the reason polio persists has to do simply with not being able to keep polio vaccine cold enough to be effective when it is finally given. (See WHO, 1996d.) A 1991 study by Mitchell et al. showed that there were major deficits in structure measures in 76 rural health centers in Papua New Guinea, such as cold chain support and maintenance, pharmaceutical supply, and management. But a 1989 Jamaica study unexpectedly found that some rural primary-care clinics had better drug supplies and overall facility maintenance than urban clinics. (See Peabody, 1994.)

Table 3.17

Common Measures of Quality—Structure, Process, and Outcomes for Prenatal Care

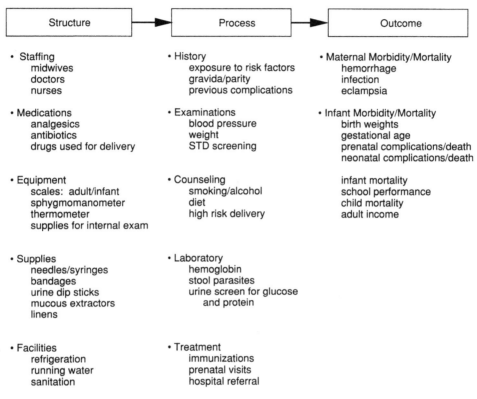

Structure	Process	Outcome

- Staffing
  - midwives
  - doctors
  - nurses

- Medications
  - analgesics
  - antibiotics
  - drugs used for delivery

- Equipment
  - scales: adult/infant
  - sphygmomanometer
  - thermometer
  - supplies for internal exam

- Supplies
  - needles/syringes
  - bandages
  - urine dip sticks
  - mucous extractors
  - linens

- Facilities
  - refrigeration
  - running water
  - sanitation

- History
  - exposure to risk factors
  - gravida/parity
  - previous complications

- Examinations
  - blood pressure
  - weight
  - STD screening

- Counseling
  - smoking/alcohol
  - diet
  - high risk delivery

- Laboratory
  - hemoglobin
  - stool parasites
  - urine screen for glucose
    and protein

- Treatment
  - immunizations
  - prenatal visits
  - hospital referral

- Maternal Morbidity/Mortality
  - hemorrhage
  - infection
  - eclampsia

- Infant Morbidity/Mortality
  - birth weights
  - gestational age
  - prenatal complications/death
  - neonatal complications/death

  - infant mortality
  - school performance
  - child mortality
  - adult income

SOURCE: Adapted from Peabody, 1994.

These findings have direct practical policy implications. In the case of the structural problems surrounding polio, Rotary International—a network of clubs for business and professionals—has raised more than $300 million for purchasing the vaccine and for dealing with the unglamorous but necessary problem of cold chain refrigeration. (See WHO, 1996d.) In Papua New Guinea, resources are now targeted to improving equipment and supplies for the EPI program; in Ghana, performance criteria were recommended for primary-care delivery; in Bangladesh, record keeping was upgraded; and in Jamaica, recommendations were made to concentrate on staff development and training. These studies suggest that many aspects of quality need to be improved, but determining which elements depends on the setting and the program.

Unfortunately, such developing-country studies are hampered by generally being cross-sectional in design and limited in scope. Another critical problem with these studies is their lack of linkage between structure or process and outcomes. This occurs for two reasons: First, the relatively infrequent occurrence of adverse events (death, morbidity, or complications) in small studies limits the conclusions that can be drawn. Second, the studies only focus on outcomes of patients who use facilities. Since patients may not elect to get care because the care is so poor, it is important that quality be assessed in the community. This, therefore, requires that population or household-based studies of outcomes be linked to facility-based studies (structure and process).

When this has been done (e.g., in Jamaica), it reveals a rich source of prescriptive policy information. This is the type of opportunity that also exists in the planned Viet Nam National Health Survey that will combine household information on outcomes with the structure and process of care from facility surveys.

Given that process and structural problems can be identified, how can quality of care be improved? Several approaches have been used in developing countries. Many of these are care-based and use *tracer* conditions. Tracer conditions are specific health care problems that provide a summary of the strengths and weaknesses of medical services. This approach can be a public policy tool when it is extended to the community. The extension allows for the measurement of prevalence (those that have the disease) or incidence (those that get the disease) by measuring the health condition of everyone living in a service area.

The strategy of health accounting is another commonly used approach, familiar to most doctors. This technique focuses on facility-based diagnoses or services and uses standards set consensually by physicians. Typically, standards are set by a panel of physician experts (e.g., WHO, specialty societies) and actual practices are then compared to the preset standards. The comparison of actual to standard practices is usually done by reviewing patient charts but can also be done by direct observation or examination. Corrective measures, such as training or censure, are then taken. Typically, these actions are taken by colleagues or licensing agencies. (Changing provider practices is taken up in detail in Chapter 6.)

A related approach is accreditation. This is generally a multistep procedure, done by external review, that looks for deficiencies in care. It usually requires establishing in advance detailed standards, such as assigning responsibilities, creating job descriptions, and collecting data on an ongoing basis. These approaches originally started in the United States and have recently been extended to Latin America and other parts of the developing world.

Facility-based approaches have recently been advanced using principles borrowed from private enterprises, such as Continuous Quality Improvement (CQI) and Total Quality Management (TQM). CQI and TQM use the clinic or specialty service system as the unit of analysis. These approaches focus on prevention and improved efficiency rather than on correcting poor quality. The organization is expected to transform itself, focusing exclusively on improving patient health and satisfaction through a process of empowering employees, integrating information and services (e.g., maintenance, pharmacy and clinical care), and decentralizing decisionmaking.

Of course, trying to fix the problems identified using any of these approaches has an initial cost. On the process side, for example, there is the cost of upgrading practices; on the structural side, there are costs for purchasing better equipment or increasing staffing. This means that, as we did for clinical interventions, costs need to be measured and the benefits of quality improvement assessed.

Still, improving the quality of care is a way to improve all interventions and can often be done without a net increase in cost. Because quality varies throughout every country, improvement in quality could improve national health outcomes and provide a more efficient use of limited resources. There is an enormous potential to improve health through better clinical practice in Asia. To realize these objectives and improve the quality of care, quality of care must be measured.

POLICY IMPLICATIONS

When we look across the findings, what can we say about prioritizing medical interventions? First, the process of establishing priorities fundamentally relies on population-based measures of morbidity and mortality. These measures can be combined into a single metric such as DALYs, and used to establish disease priorities in developing countries. The data, however, are grossly insufficient, and many more resources—from national and international sources—are needed. In a world filled with promising medical interventions, improving national health first depends on having enough information on disease and illness to choose a sensible solution.

Second, there is strong evidence, coming from well-designed studies, that there are medical interventions that are both affordable and effective. Understanding precisely how much an intervention costs is plagued by the dearth of cost data and a lack of understanding about marginal, joint, and social costs. Effectiveness is always harder to estimate because nonmonetary costs, future benefits, and externalities can be hard to estimate. Nevertheless, adapting a framework, be it cost-effectiveness or some other alternative, to a country's unique national, cultural, and social characteristics can link the realm of the technically possible with the reality of the sick and suffering.

Third, much of the improvement in national health can be attributed to advances in knowledge and technology. These advances, derived from research and development, have not always been aimed at the highest burdens of disease. As a consequence, developing countries would benefit from appropriate, low-cost, technical advances. Research and development, as public goods, should be funded by national and international agencies. The expected gains, particularly in the poorest countries, would be sizable. Given the great possibility of future benefits, research should focus on two types of technologies: aids to clinical diagnosis and treatment, and insights into how health systems finance and deliver care.

Finally, many essential and desirable medical interventions are already possible. More than 80 percent of the former and nearly 70 percent of the latter are cost-effective and can be provided in the primary-care setting. Even in the poorest countries, reallocation of resources can be used to substantially improve health. While cost-effectiveness criteria for ranking medical interventions are imperfect, policymakers can make substantive gains in health care by ensuring that the highest quality of primary care is available to the entire population.

CHAPTER 4: SUMMARY OF POLICY QUESTIONS, FINDINGS, AND IMPLICATIONS

ISSUES	EVIDENCE
• How do Asian countries finance and allocate public expenditures in the health sector?	• Financing and allocation of public expenditures are inadequate to further major health objectives.
• How much private financing can be mobilized and what is the impact on public subsidies, access to care, and the quality of services?	• Private resources can be mobilized for curative services but at a cost in reduced utilization and lower health outcomes.
• What is the optimal mix of public subsidy and private financing?	• Choosing the optimal mix of public subsidy and private financing depends on government objectives and entails trade-offs.
• How promising are social insurance plans for Asian countries?	• If designed correctly, social insurance plans hold promise, but they can introduce rapid cost inflation.
• What is the potential for managed care strategies in developing countries in Asia?	• Managed care can control costs but requires a complex infrastructure and provider competition, which generally do not exist.

POLICY IMPLICATIONS

- Because budgets are limited, government objectives for intervening in the health sector conflict with each other, and policy trade-offs will have to be made.

- Financing policy not only affects the amount of resources available, it also can shift utilization, potentially improve quality, and affect the health of the population.

- To most effectively use its public subsidies to improve health status, policymakers should follow a general pricing policy: allocate higher subsidies for services that are more effectively provided by the public sector, where demand is more price-elastic, and for which there are limited private-sector alternatives.

- Policymakers need to deal with the potential downside of user fees—decreased utilization by the poor and lower health outcomes. This requires conducting well-designed longitudinal studies with control groups and ensuring that all user fee policy interventions and pricing strategies are pilot-tested before being implemented nationally.

- Social insurance through prepayment can mitigate some of the unwanted effects of user fees. Implementing social insurance and managed care policies, however, requires that conditions be right in developing countries and that capabilities be in place. This means that policymakers should take a deliberate approach, developing the necessary infrastructure for successful implementation while waiting for conditions to develop.

FINANCING AND ALLOCATING PUBLIC EXPENDITURES: LEVERAGING PUBLIC RESOURCES TO MEET OBJECTIVES AND INCREASE PRIVATE PARTICIPATION

OVERVIEW

In Chapter 1, we discussed *when* governments should intervene and *how* values influence these judgments. Government interventions should correct market failures that cause health outcomes to be lower than they otherwise could be, cross-subsidize the poor's access to medical care, and correct health insurance market failures. In Chapter 3 we described a set of health interventions that governments can and should make available to improve the health of the population. These interventions can be prioritized, not only in terms of their cost-effectiveness, but also in terms of how well they meet the requirements for government intervention. We also noted that governments have resource constraints, which means they cannot fully subsidize all programs and activities they want to. At the end of Chapter 3, we talked about some ways that governments can work within their resource constraints to improve health outcomes by delivering care more efficiently through higher quality and by using traditional medical practices.

In this chapter, we examine how governments can achieve their objectives in the health sector by how they finance and allocate public expenditures. Public expenditures are defined as the cost of services and subsidies purchased by, and sometimes delivered through, the public sector. How these expenditures are financed is a critical element of successful health policies because financing determines the budget available for public activities. It also has implications for how expenditures are allocated.

More specifically, public expenditures are financed from both public and private sources. Public subsidies come from general or special government budgets and are the resources governments use to further the objectives of public intervention in the health sector. These are supplemented by revenues generated from private individuals through user fees—private resources paid or prepaid by individuals, families, or enterprises for their health care.[1] We will discuss how this combination affects the allocation of public subsidies across programs and who benefits from the subsidies. In particular, it affects how much the poor are cross-subsidized and, consequently, how much equity there is in access to medical care. How user fees are structured also provides financial incentives that affect utilization patterns and health outcomes. This affects how well individuals are

---

[1]User fees, simply defined, are paid when the consumer uses a service. They can be collected in many different ways. The most common is collection at the point and time of service delivery from the individual. Alternatively, individuals can be covered under an insurance plan that pays the fees for the individual, or facilities that finance care when needed may collect regular payments from individuals.

insured against the risk of large economic losses associated with unexpected illness.

Much policy debate centers around the question of *how much* governments can mobilize private resources to supplement public subsidies in financing public expenditures. Proponents of private resource mobilization argue that individuals are willing to pay for medical care and that the additional financing will allow governments to expand and improve some of the critical programs we discussed in Chapter 3. (See World Bank, 1987.) However, opponents argue that the poor are unable to pay for medical care and will be worse off if governments expand private resource mobilization. (See Cornia et al., 1987; Gilson, 1993.)

This debate grapples with the equity–revenue trade-off in government policy. But it often overlooks a key issue: Optimal policy must be based on how much the society would benefit from the policy *above and beyond* what would have happened without public intervention. In other words, the benefit of a proposed policy should be how much that policy ameliorates individual and social losses from private market failures. Thus, priorities should be based not only on the effectiveness of the policy but also on the importance governments (through the political process) place on the types of losses that are incurred.

Given these concerns, we can formulate five policy questions that need to be answered in financing and allocating public expenditures.

1.   How do Asian countries finance and allocate public expenditures in the health sector?
2.   How much private financing can be mobilized and what is the impact on public subsidies, access to care, and the quality of services?
3.   What is the optimal mix of public subsidy and private financing?
4.   How promising are social insurance plans for Asian countries?
5.   What is the potential for managed care strategies in developing countries in Asia?

The answers to these questions form the basis for the remainder of this chapter.

THE INADEQUACY OF FINANCING AND ALLOCATION OF PUBLIC EXPENDITURES

In trying to understand how Asian countries finance and allocate public expenditures and whether such financing and allocation are adequate, we must first discuss the major health objectives governments should pursue. Then, we can examine how well the current financing and allocation schemes in Asian countries further those health objectives.

The Three Major Health Objectives That Justify Government Involvement

As discussed in Chapter 1, three important market failures in the health sector justify government involvement: public goods and externalities, universal access and equity, and imperfections in health care and insurance markets. Preventing or correcting these market failures involves allocating public subsidies to them.

Public Goods. What constitutes a public good? A public good is one where a private market cannot exist because (1) beneficiaries cannot be made to pay for benefits (non-excludable), and (2) one person's benefit is not reduced by another's benefit (non-rivalrous). This means that individuals value public goods less than society does, and thus private markets will provide too little of a good and individuals will consume less than the socially optimal amount. Therefore, there is a public benefit for subsidizing the consumption of public goods. For example, in The Gambia, the use of pesticide-treated bednets reduced the high incidence of malaria even among those who do not use such bednets. (See WHO/Tropical Disease Research (TDR), 1995.) As this example illustrates, the most important health-sector public goods are preventing and treating infectious diseases.

Left to their own devices, individuals prevent and treat infectious diseases (and utilize other public health measures) less than is socially optimal. For example, individuals may be unwilling to pay the full cost of immunization because they know they will be protected if enough other people get immunized. Even if individuals do achieve worthwhile medical benefits from a treatment, the cost of seeking the treatment may cause them to postpone seeking it long enough to allow the disease to spread to other individuals; and even if they do seek the treatment in time, the cost may discourage them from completing the full course of treatment and lead to a resurgence of the disease. Treating tuberculosis is a good example. Because individuals feel better after partial treatment for tuberculosis, they tend to stop treatment long before the course of drugs is completed, especially since the treatment is expensive and time-consuming. As a result, such individuals remain a public hazard.

To get individuals to obtain the proper levels of prevention and treatment, the government can use public subsidies to lower the price of these services and thus encourage utilization. In the case of pure public goods—activities in which no one can be excluded from benefiting even if they refuse to pay—only the government can ensure provision; as a result, the government must fully subsidize the activities. Examples of nearly pure public goods include the general control of pests or vectors of disease (e.g., mosquitoes, rats, snails) and the collection and dissemination of information (e.g., epidemiological surveillance and the monitoring of food or drug safety).

Equity. Most countries recognize that poor individuals may not be able to afford health care and therefore subsidize their access to care. Overall, this use of public subsidies is based on the idea that nobody, regardless of income, should be denied access to basic minimal health care. While these commitments are not boundless, they are pervasive throughout the world. The value placed on equity, of course, varies between countries, depending not only on national resources but also on cultural perceptions of equity. This has important implications, because redistribution policies are an inseparable part of health care policy. Unless private health care and insurance markets are able to guarantee universal access, governments will intervene to varying extents.

Insurance Market Failure. The classic reason for most developed countries to intervene in health markets is that health status is inherently uncertain. (See Arrow, 1963.) No one knows what tomorrow will bring. Seemingly healthy individuals can be struck by cancer, injured in accidents, or experience bouts of severe diarrhea. The uncertainty is compounded the longer one looks into the future and the less one knows about one's current health. While most families are able to finance routine care out of their own budgets, most cannot finance the rare but expensive incidents. In fact, in all countries, expenditures on health care are highly skewed because a small proportion of the population accounts for a large fraction of total expenditures. Therefore, while most families have only small expenditures in a given year, a relatively small number have very large expenditures. Given the aversion to risk and the strong positive relationship between earnings and health, individuals would prefer to have predictable health care expenditures. If a major illness befalls a family, insurance allows it to hold onto its assets and maintain productivity. Without formal health insurance, individuals would have to informally finance the losses out of accumulated savings, assets, transfers from relatives and friends, credit markets, or help from charities.

Despite the demand, individuals often do not buy insurance from private sources. The reason is information asymmetry. Several types of asymmetry exist. Individuals, particularly the poor, are unfamiliar with the advantages of insurance and perceive it as a luxury that is administratively complex. Also, because of adverse selection, private insurance is likely to be expensive, and thus unaffordable to the poor. Adverse selection arises because insurers cannot observe differences in health status among different people. This affects both the insurers and insurees. Because individuals are born with different genetic makeups and have different life course experiences with respect to accidents and exposure to environmental contagion, there is substantial variation in the propensity to become ill. Insurers cannot observe each individual's propensity to become ill and so they are forced to make the best estimates of health and can only provide an insurance plan based on expected costs. For the insuree, the terms of these contracts can be quite unfavorable to relatively healthy individuals, since the good risks typically subsidize the bad risks. The incentive is for the good risks to drop out of the market, leaving the bad risks to insure among themselves. This substantially drives up the cost of insurance, making it unaffordable for the poor and unavailable to the sick. It is also a financially bad deal for insurers because they are likely only to enroll the sick.

A related problem is "risk-rating" or "cream skimming," which occurs when individuals of poor health *are* observable. Competing on their ability to select good risks leads insurers to avoid insuring individuals with "preexisting" conditions such as cancer or AIDS (who are "certain" bad risks) or smokers (who are "predictably" bad risks)—both of whom will have higher medical care expenditures. Instead, insurers either explicitly deny coverage or effectively deny coverage by charging an actuarially "fair" premium. As a result, insurance becomes prohibitively expensive and these individuals are effectively uninsured.

Insurance market failure also occurs when insurance is voluntary rather than compulsory. But the problems of adverse selection and cream skimming do not occur when everyone is in the insurance pool. Most countries correct the insurance market failure either through a universal public system with subsidized low prices or through compulsory social insurance (SI) in which the poor's enrollment is subsidized. Care funded by SI can be provided directly through heavily subsidized public hospitals or through the private sector, to insure individuals against large financial losses. Publicly funded systems provide less insurance if they provide lower-quality care than the SI-funded private sector.

Financing and Allocating Public Expenditures in the Health Sector

Given that governments should provide public subsidies to prevent and/or correct the market failures described above, the question is: Where do government subsidies go and what market failures do they correct? To answer this question, we start by looking at health care expenditures in levels and as percentages of GDP for selected Asian countries sorted by income (Table 4.1.)

Table 4.1

Annual Health Care Expenditures for Selected Asian Countries, Using 1990 Data

Country	GDP Per Capita 1990 (US$)	Total Expenditures Per Capita*	Expenditures as % of GDP	Public Expenditures as % of Total
Nepal	188	8	4.5	48.9
Bangladesh	204	6	3.2	43.8
Viet Nam	240	5	2.1	52.3
China	311	11	3.5	60.0
India	353	21	6.0	21.7
Pakistan	354	12	3.4	52.9
Lao PDR	364	9	2.5	40.0
Sri Lanka	473	18	3.7	48.6
Indonesia	596	12	2.0	35.0
Philippines	724	14	2.0	50.0
Papua New Guinea	839	37	4.4	63.6
Thailand	1,558	73	5.0	22.0
Malaysia	2,581	78	3.0	43.3
Korea, Rep.	5,921	390	6.6	40.9
Taipei, China	11,200	515	4.6	52.2
Singapore	13,653	546	4.0	57.9

SOURCES: World Bank, 1993a; WHO, 1995c.
* Expenditures per capita are rounded to nearest whole number.

As expected, total expenditures (both public and private) per capita rise with income. However, the percentage of GDP does not seem to be strongly correlated with income. Several very poor countries, such as India and Nepal, spend large percentages of their GDP on health, while some wealthier countries, such as Malaysia and Singapore, spend relatively small percentages.

In addition, the relationship between the percentage of health expenditures accounted for by the public sector and GDP is weak. The public sector accounts for a greater share of total expenditures in some of the poorer countries (e.g., China and Pakistan) than in several wealthier countries (e.g., Thailand and South Korea). These weak associations with income reflect different health priorities across countries, both on the part of government and private citizens.

While the data in Table 4.1 tell us about the size of public expenditures in Asian countries, they do not tell us about the source of public expenditures and how the money is spent—information that is critical in determining whether governments are adequately meeting their health objectives.

A useful method of summarizing the role of the public sector is NHAs, which make explicit how much is being spent, where the money comes from, and what is being done with the money. The NHA allows policymakers to assess whether public subsidies are being allocated in accordance with priorities and how much

> ### Box 4.1: Financing Health Care Systems and Delivering Services: The Experience in Asia
>
> Modern health care finance in Asia has its roots in the post-colonial period. During this time, Asian health care delivery systems were generally poor and disorganized. As countries grew, more of their expanding income was spent on health care. In this period, then, Asian governments had to make two critical choices about how health care systems were financed and how services were delivered: (1) whether to finance health care publicly through taxation or to allow individuals to privately finance health care; and (2) which services, if any, would be delivered through the public sector.
>
> In setting up their post-colonial health care systems, Asian countries looked to both the West and East for health care models, since the socialist and communist systems were still viable. Some countries opted for socialized medicine systems where the government financed care publicly out of general tax revenues and directly operated facilities as public institutions (e.g., China and Viet Nam). Others publicly financed SI plans that financed the purchase of medical care from the private sector (e.g., South Korea and Taipei, China). Most developed mixed systems of public and private finance and delivery.
>
> A characteristic common to most countries was the focus on improving access to medical care, especially for the poor. To this end, beginning in the early 1960s and continuing into the 1980s, most countries created large universal public health-care systems. The systems were universal in the sense that all citizens had the right to use them and fees were kept close to zero to ensure that individuals from all income groups could afford care. Many of the low- and middle-income countries that established universal public health care systems allowed individuals the choice of opting out of the public sector into the higher-priced and higher-quality private and NGO sectors. Public-sector delivery dominates some of these mixed systems (e.g., Bangladesh, Indonesia, and Nepal); in others, the private sector captures very large shares of the market (e.g., Malaysia, Pakistan, Philippines, and Thailand).

private resources must be mobilized to expand expenditures on particular programs. In addition, NHAs provide a baseline for evaluating the impact of proposed or recently implemented sector finance reforms.

Below, we examine the NHAs of four very different countries—Viet Nam, Sri Lanka, Philippines, and India. The NHAs are presented in tables using the same general format.[2] The numbers are normalized for comparison purposes into percentages of total spending. The columns represent sources of funds (how expenditures are publicly or privately financed), and the rows represent the uses of funds (how expenditures are publicly or privately allocated). The last column reports the total spent on each use, and the last row reports the total spent by each source. Each cell reports the percentage of total expenditures from a source spent on a use.

In Table 4.2, which shows the NHA for Viet Nam, we see that while the public sector accounts for a large share of total expenditures (almost 51 percent), public subsidies are relatively small (only about 16 percent) for about 32 percent of total

---

[2]National-level data vary considerably, particularly by uses (expenditures) of funds. As a result, the NHA tables have different categories of public and private allocations.

Table 4.2

National Health Accounts for Viet Nam, 1993
(% of Total Expenditures)

Uses of Funds (Expenditures)	Source of Funds		
	Public Subsidies	Private Sources	All Sources
Total Public Expenditures	16.2	34.5	**50.8**
Hospitals	14.8	2.9	17.7
Drugs	N/A	31.5	31.5
Primary care	0.4	0.0	0.4
Public health activities	0.4	0.0	0.4
Other	0.7	0.1	0.8
Total Private Expenditures	0.0	49.3	**49.3**
Providers	0.0	0.7	0.7
Drugs	0.0	48.6	48.6
All Uses	**16.2**	**83.8**	**100.0**

SOURCE: World Bank, 1995c.
N/A = Not available. NOTE: Numbers may vary due to rounding.

public expenditures.[3] The rest of public expenditures are financed through user fee charges for treatment and (mostly) drugs, collected from both insured and uninsured patients.

Where do Viet Nam's public subsidy expenditures go? As we can see, most of the money goes toward hospital care. While only 17.7 percent of total expenditures is spent on hospitals (excluding drugs), hospitals account for 35 percent of public expenditures and over 90 percent of public subsidies. Only a small amount of public expenditures goes for primary care and prevention, and all of it is financed through public subsidies.

Most of the private sources of funds are used to purchase drugs and account for about 80 percent of total spending.[4] Private purchase of drugs from the public sector accounts for 62 percent of public expenditures and 31.5 percent of total spending. Private purchases of drugs from private providers represent half of total spending and almost all of private-sector expenditures.

Except for drugs, user fees finance a trivial amount of public and private expenditures, accounting for 3.6 percent of total expenditures, 5.7 percent of public expenditures, and only 1.4 percent of private uses of funds.

In Sri Lanka (Table 4.3), as in Viet Nam, health-sector expenditures are split about equally between the public sector and private out-of-pocket payments. However, Sri Lanka finances public expenditures mostly out of public subsidies, with a

---

[3]Public expenditures are the total amount spent by the government. These are divided into government purchase of goods and services and government subsidies to consumers or producers in the form of direct transfers or lower prices.

[4]Until the breakup of the Soviet Union, most of Viet Nam's drugs were provided free as foreign aid from Moscow. After the breakup, the flow of drugs stopped and the Vietnamese government was not able to fill the gap. As a result, a private pharmaceutical sector emerged. (See Gertler and Solon, 1996, for a discussion of the role of the private health sector in Viet Nam's transition to the market.)

Table 4.3

National Health Accounts for Sri Lanka, 1991
(% of Total Expenditures)

Uses of Funds (Expenditures)	Source of Funds				
	Public Subsidies	Employers	Insurance	Household	All Sources
Public Expenditures	47.0	0.0	0.01	0.0	**47.0**
Hospitals	36.7	0.0	0.01	0.0	36.7
Primary care	10.3	0.0	0.0	0.0	10.3
Private Expenditures	0.0	0.75	0.30	52.0	**53.0**
Providers	0.0	0.70	0.29	32.5	33.5
Drugs	0.0	0.05	N/A	19.5	19.5
All Uses	**47.0**	**0.75**	**0.30**	**52.0**	**100.0**

SOURCE: Rannan-Eliya and de Mel, 1996.

trivial amount financed out of fees from insured patients. User fees are only charged by private providers. As was the case in Viet Nam, most of the public subsidies are allocated to hospitals, which account for over 75 percent of public expenditures and 36.7 percent of total sector spending. Again, as was true with Viet Nam, the public sector spends little on public health and prevention, and the private sector spends nothing.

In the Philippines, public subsidies finance about 44 percent of total health spending, with spending priorities placed on curative services rather than public health activities (Table 4.4). In fact, less than 30 percent of public funds are spent on public health activities. As expected, neither the SI fund nor individuals privately finance any public health. Most of the spending on curative health care is private out-of-pocket, suggesting that social insurance is not reducing the financial risk of unexpected illness.

India, like Viet Nam, finances only about one-fifth of total expenditures out of public subsidies (Table 4.5). In addition, like the other three countries, almost all India's public subsidies finance curative care, especially hospitalization. Only 9.0 percent of total expenditures are on public and preventive health care, and insurance contributes relatively little. Private out-of-pocket household expenditures finance the bulk of health care, indicating that there is very little protection from risk available in the system.

Table 4.4

National Health Accounts for the Philippines, 1993
(% of Total Expenditures)

Use of Funds (Expenditures)	Source of Funds			
	Public Subsidies	Social Insurance	Out-of-Pocket	All Sources
Public Health	13.0	0.0	0.0	**13.0**
Curative care	25.4	6.2	40.3	71.9
Other	5.7	5.7	3.7	15.1
All Uses	**44.1**	**11.9**	**44.0**	**100.0**

SOURCE: Herrin et al., 1996.

Table 4.5

National Health Accounts for India, 1991
(% of Total Expenditures)

Use of Funds (Expenditures)	Source of Funds			
	Public Subsidies	Insurance	Out-of-Pocket	All Sources
Primary Care	9.9	0.8	48.0	**58.7**
Curative	3.3	0.8	45.6	49.7
Preventive, public health	6.6	N/A	2.4	9.0
Inpatient Care	9.3	2.5	27.0	**38.8**
Non-Service Provision	2.5	N/A	N/A	**2.5**
All Uses	**21.7**	**3.3**	**75.0**	**100.0**

SOURCE: Berman, 1996. N/A = not available.

In summary, three patterns emerge from the four NHAs. First, private out-of-pocket payments are an important source of financing. Second, little is spent on preventive and public health, either out of public subsidies or private sources, and third, hospitals and drugs account for most of the public subsidies and private spending.

The four NHAs are useful for helping us understand how adequately Asian governments are allocating their resources to further the three health objectives described above.

Government Allocation of Resources to Meet the Public Goods Objective. While there are good reasons to subsidize public health activities, Asian governments spend very little money on them. According to the four NHAs, less than 10 percent of total sector resources are spent on preventive and public health programs in all four countries. Moreover, consistent with the definition of public goods, no private resources are spent on these activities.

The fact that so little money is spent on public health activities is surprising given the huge positive effects such spending is likely to have on health outcomes. Spending public subsidies on preventing and controlling infectious diseases is an extraordinarily productive use of public subsidies. Not only does the clinical literature suggest that there are cost-effective interventions (see Chapter 3), but there is evidence that even very poor countries can achieve huge improvements in their health indicators by subsidizing public health activities. For example, Taipei, China, used public health interventions to achieve health status indicators comparable to OECD countries, although its GDP per capita was less than $400 in today's terms. (See Peabody et al., 1995c.)

Government Allocation of Resources to Meet the Equity Objective. Many governments try to promote equity by subsidizing health care services. Because low-income countries have trouble implementing means testing (i.e., identifying the poor individually by examining their financial resources), they keep fees low for everyone. This amounts to across-the-board subsidies.

As we will discuss more in the next chapter, using across-the-board subsidies to subsidize the poor has a major cost: The subsidies leak to the nonpoor. In

Jamaica, as in Indonesia and in the four NHA countries shown above, the government heavily subsidizes hospital care. But to target one dollar to the poor, the government must give the nonpoor about $3.25 in subsidies. (See Gertler and Sturm, 1997.) Similarly, Baker and van der Gaag (1993) show that China, Cote d'Ivoire, Peru, and Tanzania, while espousing equity as a goal, also provide higher subsidies to the wealthy. Solon (1995) shows that high-income individuals in the Philippines receive much more in public health care benefits than they pay in taxes.

Moreover, the NHAs demonstrate that governments tend to allocate most of their public subsidies to hospital services, which are the services least used by the poor, and not to preventive or primary care, which are the services that are most likely to benefit the poor. As a result, public subsidies tend to benefit the wealthy more than the poor.

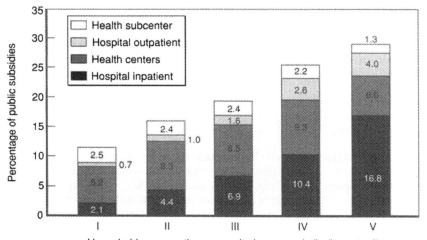

SOURCE: World Bank, 1995e.

Figure 4.1—Percentage of Public Subsidies by Income Quintile, Indonesia, 1992

Indonesia is typical of countries that try to subsidize the poor's access to medical care through low-fee public health care systems. Figure 4.1 (above) presents the percentage of public subsidies that accrue to families in each income quintile. The subsidies are calculated as the number of visits made to each public facility times the subsidy (unit cost less the user fee). The wealthiest quintile captures about 29 percent of total government health care subsidies, whereas the poorest quintile obtains only about 12 percent of total subsidies. Why do the wealthy receive more subsidies than the poor? As we discussed above, they utilize hospital inpatient and also outpatient services much more than the poor do, and hospital services are subsidized at much higher levels than are health center and health subcenter services.[5]

---

[5]In fact, the subsidies were Rp. 206,000 for a hospital inpatient visit, Rp. 8,100 for a hospital outpatient visit, Rp. 3,400 for a health center visit, and Rp. 2,200 for a health subcenter visit. (See World Bank, 1993d.) In contrast, subsidies through health center and subcenter facilities are much more equitably

Figure 4.2 shows that the story is similar for Viet Nam. (See World Bank, 1995c.) The allocation of public subsidies increases with income. Again, the overall result is driven by the fact that the wealthy capture a much greater share of both hospital inpatient and outpatient subsidies. While the poor use commune health centers at much greater rates than the nonpoor, this has little impact on the benefit-incidence distribution, because the public subsidies to commune health centers make up a very small portion of total public expenditures.

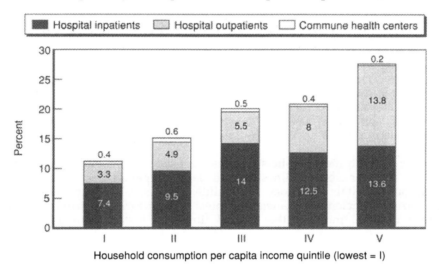

SOURCE: World Bank, 1995c.

Figure 4.2—Percentage of Public Subsidies by Income Quintile, Viet Nam, 1993

Government Allocation of Resources for the Insurance Market Failures Objective. In most countries, the allocation of public subsidies is consistent with trying to ameliorate losses from private insurance market failure. Evidence from the four NHAs and from the allocation of subsidies shown in Figures 4.1 and 4.2 shows that the bulk of public subsidies is spent on hospitals. However, the level of public subsidy does not seem to be enough to adequately insure families against the risk of financial loss from unexpected ill health. In fact, the NHAs show that, despite the large subsidy of public hospitals, individuals are still incurring large out-of-pocket expenditures. In India, for example, only 24 percent of all inpatient care is financed from public allocations. Moreover, in Indonesia—a country with a heavily subsidized public health care system—families finance the economic costs of illness by reducing consumption. (See Gertler and Gruber, 1997.)

In summary, then, the data suggest that Asian governments are using their public funds mainly to subsidize hospital services as opposed to health status and equity. The emphasis on hospital subsidies is consistent with governments' intervening to correct insurance market failure and to lower the out-of-pocket financial risk associated with unexpected, rare, and expensive major illness.

distributed, because utilization rates of these facilities are more evenly distributed across income groups.

If governments wanted to emphasize health outcomes, they would put their money into subsidizing the prevention and treatment of infectious diseases through primary care. However, few subsidies appear to be allocated to infectious diseases and other public health measures; instead, expensive curative and hospital care is emphasized. Without subsidies for these public goods, the private market will not adequately provide public health, particularly control of infectious disease; as a result, health status indicators are below what they could be.

The current pattern of funding allocations also indicates limited efforts toward improving equity. Publicly financed or operated health care facilities tend to be located in urban areas and those facilities located in rural areas tend to be of lower quality. The result is that the poor, who are in rural areas, have to travel further to obtain health care, have lower access to health care, and generally must use facilities that are of lower quality. These factors, along with the fact that most public funds subsidize high-end hospital care—which is used more by the nonpoor—mean that few public subsidies accrue to the poor.

Finally, even though most public subsidies are used for hospital care, individuals are still at risk for severe illnesses and large expenditures. This is because spending on hospital care does not fulfill the insurance function, since the subsidies are insufficient to financially protect against rare catastrophic events. To compound matters, most of the cost of illness is lost income as opposed to medical expenditures, especially in countries that have heavily subsidized public health care systems.

MOBILIZING PRIVATE RESOURCES

In most countries, governments allocate public expenditures—both public subsidies and private resources mobilized through user fees—into two general categories: (1) public health activities, such as vector control and preventing and treating communicable diseases, that benefit society above and beyond the individual, and (2) curative services, such as primary-care health centers and hospitals, that mainly benefit the individual.

Since the allocation of public subsidies is limited by a fixed allocation from general or earmarked tax revenues, the only way subsidies can be increased for public health activities is to reallocate them away from curative services. To maintain the current level of curative expenditures and lower subsidies, the government can raise user fees, thereby mobilizing private resources to replace public resources. This policy is feasible if individuals are willing to pay for curative services; moreover, since curative services benefit primarily the individuals who use them (i.e., it is a private good), it should be possible to implement.

Raising fees increases revenues by raising the revenue per visit. However, there is a limit: Patients are not willing to pay *any* amount for curative care. When prices are too high, individuals will utilize services less; in other words, price increases have the countervailing effect and at some point lower revenues by reducing visits. The real question is, at what point? From an economist's point of view, the answer has to do with "price elasticity."[6] The less sensitive (or more price-inelastic) an individual's demand for health services is to price increases for those services, the more revenue can be mobilized through increases in fees for those services, and vice versa.

Similarly, the amount of subsidies that can be reallocated to public health activities depends on the expected reductions in utilization, or on the price elasticity of demand. The more price-elastic demand is, the greater the amount of subsidies that can be reallocated. This is because the price increase not only lowers the subsidy per visit, but also lowers the number of visits that need to be subsidized. However, as noted above, fewer private resources can be mobilized for curative care when demand is price-elastic.

What Effect Do Price Increases Have on Utilization?

Given how critical the question of price elasticity is, it is not surprising that a large number of studies have tried to estimate the price elasticity of demand for outpatient services, in most cases using cross-sectional household surveys. (See Alderman and Lavy, 1996.) They typically find that higher prices are associated with lower utilization, but that estimated price elasticities are low (i.e., that individuals are willing to pay more for medical services). This says that increases in fees will mobilize substantial resources. A number of studies have found that the poor are more price-elastic than the wealthy, suggesting that fewer resources can be mobilized in poor areas and that fee increases may have their most negative impact on utilization by the poor.

However, policymakers need to view the results of these studies with caution, since the studies suffer from several methodological problems. (See also Gertler and Hammer, 1997b.) First, the countries studied typically had public institutions that charged very low fees with little geographical variation in those fees. In some of these studies, the investigators used travel costs to measure the price elasticities, since the costs of the time to travel to a facility ration the market when fees are low. These studies used estimated models of demand to conduct policy simulations that forecast how increases in fees are likely to affect utilization and revenues. However, the forecasts were based on price changes well outside the observed range of the price data and, therefore, are highly unreliable.

Second, the results of these studies likely reflect the rules that governments use to set prices and locate facilities. (See Pitt et al., 1994; Gertler and Molyneaux, 1996a.) Since government policy is trying to achieve some objective, the variation in fees and travel costs is not random. In many cases, governments set fees and locate facilities based on the characteristics of the population, such as economic status and health problems. If the multivariate analysis does not explicitly account for the government's policy rule for setting fees and locations of facilities, estimates of

---

[6]The price elasticity of demand is defined as the percentage reduction in visits from a 1 percent increase in price. Price elasticities are negative, indicating that demand falls as prices rise. If the price elasticity is small, between 0 and –1, then demand is said to be *inelastic*, since the percentage reduction in demand is less than the percentage increase in price. When demand is inelastic, price increases raise revenues, since the positive price effect is larger than the negative demand effect. When the price elasticity is large, less than –1, demand is said to be *elastic*, and increases in price reduce revenues, because the negative demand effect outweighs the positive price effect. Finally, when demand is unitary elastic, equal to –1, the percentage decrease in demand is exactly equal to the percentage increase in price, and there is no change in revenues.

how the fee affects utilization will be confounded with how government policy affects utilization. For example, if fees are set low in areas where people have serious illness problems, the observed correlation between prices and utilization reflects both the fact that sicker individuals use more health care and the effect of price on utilization. Alternatively, if facilities are located closer to urban areas where individuals are wealthier, then the correlation between travel costs and utilization reflects both the relationship between income and utilization and the effect of travel costs on utilization. In both cases, the price elasticity estimates are biased, since they are confounded with other omitted factors related to government policy choices.

Finally, most of these studies have only rudimentary controls for quality of care. While they typically distinguish between levels (e.g., hospital, health center) and sector of care (i.e., public or private), they do not control for quality variation *within* provider types, such as provider training, drug availability, and diagnostic accuracy.

Some studies have gotten around much of this problem by using longitudinal analysis of panel data to investigate how changes in fees affect changes in utilization. By looking at change over time, these studies control for geographical differences in government policy and thus can sort out the direction of causality and evaluate the impact of actual fee increases on utilization. Moreover, they evaluate fee changes in the relevant range for policy purposes. In addition, they control for unobserved sociodemographic differences in individuals and their access to medical care and for provider differences in quality.

For example, researchers and policymakers took advantage of a natural experiment of an increase in fees at public clinics in the Ashanti-Akim region of Ghana. (See Waddington and Enyimayew, 1989.) Methodologically, they compared utilization before and after the price increase at clinics and found that utilization fell dramatically at clinics serving poor patients, but that utilization at clinics serving the nonpoor did not fall.[7]

Of course, longitudinal analysis only solves the problem if the government policy rules are fixed and cannot be updated. In this case, the longitudinal analysis differences out the omitted factors that confound the estimated relationship between utilization and prices. If the government's rules are dynamic (i.e., prices, locations, and quality are updated based on new information), then even longitudinal analysis cannot isolate the effect of price changes on utilization from confounding factors.

Three studies that are not subject to these criticisms analyze the effect of experimentally designed fee increases on individual utilization in experimental and control areas. These studies, with their superior design, find much larger price elasticities than the earlier cross-sectional studies found.

Gertler and Molyneaux (1996b) estimated price elasticities for outpatient services in Indonesia using longitudinal panel data in which public-sector user fees were

---

[7]Researchers did not provide price-elasticity estimates comparing the poor with the nonpoor. Moreover, a longitudinal design does not completely control for quality bias if this is not measured before and after the intervention or change.

varied experimentally. Specifically, they evaluated the effect of increases in public facility user fees on utilization and health outcomes in two Indonesian provinces—Kalimantan Timur and Nusa Tenggara Barat.

The prospective cohort study design was integrated into the local political decisionmaking authority, which was already in the process of developing user fee increase plans. Rather than raising fees everywhere, fee changes were staggered to generate price variation based on an explicit experimental design. User fees were increased in some districts (treatment areas) but not in others (controls), and in both health centers and health subcenters.

The first row of numbers in Table 4.6 reports the estimated price elasticities of demand for health center visits. While price increases significantly lower utilization in both urban and rural markets, the effect is much larger in urban areas, where there are more private-provider alternatives. In urban markets, a doubling of fees reduced utilization by one-half. These results suggest that while increases in user fees are likely to mobilize private resources in rural markets, little revenue is likely to be mobilized in urban areas, because individuals simply switch to private providers when prices rise too much.

Table 4.6

Estimated Price Elasticities of the Demand for Public
Health Center Visits and for Visits to All Providers

Price Elasticity	Children		Adults		Seniors	
	Urban	Rural	Urban	Rural	Urban	Rural
Visits to health centers	−1.07	−0.63	−1.04	−0.01	−0.45	−0.47
Visits to all providers	−0.48	−0.49	−0.70	−0.01	−0.22	−0.39

SOURCE: Gertler and Molyneaux, 1996b.

Similarly, Cretin et al. (1990) used longitudinal data from a rural health insurance study in China in which copayments were experimentally varied to estimate price elasticities of demand. They found outpatient demand price elasticities in the same range as Gertler and Molyneaux, although they also found inpatient demand was much more price-inelastic.

Another study in Niger examined how introducing fees for curative services in government health facilities would affect preventive services. (See Yazbeck and Gemmen, 1995.) The study was implemented in two districts at the primary care (nonhospital) level—Boboye and Say—with household and facility data collected from the two districts and from a control district—Illela—where no fees were instituted. The study showed that in terms of the measure of utilization used—enrollment in prenatal care programs—overall enrollments were not adversely affected. It also found that in Boboye, quality improvements actually encouraged utilization. Moreover, in line with other studies, the increases in utilization were higher for the nonpoor than for the poor. (See also the discussion of quality in this chapter.)

What Effect Do Price Increases Have on Access to Care?

While knowing the price elasticity of demand for curative services at public facilities is needed to forecast expected revenues, it is not sufficient to evaluate the

> **Box 4.2: Measuring the Elasticity of Demand for Health Services: Findings from the China Rural Health Insurance Experiment**
>
> During 1989 and 1990, 26 villages in two rural counties of Sichuan Province, China—Meishan and Jianyang—participated in a prospective experimental study to provide an analytic basis for developing sound health care financing mechanisms in China. Specifically, Chinese policymakers were afraid that offering generous inpatient insurance would open a flood of utilization similar to their experience of outpatient insurance. To test this concern, each village was assigned two different health insurance plans, one to operate in 1989 and one in 1990. A total of eight different plans were assigned, with outpatient and inpatient coinsurance rates ranging from 30 percent to 75 percent. Three of these plans emphasized the coverage of outpatient care; three emphasized the coverage of inpatient care; and two represented a "balanced" coverage of outpatient and inpatient care. Although participation in the insurance plans was voluntary, each household had to enroll as a unit. Initial-year participation rates were over 95 percent in Meishan and 85 percent in Jianyang, and by the second year, the overall participation rate was over 95 percent in both counties.
>
> The findings of the study were rather surprising to policymakers. As expected, for outpatient services (used by about two-thirds of the population each year), higher coinsurance rates were associated with significantly lower probability of use and significantly lower expenditures. For inpatient services (used by only 3 percent of the population each year), the higher coinsurance also led to less utilization and less expenditures; however, contrary to policymakers' expectations, this effect was weaker than in the outpatient case.
>
> Why did utilization and expenditures not go up as policymakers had feared? Part of the reason is that in rural China, inpatient stays have particularly high nonmonetary costs for families. Hospitals expect families to tend to patients' routine needs, thus keeping both the patient and family away from doing productive work. Since health insurance only covers the direct monetary part of obtaining care and since the nonmonetary costs are so high, health insurance does not lead to increased demand for inpatient care.
>
> This less-elastic demand for inpatient care means that inpatient expenses are actually *more* insurable than outpatient ones. The relative rarity of inpatient admissions also makes it easier to design efficient management systems that control fraud and inappropriate use. As shown in Figure 4.2.1, Jianyang, as opposed to Meishan, instituted an aggressive utilization review procedure and was able to moderate the increased demand induced by better insurance. Furthermore, exit survey results showed that farmers understood the value of catastrophic insurance and were willing to pay for

impact of price increases on individual welfare. A step toward such an evaluation is to assess the effect of price increases on access to care. In other words, did the individuals who chose not to obtain treatment switch to self-treatment or to treatment from the private sector? Thus, to measure the effect of price increases on access, we need to examine how price increases affect the utilization of all providers, both public and private.

In the user fee study in Indonesia, investigators examined the effect of public health center fees on total visits, including visits to all public and private providers. The second row of numbers in Table 4.6 reports the elasticity of total demand with respect to an increase in public health center fees. The total demand price elasticities are less than health center demand price elasticities, implying that some individuals did indeed switch to other providers as opposed to self-treatment. In urban areas, where there are more private-sector alternatives, the it. Thus, contrary to what policymakers initially feared, the results suggest that inpatient insurance is a viable means of offering rural families help with the large expenses associated with inpatient admissions.

The data also confirmed the finding that health expenditures are not very predictable. Although 10 percent of the population accounted for about two-thirds of the spending in each year, the year-to-year correlation between expenditures was only 0.13. The best models could only predict about 6 to 8 percent of the variance in expenditures. Thus, while understanding how to adjust insurance premiums and benefit packages to account for elasticity of demand is important, it is not sufficient to guarantee fiscally sound insurance plans. In China, as in the United States, adequate risk pooling and careful ongoing monitoring are essential components of sound insurance systems. (See Cretin et al., 1990; Cretin et al., 1997.)

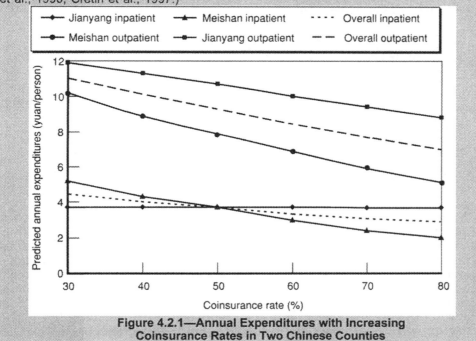

Figure 4.2.1—Annual Expenditures with Increasing Coinsurance Rates in Two Chinese Counties

total visit elasticity is about half the health center elasticity, implying that about half of those who stopped using health centers switched to other providers and about half to self-treatment. In rural areas, the total elasticity is about two-thirds the health center elasticity, implying a much larger percentage switched to self-treatment than in urban areas. These results suggest that public-sector fee increases reduce access more in rural areas where there are fewer private-sector alternatives.

In trying to understand how public fee increases affect public facility and total utilization, we also need to know how competing private-sector providers respond to the increased prices charged at public facilities. When government providers raise their prices, some patients may shift to the private sector, which may lead private providers to respond by raising their prices. The larger the private-sector price response, the fewer the number of people who will switch to the private sector; this implies that more individuals will choose self-treatment or will remain in the public sector.

Table 4.7 shows that when public user fees were increased experimentally in Indonesia, both private doctors and private nurse/paramedics significantly increased their prices in response to the increase in public-sector fees. In general, the private-sector responses were greater in semi-urban and rural areas, where there is more direct competition between the public and private sectors. Similarly, private nurses/paramedics, who are closer substitutes to public primary care facilities, had larger relative price responses than private doctors. The price elasticity estimates reported in Table 4.6 reflect both the fee increases in public sector and the consequent fee increases in the private sector.

Table 4.7

Private Providers' Price Responses to Increases in Public-Sector Fees (%)

	Urban Areas Health Center Only	Semi-Urban: Both Center and Subcenter	Rural Areas: Health Subcenter Only
Change in private doctor prices in response to a 100% increase in . . .			
Health center fees	4.4	18.4	...
Health subcenter fees	..	3.5	20.1
Change in private nurse/paramedic prices in response to a 100% increase in . . .			
Health center fees	23.8	9.5	...
Health subcenter fees	..	16.7	57.9

SOURCE: Gertler and Molyneaux, 1996a.

The reductions in total utilization associated with the fee increases can have negative affects on health outcomes. The Indonesia user-fee experiment showed that the observed reductions in utilization were not only for minor illnesses, but for medical problems that measurably affected health status indicators. For example, the fee increase caused increases in illness symptoms associated with infectious diseases and the duration of illness for all age groups. In addition, the fee affected outcomes by reducing the ability of older Indonesians (50 or older) to function physically. Outcomes in the population were measured by a series of Activity of Daily Living (ADL) measures and by increased days of restricted activity from illness.

The implication of these decreases in utilization and outcomes is that there are real returns to public subsidies and that removing them can have negative consequences. If governments choose to raise fees, then unless the freed subsidies are reallocated to more efficacious programs, health outcomes may deteriorate. We now have better ways to measure health status—ADLs, QOL measures, and DALYs—and processes of care linked to outcomes are available and validated. So policy interventions should be evaluated against outcomes and processes, not just against intermediate determinants such as access and utilization.

What Effect Do Price Increases Have on Improving Quality of Care?

Governments can also use the price increases to improve the quality of care and, hopefully, the health outcomes of those treated. However, exactly how much such a policy improves welfare depends on how willing individuals are to pay for the quality and access improvements. If individuals are willing to pay the full cost of the improvement, then the improvements can be fully financed through increased user fees without reducing utilization. However, if the wealthy are willing to pay but the poor are not, then this policy could lead to a reallocation of public subsidies from the poor to the wealthy.

There is some empirical support that individuals are willing to pay at least a share of the cost of improvements in access and quality, especially for drugs. For example, a few studies of cross-sectional household data show that individuals are willing to pay to improve their access to medical care as measured by the distance they have to travel to reach the closest public facility.[8] In addition, four studies that analyze cross-sectional data find that a number of structural quality indicators, especially drug availability, significantly affected demand in Ghana, Nigeria, Kenya, and the Philippines. (See Lavy and Germain, 1994; Akin, et al., 1993b; Mwabu et al., 1995; and Hotchkiss, 1993, respectively.) Another study, a 1994 Health, Financing and Sustainability (HFS) household survey in Burkina Faso, showed that higher charges tended to stimulate utilization, with the possible explanation being that the charges were perceived to be a measure of quality of care. (See Barlow and Diop, 1995.)

The magnitudes of the estimated quality effects are quite large. For example, in Ghana, if the percentage of public facilities with drugs increased from its present 66 percent to 100, utilization of public facilities would increase by nearly 44 percent. Simultaneous improvements in drugs, infrastructure, and services would increase the use of public facilities by 127 percent. However, much of the increase in utilization comes from substituting public care for private care. The same quality improvements that increase public utilization by 127 percent only increase utilization of nonusers by 14 percent. Therefore, the net effect on utilization is quite small. Since most of the effect of quality improvements centers on the choice among providers rather than on whether to obtain treatment, the net effect on health outcomes is likely to be small.

These studies all use estimated parameters from demand models to calculate the willingness to pay for the quality and access improvements. Methodologically, this is like asking: How much would the fee have to increase to offset the increase in utilization that results from improved quality or access? In Peru and Cote d'Ivoire, individuals were willing to pay an average of about 20 percent of the cost of operating a health facility to reduce the distance from public health centers from two hours travel time to less than 30 minutes. (See Gertler and van der Gaag, 1990.) However, the poor were willing to pay substantially less than the wealthy. In Ghana, wealthy individuals were willing to pay on average half of the cost of operating a facility to reduce travel time by two hours, but the poor were willing to pay substantially less. Therefore, if the government asked consumers to pay the "average willingness to pay" fees for improved access, utilization by the nonpoor would increase, while utilization by the poor would decline.[9]

The poor's utilization may even fall if user fee revenues are reinvested to improve quality. Under this scenario, fee-financed expansion would lead to a redistribution of public subsidies from the poor to the nonpoor. For example, suppose that

---

[8] See Gertler and van der Gaag, 1990, and Alderman and Lavy, 1996, for reviews of the literature.

[9] See Kartman et al., 1996, for a theoretical discussion on two methods of measuring willingness to pay.

households are, on average, willing to pay for the full cost of better medical equipment and drugs, but poor households prefer lower fees with worse equipment and fewer drugs. Therefore, increasing fees to pay for higher-quality equipment would reduce the use of medical care by the poor while increasing use by the nonpoor. The extent to which such a redistribution takes place depends on how willingness to pay varies by socioeconomic status. Unfortunately, there are very little data comparing price elasticities by income group.

While these studies do demonstrate a significant statistical correlation between quality and utilization, there are questions about the direction of causality. First, the studies used cross-sectional household data to investigate the effects of price, travel time, and quality on utilization and then use the estimated models to simulate the effects of price and quality changes on utilization. Thus, they suffer from the same problem as the cross-sectional demand studies discussed earlier: The results confound the effects of prices and quality on utilization with the effects of utilization on government geographical pricing and quality policy. (See Alderman and Gertler, 1989.) Second, the policy simulations ignore the likely private-sector response. As we saw earlier in Indonesia, private-sector price responses are likely to be significant and thus to greatly affect the simulation results.

A third problem with these studies is how they measure quality itself. Most of the studies use structural measures of quality, such as the availability of drugs, personnel, physical infrastructure, and equipment. However, it is not what you have—it is what you do that matters. Indeed, as we pointed out in Chapters 2 and 3, several studies show that process measures of quality are better predictors of health outcomes than structural measures. (See Peabody et al., 1998a.) Moreover, the most important structural measure, the availability of drugs, confounds supply-and-demand effects. Facilities may have shortages of drugs *because* they are high quality and, as a result, have high utilization that depletes the drug stocks.

One study that does not suffer from the methodological problems of the cross-sectional studies is a prospective controlled field experiment done in the Adamaoua province of Cameroon, where researchers investigated the willingness to pay for drugs. (See Litvack and Bodart, 1993.) In the treatment area, the facilities charged user fees to finance a revolving drug fund that increased drug availability. The researchers found that utilization increased in the treatment area after the revolving drug fund was introduced, compared to the change in utilization in the control area. The conclusion is that the consumers in the treatment area were willing to pay for the drugs; hence, their utilization increased.

Finally, there is empirical evidence suggesting that increases in access and quality do improve health outcomes. In a cross-sectional analysis of household data, researchers found that child mortality was lower among families that lived closer to government health facilities in Cote d'Ivoire and in Ghana. (See Benefo et al., 1994.) They also found that a doubling of drug prices was associated with a 50 percent increase in child mortality. An analysis of cross-sectional data from another study in Ghana showed that improving drug supplies significantly improved the nutritional status of children. (See Thomas et al., 1996.) In an analysis of cross-sectional data from Jamaica, the birthweight of babies was 128 grams higher in communities that offered better prenatal care services using process measures of quality. (See Peabody et al., 1998a.)

However, as with the cross-sectional studies of demand, one is not sure how much the associations between health outcomes and quality of care reflect the impact of quality and access on health outcomes or the effect of outcomes on the government policy toward the geographical allocation of facilities and quality. One of the few explicit attempts to sort out the direction of causality is a study that used longitudinal data from Indonesia to show that infant mortality was lower in families located closer to public health centers.

In summary, user fees can be used to finance curative care, allowing governments to reallocate public subsidies to public health programs. However, there is strong evidence that increases in fees lower utilization and some evidence that increases in fees negatively affect health outcomes. Therefore, governments need to ensure that the subsidies pulled out of the curative sector have a more efficacious use in public health activities. In general, user fees serve an important role in cofinancing health care, but *not* as the primary means of finance.

In addition, there is some evidence in favor of using revenue generated from user fees to finance improvements in quality and access to curative medical care. There is some empirical support to the notion that individuals are willing to pay at least a share of the cost of improvements in access and quality, especially for drugs. However, the wealthy are willing to pay a lot more than the poor. Therefore, if governments charge the "average willingness to pay" fees to finance quality improvements, utilization by the wealthy will increase and utilization by the poor will fall.

CHOOSING AN OPTIMAL MIX OF PUBLIC SUBSIDY AND PRIVATE FINANCING

Above, we considered the possibility of charging user fees to generate revenue and supplement the public subsidies allocated from general tax revenues for publicly financed programs. Here, we consider the joint problem of how governments should set user charges and allocate the total budget (public subsidies plus user-fee revenues) while maximizing government objectives. As discussed in the Overview at the beginning of this chapter, three general groups of objectives are often cited: (1) improving health status or outcomes, (2) improving equity in terms of access to medical care, and (3) improving individuals' insurance against the risk of large financial losses from unexpected ill health. (See Hammer and Berman, 1995.) Regardless of which objectives a government pursues or emphasizes, most countries have limited public resources to invest in health. Thus, in allocating their limited budgets, MOHs must use the resources wisely to get as close as possible to their goals within a fixed budget.

We first consider improving health outcomes as the single objective of public policy, and then discuss how optimal policy would be adjusted when equity and insurance considerations are added.

Improving Health Status

One of the major policy levers by which the MOH can improve health status is to encourage or discourage utilization by how it sets the price of health care services. For example, the MOH may want to stratify its price subsidies to encourage utilization of specific services (e.g., immunizations, prenatal care) or by specific groups (e.g., the poor). However, not all increases in utilization are from new utilization. Some may be substitution for private-sector services (or other less-public services). The degree to which the increased utilization improves health depends on the efficacy of the additional health care consumed. In calculating additional care consumed, however, we have to subtract any reduction in private-sector services the individual would have purchased had there been no subsidy.

The MOH's policy objectives are valued in terms of the population's health, but its policy levers are in terms of the prices it sets that determine both the level of private resources and the allocation of public subsidies. So to understand policy impacts, we need to establish the linkages between health and prices. Prices affect utilization of medical care and the amount of money spent on public health activities. Utilization of medical care and public health programs, in turn, influence health outcomes in the population.

With improved health as the objective, and the links between policy and objectives established, we identify four pricing principles that need to be balanced for the government to get the most health out of its available budget for subsidies.[10]

1. *Subsidies should be higher for those services where public care is better than private (i.e., medical care yields better health outcomes).* If the alternative to public care, for example, is an untrained pharmacist of dubious quality, fees should be raised with great caution. If the alternative is a reasonable private sector, then raising fees may make more sense. Obviously, if health is the objective, then it is better to encourage the use of the most productive services by raising or lowering subsidies.

2. *Subsidies should be higher for those services for which demand is most elastic.* Governments cannot mandate the use of health care; they can only provide incentives for use. Subsidies encourage the use of a service by lowering its price. And the more price-elastic demand is, the larger the increase in utilization will be for a given price subsidy. Demand, however, may be more price-elastic for less efficacious services. Therefore, the subsidies should be higher for those services that produce the most health. Services that are most successful in producing the most health are thus a combination of efficacy and the volume of patients generated by introducing the subsidy.

3. *Subsidies should be higher for those individuals whose demand is more price-elastic.* For similar reasons as in (2), subsidies produce more health for individuals for whom the subsidy is more likely to encourage use. This implies that subsidies should be higher to poor individuals, whose

---

[10] See Hammer, 1997a, and Gertler and Hammer, 1997, for a more detailed discussion of pricing rules.

demand is more price-elastic. An interesting implication of this pricing principle is that it is optimal to lower prices to the poor even if the government is *not* concerned with equity.

4. *Subsidies should be higher for those services and in those areas where there are limited private-sector alternatives (i.e., competition).* Subsidies will produce substantially less health if they *only* cause individuals to shift from the private sector and into the public sector. The most health will be produced when subsidies encourage *new* utilization so that illnesses that would not otherwise have been treated are now treated. This implies that certain types of preventive services and health care services in rural areas should be more heavily subsidized.

In essence, the first three principles argue that setting prices for services or for particular groups must balance two competing needs: (1) limiting the adverse health effect from a reduction in utilization, and (2) mobilizing resources that can be used to subsidize activities or groups, thereby providing more services. This implies that price subsidies should be assessed in terms of their effect on health outcomes and their impact on the budget, rather than relative to the costs of service delivery. Services or groups for which prices discourage large numbers of individuals from getting treatment, either from the private or public sector, should have lower prices. Conversely, when demand is more price-inelastic, higher prices mobilize more revenue (which can be used to cross-subsidize other activities) and affect health status less. The basic idea in setting prices is to push the public budget as far as it can go to achieve health gains.

The first and fourth principles point out that the interaction between the public and private sectors is critical in setting prices. If the private sector offers comparable quality services and individuals are willing to pay the private-sector price, then the government subsidies will not improve health. All they will do is cause individuals to substitute public-sector care for private-sector care. In this case, the MOH should not provide the care—or at least should price the services so that few subsidies are absorbed. This is clearly the case for VIP rooms in public hospitals, which are used only by the wealthy.

Two behavioral responses need to be measured to determine the implications for pricing policy of competition between the public and private sectors. The first is how much price differentials between the sectors induce individuals to switch from private to public care. The second is the response from new users. The effect of an increase in public-sector price subsidies on health, then, is the number of individuals who switch from the private sector to the public sector times the difference in efficacy (quality), plus the number of new users times public-sector quality. The extent to which the first effect is larger (switches versus new users), the lower the total impact of the price subsidy on health. The extent to which public-sector price increases cause substitution of the private sector is measured by the cross–price elasticity of demand.

In addition, when the public sector lowers its prices because of subsidies and draws patients away from the private sector, it is in essence competing with the private sector. This is because the availability of subsidies to public-sector providers lowers the profitability of private-sector providers. Public subsidies affect the prices that the private sector can charge and raise speculation on whether it is profitable to locate in the same area. The fact that there are no private providers in an area is not necessarily an indication that the area would not be served by private providers if no public services were available. It is only a statement that the private sector does not currently find the area profitable. As the public sector raises its prices, however, the competitive constraints on the private sector are eased. As a result, we may see new private-sector entry into the market or a rise in private-sector prices. These supply responses will affect the demand for public- and private-sector services and, thus, affect health outcomes and resource mobilization. Therefore, these supply responses need to be factored into the setting of public-sector prices.

Adjusting Resource Allocation to Use Facilities More Effectively. Where health care is provided makes a difference to both health outcomes and the budget. With constrained resources, the objective is to use enough inputs—but just enough—to improve health. Adjusting copayments or coinsurance can direct patients toward facilities that progressively screen, treat, and refer them to the most-appropriate facility. In practice, this means that people should go to primary-care facilities—public or private—and be referred to higher levels of use as clinically indicated. Table 4.8 describes the spectrum of facilities where care is provided. Typically, facilities are divided into outpatient clinics staffed by primary care providers using a limited amount of equipment and inpatient hospitals (either district or referral), which require more-extensive amounts of equipment, supplies, and specialized staff.

Governments can vary the resources they invest in these facilities, either explicitly by policy mandates and regulation or implicitly by funding decisions. Too often, however, the decisions are made implicitly. Even worse, explicit regulatory incentives and policy mandates often compete with funding decisions that are not explicit. Funding decisions emphasize types of care and thus where patients will want to go for care by virtue of where public subsidies go. Hospitals and inpatient curative care, as we saw earlier, are the places that capture resources in the health sector.

To match policy objectives with funding decisions, governments can use two approaches. Since demand for outpatient care is generally more price-elastic, governments can balance the costs of improving the quality of clinic facilities with the regulatory costs of administering a sliding scale of user fees. Both approaches provide incentives for patients to first go to outpatient clinics. The right balance between the two depends on the behavioral response to the perceived quality of primary care and the cross-price elasticity between primary- and advanced-care facilities. Government subsidies, as we discussed above, can improve quality in primary-care settings and thus will increase utilization.

Similarly, better-quality care in the outpatient setting will increase responsiveness to user-fee incentives.

Adjusting Resource Allocation to Better Target Subsidies to the Poor

One of the major factors motivating the government to charge very low prices is to ensure that all individuals have access to health care, regardless of income. Such equity concerns may limit the desirability of increasing curative care fees to

Table 4.8

Clinical Interventions: Level of Clinical Facility and Mode of Intervention

Level of Clinical Facility	Typical Conditions Addressed and Duration of Care	Mode of Intervention		
		Medical	Surgical	Physical or Psychological Therapy
Clinic—outpatient care (community, private, and school- or work-based)	Minor trauma; simple injections; support of population-based interventions; uncomplicated childbirth; family planning; traditional medicine Care typically definitive; visits typically short/often done in ambulatory setting	Short list of essential drugs (about 20)	Simple suturing, incision and drainage and simple fractures	Important potential role for integrating traditional medicine and rehabilitative treatment
District hospital— inpatient care	Complicated childbirth, fractures, and burns; complicated infections; cataract; hernia; appendectomy; diabetes, hypertension, and similarly complex condition Care either definitive or requires limited follow-up treatment; visits may require brief stay at facility	Longer list of essential drugs (about 200) Basic radiologic diagnosis	Capacity for dealing with abdominal surgery, many fractures, cesarean sections, some rehabilitative surgery	Design and management of more-complex regimens of physical and psychological therapy
Referral hospital— specialist	More-complicated medical and surgical conditions Care may not be definitive or effective; Prolonged treatment may be necessary	As above, but also specialized drugs, chemotherapy, and radiotherapy	As above, but also capacity for more-complicated head/chest surgery; orthopedics and specialty care (such as high-risk obstetrics)	Support teaching, and referral capacity for district hospitals

SOURCE: Adapted from Jamison, 1993.

subsidize infectious disease control or public goods. This may cause the government to subsidize curative services that might already be efficiently provided by the private sector. This is because large curative care fees may disproportionately reduce the access, affordability, and ultimately the utilization of curative care by the poorest segments of the population.

How much the government is able to price-discriminate and only raise fees that the nonpoor pay mitigates the severity of this efficiency-equity trade-off. This involves developing a policy that lowers the price paid by the poor relative to that paid by the nonpoor by even more than is indicated by the optimal pricing policies developed in the last section. Four common types of price discrimination—individual, geographic, self-selection, and indicator targeting—are used to do this. These are discussed in detail in Chapter 5.

Governments can vary the resources they invest in these facilities, either explicitly by policy mandates and regulation or implicitly by funding decisions. Too often, however, the decisions are made implicitly. Even worse, explicit regulatory incentives and policy mandates often compete with funding decisions that are not explicit. Funding decisions emphasize types of care and thus where patients will want to go for care by virtue of where public subsidies go. Hospitals and inpatient curative care, as we saw earlier, are the places that capture resources in the health sector.

Adjusting Resource Allocation to Insure Against Financial Risk

Major illness is one of the most sizable and least predictable shocks to the economic opportunities of families in developing countries. Two important costs are associated with illness: (1) the cost of the medical care used to diagnose and treat the illness, and (2) the loss in income associated with reduced labor supply and productivity. This loss of income is especially important in developing countries, where there is little sick leave and other forms of formal insurance against lost work time. The size and unpredictability of both these costs suggest that families may not be able to use formal or informal insurance markets to tide them over during periods of major illness.

The debate over whether to increase user fees has ignored the crucial role public subsidies serve as insurance. Subsidies can reduce uncertainty in two ways. First, they can make the costs more predictable by spreading the medical care costs of uncertain illness across healthy and sick times (i.e., taxes incurred in all states of health finance medical care purchased when sick). As a result, raising user fees in a world of imperfect consumption insurance has an important welfare cost: Higher user fees "tax families while they are down," imposing higher costs at exactly the time they need the money most. Second, subsidies may help mitigate the loss of income from the illness by financing the use of medical care that improves health and productivity. In essence, the public subsidies relax credit constraints on the purchase of medical care that may help individuals get back to work faster.

Public subsidies for medical care can correct failure in the insurance market, because, given the issue of adverse selection, private markets are unlikely to supply adequate insurance. Insurance principles suggest that the subsidies should go to the services that provide care for the rare, high-cost illness that wreak the most havoc on family budgets. The implication is that hospital care must be subsidized if the government is to insure against financial risks.

THE PROMISE OF SOCIAL INSURANCE PLANS

From the above discussion, we see that while mobilizing resources through user fees can improve welfare, there are still potentially large costs to such a policy: (1) reduced insurance coverage against the risk of financial loss from unexpected illness, and (2) reduced utilization with the possible consequence of worse health outcomes, especially for the poor. However, these costs are much lower in health systems financed through social insurance.

In terms of mitigating the losses associated with reduced or nonexistent private insurance coverage, under social insurance individuals prepay their medical care expenditures (i.e., premiums) into a fund. This fund is used to pay for their medical care if and when they become ill or injured. They thus avoid unexpected medical costs and are therefore insured against the risk of financial loss from illness. Governments mobilize these private resources by raising the fees charged by insurance plans for health services provided to the plan's beneficiaries. Because increases in medical costs can raise premiums but do not entail out-of-pocket charges at the time of treatment, there is no loss in the insurance value of higher premiums. Of course, higher insurance fees still cause a loss in welfare, since families must pay the increased premiums at the expense of other consumption or savings; however, that loss is predictable and can be spread throughout the year and across individuals.

Social insurance can also address the problem of equal access to medical care and the associated health consequences. Indeed, using government subsidies to improve equity in access to medical care is fundamentally easier to deal with in the context of social insurance. The policy mechanism is for the government to subsidize the enrollment of the poor into the insurance plans. For this to be budget-neutral, subsidies directly provided to facilities would have to be reduced concurrently to finance the costs of enrolling the poor in the insurance plan. Facilities would then recoup the lost revenues by providing care for the poor, who are now insured patients; the facilities are now assured of reimbursement. In this way, public subsidies would be better targeted to the poor, and the facilities that get the indirect subsidies would be the ones that care for the poor. Using such a program would be easier to administer than having facilities price-discriminate at the time care is needed. This is because the program would be centralized, enrollment would be periodic (outside the pressure of having to treat an illness), and the program could be administered by a trained, dedicated staff who did not have other responsibilities.

While social insurance holds promise for correcting some of the problems created by a resource mobilization policy, it creates a host of other problems that, if not addressed as part of insurance design, could outweigh its benefit. The most obvious problem, already raised earlier, is that social insurance must be compulsory to be financially viable, since voluntary insurance markets fail because of adverse selection. This does not mean that SI plans need to enroll the whole population; rather, they must enroll segments of the population such as the wage sector. In fact, most countries already have compulsory social insurance for civil servants, many have expanded compulsory coverage to wage-sector employees, and a few have achieved universal coverage.

In addition to adverse selection, there are a number of other important design issues. Below, we discuss those problems, including SI financing, private-sector benefits, and moral hazard, before examining whether social insurance makes sense for low- and middle-income countries in Asia.

Financing Social Insurance

Typically, social insurance (for wage-sectors employees) is financed through earmarked payroll or wage taxes, because low administration costs and ease of collection from wage-sector employees make these taxes attractive to governments. Because the taxes are earmarked, the revenues are placed into a trust fund that can only be used to pay for the beneficiaries' medical care costs. Such earmarking serves an important political purpose. First, it is easier to introduce a tax if people know what it is for and value what they are getting for the tax. Second, earmarking creates a feeling of entitlement in the public's eyes that makes it politically difficult for a government to downsize the program in later years by reallocating the revenues to other purposes. The current debate in the United States over Medicare and Social Security illustrates this point.

However, despite these advantages, wage taxes introduce an important economic inefficiency: They distort wages relative to other prices. If workers are taxed and do not fully value the insurance they are being forced to purchase, they will reduce labor supply or switch into the informal sector, where they are not taxed. Under Colombia's old pension system, for example, the formal employment sector shrunk from 47.5 percent to 39.5 percent between 1980 and 1992.

This pattern was repeated in the rest of Latin America, except for Chile.[11] If firms are taxed for health insurance, they will try to pass the taxes onto employees. Unless workers are willing to take a cut in wages, the taxes translate into an increased cost of labor. In this case, firms substitute capital for labor, thereby reducing formal employment. In both cases, there is a loss in productivity that is never recouped.

There is an additional problem in certain systems where there is both a public sector financed out of general tax revenues and social insurance; in this case, wage earners are taxed twice. Payroll taxes are collected for social insurance, and revenues from other taxes finance the maintenance of public facilities. Because of the limited tax capacity of developing countries, the burden may fall on a smaller number of people who are taxed more heavily. Also, since many countries use income and not wealth as the base for general tax revenue, those with substantial capital assets can escape paying their share, which concentrates the tax burden on the middle class.

Another potential problem with SI plans is that governments may end up at the end of the year with large deficits that have to be made up by deficit spending. Revenues need to cover expected expenditures, which are largely determined by the SI plan benefit design. However, unexpectedly large expenditures that exceed revenues and reserves will need to be financed out of the general tax fund, which will further increase the size of the government budget deficit. Therefore, it is critical to obtain actuarially accurate forecasts of expected expenditures and compare these forecasts to expected income. In this way, governments can make explicit decisions about benefit design and about how much to subsidize the plan. The design of an appropriate benefits package is an important challenge. It may

---

[11] During this period in Chile, the country had a fully funded system of payroll benefits, closely matched to contributions; and this likely contributed to the shrinking of the informal sector. (See Schmidt, 1995.)

be politically engaging to promise coverage, but more-generous benefits require higher taxes. Higher taxes, in turn, place larger efficiency costs on labor markets and cause larger losses in economic productivity. Governments need to take these costs into account when they choose a benefits package.

Finally, most SI plans are pay-as-you-go systems, which means they use current revenues to cover current expenditures. While in principle everyone benefits from social insurance, the burden of financing is placed on the current workforce through earmarked taxes. This means that population aging reduces premium revenues and increases expenditures per beneficiary. More specifically, as the population ages, the ratio of the number of workers contributing premiums to the number of elderly dependents falls—implying that revenues per beneficiary will fall.

This problem is exacerbated in Asia, which (as discussed in Chapter 3) is undergoing a rapid demographic transition as fertility rates drop. Table 4.9 shows the effect of Asia's demographic transition on the support ratio mentioned above. As the last two columns show, the population is expected to age dramatically, especially in the poorer countries that are still in the midst of the demographic transition. The support ratio changes are expected to be equally dramatic for these poorer countries. For example, in Bangladesh, there were 110 workers supporting each elderly dependent in 1991; by the year 2025, this ratio is predicted to drop to a ratio of about 20 to 1.

In addition, since older individuals spend more on health care, aging will lead to increased expenditures per beneficiary. This implies that as a population ages, insurance liabilities will outpace insurance premium revenues, forcing insurance fund managers into deficit financing if they intend to maintain benefits without raising taxes. Deficit financing is not sustainable without government subsidy. In fact, South Korea's pay-as-you-go national health insurance plan is expected to start deficit financing in the middle of the next decade, which will erode asset reserves by the end of that decade. (See Peabody et al., 1997.)

In dealing with aging populations, governments have several policy options in using SI funds. The first two are to cut benefits and raise taxes. Of course, these options are not always politically feasible and create intergenerational conflict. Older populations who supported their parents' health care through taxes expect their children to do the same. Children who have to pay the increased taxes, however, are forced to make a much larger intergenerational transfer to their parents than their parents made to their grandparents. An alternative is to have each generation prefund their insurance through savings before they retire.

Private-Sector Benefits

Shifting the burden of financing and delivering medical care from the public sector to the private sector can also be done with social insurance. Social insurance lowers the out-of-pocket price for private providers relative to the price of public providers at the time of treatment. This provides an added incentive to choose the private sector over the public sector for those individuals with social insurance. Thus, expanding social insurance shifts individuals out of the public sector into the private sector, thereby reducing the government's financial

Box 4.3: The Effect of Aging on South Korea's National Health Insurance

Just six years after attaining universal coverage, South Korea's National Health Insurance (NHI) program is now faced with the burden of providing benefits for a rapidly increasing elderly population. While the percentage of people age 65 and over was constant at about 3.3 percent until 1975, it has begun to increase at a faster rate. By 1995, it had risen to 5.3 percent and is expected to rise to about 9.8 percent by 2015. This has implications for both program revenues and expenditures.

As a pay-as-you-go system funded through a combination of earmarked payroll taxes and government subsidies, the NHI uses current revenues to cover current expenditures. As the population ages in South Korea, the ratio of the number of workers contributing premiums to the number of elderly dependents falls. This means that NHI revenues per beneficiary will fall. In 1991, South Korea had a worker-to-elderly dependent support ratio of about 25 to 1; by 2025, the ratio is projected to drop to about 6 to 1.

In addition, the elderly also spend more on health care. Not only do older South Koreans have greater outpatient and inpatient utilization rates, but the rates for the elderly have been growing at a faster pace than those for the young. In 1994, older South Koreans' outpatient visit rates were close to 40 percent higher and inpatient admission rates were almost twice those of younger South Koreans. Moreover, while the outpatient visit rate for young individuals grew on average about 4 percent per year, the visit rate for older individuals grew over 9 percent per year. Similarly, where the inpatient admission rate grew at about 1 percent on average per year for the young, the admission rate grew by over 5 percent per year for the elderly. Thus, NHI expenditures are also expected to increase.

While the NHI is currently in a strong financial position, the burden of population aging is beginning to be felt. In fact, NHI can expect annual budget deficits in the near future. Driven by the exponential increase in the proportion of the elderly, expendi-tures are rising exponentially; but revenues are only rising linearly. As a result, while revenues will continue to exceed expenditures through 2004, the NHI will experience annual budget deficits starting in 2005. Since expenditures are rising exponentially and revenues linearly, the budget deficit grows each year. When NHI experiences annual budget deficits, it must finance the deficit out of its asset reserves. As Figure 4.3.1 shows, the forecasts indicate that the NHI asset reserves will continue to increase through 2004 and decline thereafter. This deficit financing will erode NHI reserves by 2008.

obligation out of the general budget. Moreover, since social insurance is usually mandated for the wage sector, it is middle- and upper-income individuals who are pulled out of the public sector. The remaining individuals tend to be lower-income individuals, implying that public subsidies will be better targeted to the poor.

Some empirical evidence suggests that an expansion of social insurance increases the demand for private-sector care. Cross-sectional household survey data from Jamaica show that, controlling for income, demographic characteristics, and location, individuals with insurance demand 30 percent more outpatient care from the private sector. (See Gertler and Sturm, 1997.) In a similar analysis, using longitudinal panel data from Indonesia, researchers found a 43 percent increase in private-sector demand with the expansion of insurance. (See Dow et al., 1997.)

However, these two studies differ on the implications for public subsidies. While insurance in Jamaica was found to lower demand for public-sector services, there was no effect on public demand in Indonesia. In Jamaica, insurance did not increase the number of visits, but rather caused individuals to transfer out of the

Fundamentally, the best option is to break the pay-as-you-go system and ask workers today to save for their medical care spending in retirement. This can be done by increasing contributions to social security funds and having individuals pay health insurance premiums out of their social security when they retire. Since individuals have saved for this, it is not an extra burden. Having individuals save when young to pay premiums when old makes insurance revenues move procyclically with liabilities, thereby removing the need for increased taxes on workers or reduced benefits for retirees.

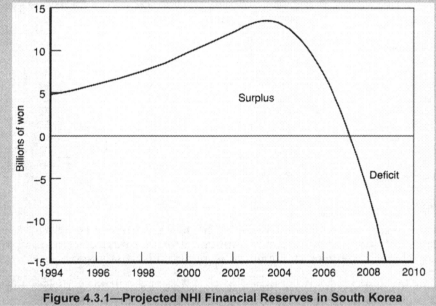

Figure 4.3.1—Projected NHI Financial Reserves in South Korea

public sector and into the private sector. Using these estimates, if compulsory social insurance were expanded to the top half of the income distribution, it would reduce public expenditures by 33 percent and improve the share of public expenditures captured by the poor by 25 percent. In the Indonesian study, which used a better research design, insurance expansion had no effect on demand for care at public facilities. The implication is that expansion allowed individuals access to services provided in the private sector that were not available in the public sector. As a result, expanding insurance did not reduce public subsidies—it only increased private expenditures. Supporting this notion, a simulation model in the Philippines that examined the expansion of social insurance showed that total health expenditures would quickly increase with SI coverage. This is in part because of the shift out of the public sector into the higher-priced private sector. (See Solon et al., 1995.)

Of course, these studies assume that private providers will not adjust in response to the SI expansion. However, in response to increased demand for private-sector care, private-sector providers are likely to increase their prices. There was evidence for this in the user fee experiment in Indonesia, illustrated in Table 4.7. There, increases in public fees lowered the price of private care relative to the price of public care, thereby providing an incentive to substitute out of the public sector into the private sector. In areas where public-sector fees were increased,

Table 4.9

Demographic Transition and Its Impact on Support Ratios in
Selected Asian Countries

Country	GDP Per Capita (US$) 1991	Total Fertility Rate 1991	% Population Age 65+ 1991	2025	Support Ratio (# of workers per elderly dependent) 1991	2025
Nepal	170	5.5	2.9	4.5	33.5	21.2
Bangladesh	220	4.4	.9	4.8	110.1	19.8
India	310	3.9	4.0	8.0	24.0	11.5
Pakistan	420	4.6	2.5	4.9	39.0	19.4
China	450	2.4	6.6	11.7	14.2	7.5
Sri Lanka	540	2.5	4.1	12.6	23.4	6.9
Indonesia	670	3.0	1.3	8.0	75.9	11.5
Philippines	770	3.6	1.7	7.5	57.8	12.3
Papua New Guinea	950	4.9	2.5	4.5	39.0	21.2
Thailand	1,840	2.3	1.7	9.7	57.8	9.3
Malaysia	2,790	3.7	2.9	8.5	33.5	10.8
Korea, Republic of	6,790	1.8	3.9	15.2	24.6	5.6
Singapore	15,730	1.8	6.4	18.2	14.6	4.5
Japan	28,190	1.5	12.3	25.7	7.1	2.9

SOURCE: World Bank, 1993a.

private-sector prices also increased. The increase in private prices lowered the number of patients who actually shifted out of the public sector into the private sector, thereby reducing the amount of public subsidies saved.

An even greater concern is that private providers will price-discriminate. In the Philippines, where the SI fund pays providers fee-for-service (FFS) and benefits are capped, private hospitals charge SI patients a higher price for the same services. In fact, private providers captured almost all the social insurance as profits by increasing the prices charged to SI patients. (See Tan et al., 1996.) Private hospitals charged a 23.4 percent price markup and that price markup accounted for more than 85 percent of total Medicare benefit payments. Therefore, less than 15 percent of Medicare payments actually financed health care utilization.

Finally, relying on the private sector to deliver care to the middle- and upper-income classes has its dangers. Once these politically influential groups leave the public system, the political will to sustain funding in the public sector, which is the only source of care for the poor, may not remain. Hence, a movement to a mixed public-private system will make the poor worse off if it leads the nonpoor to pressure governments to substantially lower public health care spending. (See Pritchett and Summers, 1996.) Indeed, in the United States, there is strong political pressure to reduce Medicaid—the program that subsidizes health care for the poor.

The Insurance Value of Social Insurance

The movement toward social insurance has been motivated more by fiscal pressure than by the desire to insure against the out-of-pocket financial risk associated with uncertain health status. In fact, the SI plans are, in part, replacing large public health-care delivery systems modeled after the British National

Health Service (NHS). These NHS-like systems deliver medical care through publicly operated networks financed by general tax revenues. They typically charge nominal user fees to ensure that income is not a barrier to medical care. (See World Bank, 1987.) Since the "free" public systems already provide insurance against the financial risk associated with uncertain illness, there is little insurance gain from switching to social health insurance.

As in many OECD countries, most of the SI plans in low-income countries typically finance medical care benefits through mandatory earmarked payroll taxes. However, unlike OECD countries, low-income countries have limited abilities to tax. Therefore, the resources available for social insurance are severely constrained, which greatly diminishes their ability to provide insurance. In such poor environments, there is a strict budget constraint on SI benefits. SI funds thus face the trade-off between providing a large number of individuals with a small benefit and providing a small number of people with a large benefit. This means a very large deductible (and possibly a large copayment) is required to provide uncapped benefits for rare large financial risks an individual faces (e.g., those associated with a rare catastrophic illness, such as major trauma). A high deductible ensures that benefits are available for expensive catastrophic illnesses and are not used up on less expensive higher-probability events (e.g., influenza). Because of the budget constraint, lowering the deductible requires capping benefits. At its extreme, a zero deductible implies the lowest possible benefit cap and the least-effective insurance against catastrophic illness.

All the same, this is exactly what many countries have done. Table 4.10 shows that many low-income countries using social insurance—in Asia and elsewhere—have adopted first-dollar coverage and therefore have placed the smallest cap possible on benefits.[12] In essence, governments, and people for that matter, have chosen to provide the minimum benefits for all illnesses rather than full insurance for rare high-cost illnesses.

These capped-benefit plans have provided little insurance against the large financial cost associated with illness. For example, the maximum benefit for a hospital inpatient episode for someone in Medicare—the SI program in the Philippines—covers about 15 percent of the average cost of the total bill and only a small fraction of the rare costly hospitalizations. In South Korea, where there is universal social insurance, individuals still pay about 66 percent of medical care expenses out-of-pocket. (See Gertler, 1996.)

If capped first-dollar coverage provides minimal insurance, why is it so widely used? Diverse political interest groups have come to support first-dollar coverage, each for a different reason. However, the combination of these political forces has made it difficult for governments to adopt more-rational benefit structures.

One common explanation is redistribution. (See Besley and Gouveia, 1994.) First-dollar coverage ensures universal access to medical care, regardless of income, thus alleviating the widespread concern that even small out-of-pocket costs may

---

[12] First-dollar coverage refers to insurance benefits where there is no deductible, so that all expenses are covered as soon as they are incurred.

Table 4.10

Features of Social Health Insurance Programs in Developing Countries

Country	Coverage	Financing Sources	Benefits	Provider Payment
Costa Rica	48%	Payroll tax and share of sales tax	First-dollar with capped benefits	Fee-based reimbursement
Egypt	33%	Payroll tax and sin taxes (cigarettes)	First-dollar with capped benefits	Fee-based reimbursement
Indonesia	17%	Payroll tax and general tax revenues	First-dollar with capped benefits	Fee-based reimbursement
Morocco	15%	Payroll taxes	First-dollar with capped benefits	Fee-based reimbursement
Korea, Republic of (S. Korea)	Universal	Payroll tax and general tax revenues	Inpatient 20% copay; outpatient 30-50% copay	Fee-based reimbursement
Philippines	38%	Payroll tax and general tax revenues	First-dollar with capped benefits	Fee-based reimbursement
Thailand	22%	Payroll tax and general tax revenues	First-dollar with capped benefits	Fee-based reimbursement
Viet Nam	38%	Payroll tax and general tax revenues	Inpatient with 50% copay	Fee-based reimbursement

SOURCE: WHO, 1995d; Herrin et al., 1996.

deter utilization, especially among the very poor. (See Cornia et al., 1987; Gilson, 1993.) Indeed, a good portion of public intervention in health care markets is justified on the tenet of universal access to basic minimum medical care, regardless of income, as embodied in WHO's slogan "Health for All by the Year 2000." Most countries recognize that poor individuals may not be able to afford health care and, therefore, subsidize the participation of poor individuals in universal insurance schemes. This partly explains why most countries have set up large universal public health care delivery systems that charge only nominal user fees. (See Jimenez, 1987; World Bank, 1987.)

The lack of deductibles and copayments in first-dollar coverage plans is consistent with the social solidarity objective to ensure access to medical care regardless of income. First-dollar coverage also readily complies with recommendations that SI benefits be integrated with primary, preventive, and promotive health care services. (See Abel-Smith, 1994; Ron, 1993.) Finally, since social insurance is typically financed by an income tax (i.e., a percentage of income) rather than by a flat actuarially fair premium, benefits are redistributed from rich to poor.

First-dollar coverage is also enthusiastically supported by politicians. While politicians may have altruistic redistribution goals, they are also concerned with re-election. First-dollar coverage puts money into more individuals' pockets, and politicians hope that people will remember that at election time.

Finally, employers also have strong financial incentives to support capped-benefit first-dollar coverage. Typically, SI premiums are cofinanced by employers. In many countries, large employers historically have provided workers with limited

Box 4.4: The Political Difficulty of Achieving SI Reform: The Example of the Philippines

In the early 1970s, with the economy starting to stagnate and civil unrest growing, the Filipino government began to rethink its existing policy of publicly financed and delivered health care. With the institution of the Philippine Medical Care Program (Medicare) in 1972, the government turned to social insurance as a way to shift a good portion of the public burden of delivering and financing health care to the private sector. By reducing the out-of-pocket prices of higher-quality private care relative to lower-quality public care, Medicare provided an incentive to choose the private sector over the public sector. Medicare was designed to finance inpatient hospital services for wage-sector employees and their dependents through a compulsory, earmarked payroll tax of 2.5 percent (up to a ceiling of $115 a month), equally shared by workers and employers.

Medicare provides limited coverage for inpatient hospitalization purchased either in the public or private sectors, but provides no coverage for outpatient services. Its inpatient benefits are first-dollar (peso) coverage up to a cap, which varies with the type of care needed (surgical and non-surgical), with severity of illness (ordinary versus intensive, or catastrophic), with the level of facility (primary, secondary, and tertiary), and with physician certification (general versus specialist). Providers are paid FFS up to the benefit caps. The end result of the 1972 policy has been that private providers have been able to price-discriminate.

In the 1980s, the country again experienced a severe economic crisis, which effectively cut real public health-care spending in half by 1992. The financial crisis reawakened political interest in an effective social health insurance program as an alternative to reduced public health-care spending. In 1992, the government began actively debating Medicare reform, and, in February 1995, the National Health Insurance Act was passed into law, expanding benefits to the whole population.

While the government is committed to expanding Medicare, strong political forces may induce it to keep the features of the program that have allowed private providers to capture most of the program's benefits. The issues being fiercely debated concern program benefits and FFS payment. During congressional hearings, a number of nongovernment organizations expressed concern that preventive and promotive health services were not given enough priority in the deliberations and argued that for equity reasons, social health insurance should cover not only inpatient hospital services, but also outpatient curative, preventive, and promotive care, including vaccinations and family planning. On the other side, institutions representing provider, employer, and "public and primary health" interests endorsed the current capped-benefit, first-dollar benefit package. The Philippine medical and hospital associations argued that if Medicare deviated from first-dollar coverage, providers would "...move out of the business of providing basic health care and into the business of providing financial relief." They endorsed first-dollar coverage, but advocated higher benefit ceilings. Representing employers, The Personnel Managers Association advocated that Medicare provide first-dollar coverage for a basic package of benefits most needed by workers.

The confluence of political forces united behind the current Medicare structure has made it virtually impossible to adopt a more rational structure, reduce the windfall for private providers, and increase the insurance benefits of Medicare for catastrophic illness. (See also Solon et al., 1995; Solon et al., 1997.)

health benefits as a means of reducing absenteeism. However, the reductions in absenteeism resulted from the quick treatment of minor illnesses. Employers typically capped benefits, since it was cheaper to fire severely ill individuals who had little chance of returning to work.

Medical Care Cost Inflation from Moral Hazard

While health insurance increases family welfare by reducing the financial risk of unexpected illness, it also introduces "moral hazard." Since health insurance lowers risk by spreading the cost of health care across the healthy and sick times of all individuals, it lowers the out-of-pocket price of medical care at the time of purchase. Because of the price reduction, consumers demand more services than they otherwise would. This extra consumption is inefficient, since individuals are purchasing health care beyond the point where the marginal benefit equals the marginal cost. (See Pauly, 1968.)

In addition, insurance facilitates the introduction of new, more-expensive medical technology, especially pharmaceuticals, before they are known to be cost-effective, which further fuels medical-care cost inflation. Technological change plays a key role in health care markets and is the root of the cost/quality trade-off in health policy. (See Weisbrod, 1991; Newhouse, 1992). If health care allocation decisions were driven by market prices, as is technology in other sectors (e.g., computers), the market would introduce them efficiently and we would not be concerned about the expansion of a sector in the economy (e.g., information technology).

However, health care is different for two reasons. First, in societies with health insurance, consumers almost never have to pay the true price of the medical care resources they use; in fact, in most cases, they pay very little at the time care is received. As new therapies become available and can treat (or promise to treat) illnesses that were incurable 10 years ago, individuals will demand those therapies; because of insurance, they will consume more of them than is efficient or even medically indicated. Second, while technological change in most industries reduces the amount of labor needed to produce a given amount and therefore saves costs, adopting new technology in health care increases the costs of treating illness and therefore uses more labor. This increase, in combination with the incentive to consume more care and technology than is efficient, leads to a technologic spiral of inefficient medical care cost inflation.

Moral hazard—both in terms of the increased utilization and the increased costs of utilization through faster-than-optimal adoption of technology—may explain the sudden and rapid medical cost inflation seen in South Korea and Taiwan after they adopted SI plans with universal coverage and regulated FFS payment. Before South Korea adopted universal insurance coverage, medical care expenditures were growing at the same rate as GDP and accounted for about 3 percent of GDP. As South Korea expanded social insurance, the growth in medical care spending began to outpace economic growth. As a result, by 1993, medical care expenditures accounted for about 5.7 percent of GDP. (See Yang, 1995.)

In Taiwan, medical expenditures started to grow faster than the economy as the country's SI program expanded its coverage. Between 1990 and 1993, health care expenditures increased 66 percent compared to a 45 percent increase in per-capita GDP.

It is important to note that in both countries, the period in which medical care expenditures were rising as a percent of GDP was the same period in which GDP

Box 4.5: Value of Medical Savings Accounts: The Example of Singapore

Unlike the usual form of health insurance, medical savings accounts (MSAs) provide less moral hazard because consumers are spending their own money. Therefore, the full cost of care is internalized at the time of purchase, which introduces discipline into the market. Singapore provides a good example of how MSAs can work.

Singapore achieved universal health insurance coverage in 1984 through the introduction of an MSA plan called Medisave.[13] Medisave mandates that individuals place 6–8 percent of their monthly income into an MSA, which they can draw on when they become ill. This compulsory savings accumulates over time and acts as insurance by spreading the cost of care over time. Medisave includes some limits that further retard expenditures. In particular, it has limits on withdrawals for some services, such as limited payments for each day of hospitalization and a maximum amount for each surgery. In this way, Medisave has a copayment for some services, which acts to help preserve lower expenditures and preserve the funds. A similar approach has been taken to pay for new, expensive technologies.

While MSAs seem to provide powerful cost-containment incentives, they provide limited insurance against catastrophic illness. MSAs only let an individual risk-pool over time, which is not enough to completely diversify the risk. In fact, individuals are usually not able to save enough to offset the costs of a serious long-term illness. Insurance usually spreads risk by including a large number of individuals in the pool so as to smooth the payments over *individuals* as well as over time. For MSAs to provide sufficient individual insurance against catastrophic illness, the mandated savings rate would have to be so high as to take a very large portion of income away from consumption and other activities.

Singapore recognized this problem and introduced Medishield in 1990. Medishield is a privately supplied insurance that provides coverage for costs associated with catastrophic illness. Except for a few groups, participation in Medishield is voluntary. The premiums are age-adjusted and are low relative to incomes, ranging from $12 per person under age 30 to $96 for a person between 60 and 65. Since the plan is meant to insure against only catastrophic illness, deductibles and copayments are kept high. Medisave accounts can be used to pay for Medishield insurance premiums and for the copayments and deductibles.

The combination of incentives from MSAs and copayments seems to have controlled medical care inflation in Singapore. Since the introduction of Medisave, medical care expenditures have remained at their pre-Medisave level of about 3 percent. However, this interpretation of the data must be taken with some caution, since Singapore has experienced substantial economic growth in the last 20 years. During periods of economic expansion, medical care expenditures have greatly expanded, but they have expanded at the same rate as economic growth. It is not clear that these policies will have the same effect in periods of slow growth.

---

was growing at a rate of over 10 percent per annum. Thus, South Korea and Taiwan were able to absorb both the increased demand for care as income rose and the high moral hazard costs associated with expanded insurance.

Examining the trade-offs between risk-bearing and moral hazard in providing medical insurance is one of the most studied problems in the insurance literature. (See Zeckhauser, 1975; Feldstein and Friedman, 1977.) Better insurance lowers the out-of-pocket payment at the time of illness. However, the greater the moral hazard, the larger the economic loss in terms of inefficiency. Losses from moral hazard occur because insurance lowers the price of medical care at the time of

---

[13]At the same time, Medicare, a government-funded insurance plan, was introduced to provide insurance for the poor.

purchase. Therefore, the bigger the price elasticity of demand for medical care, the greater the loss from moral hazard.

The demand studies reviewed earlier suggest that the price elasticity of demand is in the range of −0.5 to −1.0. This suggests that there is likely to be substantially more moral hazard in developing countries than in developed ones, where the price elasticity of demand is about −0.2. (See Newhouse, 1993a.) A number of examples bear this out. In an experimentally designed introduction of insurance in rural areas in China, insurance increased demand for outpatient care significantly, suggesting substantial moral hazard. (See Cretin et al., 1990.) Similarly, a cross-sectional analysis of Jamaican household data found that insurance dramatically increased health expenditures. (Gertler and Sturm, 1997.) Finally, a longitudinal analysis of Indonesian household data also found that insurance dramatically increases expenditures. (See also Dow et al., 1997.)

The threat of moral hazard means that governments need to adopt cost-control measures as part of any SI plan. One of the most important ways of controlling costs is the way providers are paid. Provider payment policies are discussed in detail in Chapter 7; here we examine one of the problems that can occur within SI plans when governments attempt to control costs by limiting benefits. South Korea's NHI has tried to control costs in the past by not covering low-probability, albeit expensive, services such as CT (computerized tomography or sometimes computerized axial tomography) scans, magnetic resonance imaging (MRIs), radiotherapy, ECGs (electrocardiograms), and ultrasonography. At the same time, South Korea uses a uniform fee schedule to reimburse providers, wherein providers receive the set fee for services covered under NHI and cannot balance bill,[14] but are free to charge what the market will bear for noncovered services.

While profit margins are low and in some cases negative for covered services, profit margins for the noncovered technologies mentioned above are quite large. Table 4.11 presents price markups over cost for a sample of noncovered NHI services. Not surprisingly, a strong provider lobby in South Korea exists to exclude new technologies from coverage.

The classic demand-side means of controlling moral hazard from insurance is to introduce out-of-pocket cost-sharing in the form of annual deductibles and copayments. (See Newhouse, 1993a.) The RAND Health Insurance Experiment, a randomized experiment done in the United States with 7,791 patients enrolled in different FFS (copayment) plans and prepaid plans, showed that the use of services responded to changes in the out-of-pocket expenditures. (See also Manning et al., 1988.) The larger the price elasticity of demand, the greater the copayments need to be. Since the price elasticity of demand appears to be bigger in developing countries than in developed countries, cost-sharing probably needs to be significant to control moral hazard. To get an idea of the range, copayments for indemnity insurance in the United States are in the range of 20 percent, with a cap on total out-of-pocket payments. Cost-sharing for hospitalization may need to

[14] Balance billing refers to the practice of providers charging an additional amount to the individual above what is reimbursed by insurance.

Table 4.11

Price Markups over Cost for Selected Service Not
Covered by NHI, South Korea

Service	Cost ($)	Market Price ($)	Markup (price/cost)
CT scan	57	240	4.21
MRI	163	475	2.91
Ultrasonograph	10	63	6.30

SOURCE: National Federation of Medical Insurance, 1994.

be higher, but with a lower cap on total out-of-pocket payments to maintain insurance against the financial risk of rare but expensive illness. Moreover, cost-sharing probably needs to be much higher for drugs and outpatient care than for inpatient care, since the demand is much more elastic for drugs and outpatient care than for inpatient care.

Managed-care strategies—whereby payers exert pressures to control utilization—are another way to reduce moral hazard. Both governments and private payers contract with providers, encouraging them to reduce costs. This effectively transfers some of the risk from the insurer to the provider plan and has been effective in reducing expenditures in the United States. The potential effectiveness of managed care in developing countries is discussed in the last section of this chapter.

Another demand-side policy mechanism for controlling moral hazard cost is the medical savings account. In this system, individuals are required to regularly contribute some percentage of their income into an MSA, which is used to finance medical care when they are sick. Because MSAs are composed of funds accumulated from personal savings and can only be used for individual care, they provide demand-side incentives to keep costs down. However, because MSAs do not pool risks across individuals, they are not effective insurance against catastrophic illness. Therefore, individuals need additional catastrophic insurance, although this can be financed cheaply. MSAs have the additional advantage of using market incentives to control costs and of being administratively simple. But they do not allow income redistribution, and, for MSAs to work, individuals must be forced to save much more than is necessary to finance health insurance. Poorer economies may not want to devote this much income to health care. While there is some positive experience with MSAs in Singapore, they are difficult to implement without other insurance strategies and should be extensively pilot-tested before they are universally adopted. If MSAs are voluntary, they suffer from the same adverse selections as indemnity insurance. To be effective, MSAs must be mandatory, thus requiring complex management and information systems.

Should Low- and Middle-Income Countries Adopt Universal Social Insurance?

Assuming that the problems discussed above can be addressed in designing the SI plan, how promising are SI plans for low- and middle-income countries in Asia? While the lure of social insurance is great, there has been limited experience with universal social insurance in low- and middle-income countries. However, there has been substantial experience in the high-performing Asian economies of Japan,

South Korea, Singapore, and Taiwan. Based on that experience, we can identify a number of lessons for low- and middle-income countries as they proceed down the path of implementing and expanding SI.

The above-mentioned countries successfully implemented SI only when they had relatively high income levels, were largely urbanized, and had large wage sectors relative to informal sectors. Table 4.12 compares the conditions in those countries at the time they introduced universal insurance to the conditions today in other countries that are in the process of implementing SI or considering it. The information in parentheses represents conditions in the year universal insurance was instituted for the four countries that have SI. The three columns are the real-dollar GDP per capita, the real GDP growth, and the percentage of the country that is urban. For example, South Korea had a GDP per capita of $5,371 and was 65.9 percent urban when universal health insurance was completed in 1989.

Table 4.12

Economic Conditions When Universal Health Insurance was Instituted in Wealthy Countries Compared to Other Asian Economies Today

Country (year universal insurance instituted)	Real-Dollar GDP per Capita, 1992 (when universal insurance instituted)	Real GDP Growth 1960–1992	% Urban, 1994 (when universal insurance instituted)
Bangladesh	220	1.85	17
China	450	5.05	28
India	310	1.90	26
Indonesia	670	3.50	32
Japan (1961)	28,190 (9,290)	6.02	—
Korea, Rep. of (1989)	6,790 (5,371)	10.49	74 (65.9)
Malaysia	2,790	3.39	44
Pakistan	420	2.50	33
Philippines	770	1.54	44
Singapore (1986)	15,730 (8,464)	7.90	100 (100)
Sri Lanka	540	2.19	22
Taipei, China (1995)	9,750 (9,750)	9.17	57 (57)
Thailand	1,840	5.04	35

SOURCE: Gertler, 1995a.

Notice that the four countries all waited until their GDP per capita was between $5,000 and $10,000. The GDP in most of the other countries in the region is about half that amount. Similarly, the four countries experienced much faster economic growth than the other countries. Finally, they were much more urbanized and had much larger wage sectors than the other countries have today. The fact that low- and middle-income countries are at much lower stages of development will make implementing social insurance more difficult for two reasons: macroeconomic costs (ability to pay and ability to absorb cost inflation) and administrative feasibility.

Macroeconomic Costs. The question is whether poorer economies can absorb the forced savings necessary to finance social insurance. The wealthier countries adopted universal insurance at income levels where relatively small portions of national income could finance health care delivered in the private sector. Today, the earmarked marginal income tax rates required to fund social insurance and purchase high-quality care from the private sector will require a much larger percentage of income in poorer countries. If these marginal tax rates reach a high enough level (e.g., Mongolia is considering a 30 percent rate), it would place a serious drag on the labor demand and thus on economic growth.

Associated with the introduction of insurance is rapid and allocatively inefficient medical-care cost inflation from moral hazard incentives. The wealthier countries were able to absorb this inflation because of tremendous real economic growth. It is not clear whether the slower-growing low- and middle-income countries can absorb the expected inflation and whether the health sector will significantly increase its share of the national economy.

Administrative Feasibility. The wealthy countries were largely urbanized and had large wage sectors when they moved to universal coverage. Enrollment compliance and administration is easier in a wage sector where individuals are already paying taxes. Administratively, this facilitated the expansion of coverage. Also, it is extremely difficult to get private providers to locate in rural areas. Therefore, even if one could enroll individuals in the rural areas, it is not clear that enough providers would exist to meet demand without special incentives.

These results do *not* say that low- and middle-income countries should abandon social insurance as a mechanism to achieve universal insurance and access. Rather, the results lend a word of caution about when to introduce social insurance with private-sector delivery and when the public sector needs to intervene. It is important to remember that even South Korea and Taiwan did not jump to universal coverage immediately. Rather, they expanded insurance sequentially, sector by sector, starting with those most able to pay and those easiest to administer. In South Korea, the strategy for universal coverage involved starting in those sectors (like the wage sector) that were administratively simple, whose participation would be easiest to enforce, and that (in the eyes of the government) could afford the extra taxes. Initially, in 1977, individuals employed in firms with more than 500 employees were enrolled. NHI was expanded to include civil servants, teachers, military personnel, and pensioners in 1980. In 1983, NHI included firms hiring 16 or more workers. Finally, in 1989, NHI began to cover the self-employed informal and agricultural sectors. A separate program for means-tested poor individuals, Medicare, was enacted along with the initiation of NHI in 1977. (See Peabody et al., 1994.)

The experience of the wealthier countries suggests that most low- and middle-income countries should consider first introducing social insurance into the wage sector where income levels are relatively high, where economic growth is the fastest, and where they are able to enforce enrollment through the existing income tax collection systems. The experience also suggests there is a key role for the public sector in terms of financing and delivering care in poor rural areas where ability to pay is low and where it is hard to induce private providers to live. The major conclusion is that most low- and middle-income countries are best off moving to mixed systems, with some social insurance and private delivery in urban-area wage sectors and public finance and delivery in poor rural areas.

In summary, there seems to be a razor's edge in the transition to social insurance. In societies without insurance and large public sectors, fiscal and political pressures on the public budget generally lead to underfunded systems. However, as societies switch to social insurance, more resources are mobilized than are efficient and the result is rapid cost inflation. Whereas in public systems it is easy to maintain a global cap on expenditures through public and individual budget constraints, market incentives take over under SI plans with private-sector delivery. Moral hazard induces individuals to demand more medical services than is efficient. Such plans also provide an incentive for health sectors to adopt new expensive technologies more quickly. Since technology in medical care tends to be labor-using rather than labor-saving, the effect is to greatly increase costs rather than to reduce them, as is the case with other labor-saving technology. Therefore, cost-containment policies must deal explicitly with techno-logical adoption, since it embodies the cost-quality trade-off facing societies.

Community Financing

What other alternatives exist? Community financing schemes—which are collective efforts for local insurance funds—are used to pay for a variety of medical services, such as outpatient care, curative services, and drugs. They are sometimes proposed as an alternative to national-level social insurance or introduced as an additional way to mobilize resources at the local level. Like other forms of insurance, they can expand access to service and increase demand by reducing costs and insure against catastrophic illness (although this is not usually their function). They can also suffer from adverse risk selection if enrollment is voluntary and from overutilization because of moral hazard. Unlike other forms of insurance, they depend on using local, community-level infrastructure. And while community financing may be free from excessive dependency on national resources and can establish a better linkage of expenditures with local knowledge and needs, it also introduces more reliance on local expertise and workforce contributions that may not be adequate.

Developing countries in Asia have tried community financing schemes. As an alternative financing mechanism, such schemes have had mixed results. Based on a study of community financing in Thailand, researchers found that village drug funds were very successful, with a continuation rate of up to 81 percent. Sanitation and health care funds were also fairly successful, because they had higher capital appreciation and a diverse source of income. Nutrition funds turned out to be the least successful scheme because of their particular activities, low acceptance among the people, and limited capital appreciation. The study determined that four factors contributed to the success or failure of a community financing scheme. First, there must be a strong government policy commitment. Second, support from government health personnel was critical, especially in terms of managerial capability and supervision of local personnel. Third, good community infrastructure, such as strong village leadership and a relatively high level of economic development, was found to be a necessary condition for success. Finally, the types of funds also mattered, because funds varied in terms of popularity, managerial difficulty, and necessity. (See Wilbulpolprasert, 1991.)

Another study in Nepal showed less success in improving access and service delivery. Drawing on a stratified sample of households and personal interviews in two villages—one with a community-run and financed system; the other, state-run and financed—the study showed that community financing did not appear to widen the scope and the extent of participation. Community involvement, outside of district participation, was very limited. (See Sepehri and Pettigrew, 1996.)

When used as an insurance function, community financing schemes have met with only limited success. For example, a study on rural health insurance in China examined the relationship between rural cooperative health insurance and health care expenditure, based on a controlled natural experiment in "twin" counties in the Jiangsu province of China. One county had a health financing system built on health insurance, and the other had a predominantly user-fee–funded system. (See Bogg et al., 1996.) The findings support the hypothesis that cooperative insurance, like social insurance, induces higher growth of health care expenditures and leads to a shift from preventive medicine to curative medicine and to higher expenditure levels on technologically based tertiary curative care.

A second study in China—which used a household survey to review a pilot experiment of reestablishing rural cooperative medical systems in 14 counties in 7 provinces—determined that patients would still have to pay about 80 percent of clinic charges. A simulation found that lowering copayments would cause financial shortfalls to the scheme. The study concluded that because of variation among the 14 counties, successful implementation required that each county develop its own model and have clear written plans and regulations about the scheme.

One of the large problems with community financing is that it only insures against the financial costs of idiosyncratic illnesses within communities. That is to say, insurance works best if the probability of illness is uncorrelated among the beneficiaries of a plan. That way, when one person is ill the others are likely to be healthy, so that plan expenditures can be smoothed over time. However, if illness is highly correlated, as is the case of infectious diseases in a village, then the insurance value of community financing is small. Large epidemics can quickly bankrupt community financing schemes. To be finally secure, community financing schemes need reinsurance across communities as provided in a nationally based insurance scheme.

COST CONTROL VIA MANAGED CARE

The moral hazard from insurance coverage has fueled significant medical inflation. Developed countries with universal health systems have attempted to control health care cost inflation through a variety of mechanisms. Global budgets, whereby hospitals or medical groups are given their own fixed budgets, are one mechanism. Within this global budget, decisions about utilization of specific services are made explicitly by providers and administrators. Payers—the government, private insurers, and large employers—also exert pressure on health plans and providers to control costs. Health care plans have responded to these pressures by implementing a variety of mechanisms to control the utilization of specific health care services. These are collectively known as managed care. (See Kongstvedt, 1993; Iglehart, 1992.) In the United States the pressures from payers and the savings to individuals have now moved most Americans into some type of managed care plan. (See Weiner and Lissovoy, 1993.)

This section describes managed care and considers the potential for its application in developing countries. To date, there has been very little experience with managed care in low- and middle-income countries. As with social insurance, there are a number of challenges that need to be considered before implementing managed care outside of higher-income countries.

The "purest" form of managed care organization (MCO) is the health maintenance organization (HMO), an organization that agrees to provide all of a specified range of health care services—such as outpatient physician services, inpatient medical care, and prescription medications—through its own network of providers and hospitals, in return for a set premium per enrolled member per month. Since it is accepting the risk of providing all care for its enrollees, an HMO has strong incentives to provide services cost-effectively; in addition, HMOs emphasize preventive care as a way to reduce long-run health care costs for their enrollees.

How specifically do HMOs control costs and utilization? The techniques vary by the various types of HMOs. The group or staff model HMOs (such as Kaiser Permanente in the United States) employ a staff of full-time physicians who provide care exclusively to enrollees. This helps control cost in two ways. First, the fraction of primary-care providers on the HMO panels is much higher than it is for the country at large. (See Dial et al., 1995.) Second, the group practice environment fosters a conservative, cost-effective style of medical practice. (See Smillie, 1991.) Group/staff model HMOs also own their own hospitals, so they can tailor facility sizes to the needs of their enrolled population and can tightly control utilization of hospital services.

Another MCO model—the Independent Practice Association (IPA) model—contracts with associations of independent physicians or small group practices.[15] Providers are usually reimbursed based on capitation; that is, a doctor receives a set fee per member per month in return for providing a defined range of services. This gives the provider a strong incentive to provide only appropriate services. Specialty physicians are usually reimbursed on an FFS basis, but utilization is controlled by requiring patients to obtain an authorization from their primary-care provider (often called a "gatekeeper") to obtain an appointment with a specialist. The MCO also provides contracts with hospitals to care for enrollees. Utilization rates are controlled by utilization management tools, such as preauthorization of admissions and elective procedures, and with concurrent review to control length of stay and the intensity of inpatient services. (See Gray and Field, 1989.)

Managed care features can also be incorporated into FFS plans. A preferred provider organization (PPO) is a type of FFS plan that contracts with physicians and hospitals to provide services to its members at a discounted price and that influences utilization rates by offering enrollees a reduced copayment for using

---

[15]Network model HMOs contract with large physician groups; many MCOs contract with both IPAs and groups.

these providers. These strategies, it is worth pointing out, are similar to the user fee and subsidization policies discussed in the earlier sections of the chapter. In addition, utilization management tools can be employed by PPO or standard FFS plans to preauthorize expensive procedures and inpatient admissions and to concurrently review hospitalizations. Another mechanism for reducing inpatient expenditures under FFS is prospective payment, that is, setting a fixed price for all inpatient services for a given diagnosis. This mechanism has been instituted by the U.S. Medicare plan, and has succeeded in reducing the growth rate of Medicare inpatient expenditures. (See Coulam and Gaumer, 1991.)

Given the various types of MCOs and the techniques they use to control costs, how well does managed care actually work, and what is the potential for applying it in developing countries?

Evaluating the Effectiveness of Managed Care

Even though managed care has become the predominant model in the United States, relatively few well-designed studies, containing a comparison group and risk adjustments for differences in illness, have evaluated the performance of managed care. (See Miller and Luft, 1994a, 1994b.) However, based on the few good studies that have been done, we find that MCOs do reduce utilization and costs. They have lower hospital utilization than FFS plans, which accounts for most of their cost reduction. (See Luft, 1978b.) The RAND Health Insurance Experiment, an RCT that compared utilization in HMO and FFS plans, found a 40 percent lower rate of hospital admissions in the HMO, but similar rates of ambulatory visits. Interestingly, the rate of preventive visits was higher in the HMO. (See Manning et al., 1984.)

Another way to assess the effect of managed-care plans on costs is to examine premium levels and growth rates. (See Miller and Luft, 1994b; Higgins, 1994–95.) HMOs appear to charge lower premiums than FFS plans, but caution is warranted because the available data are not adjusted for differences in plan design or enrolled population. Premium increases have also slowed markedly in recent years, coincident with increases in managed-care prevalence, but a causal relationship is not certain. It is also not clear whether premium growth rates will remain so low, once managed care becomes nearly universal among employer-financed insurance, as it has in California in the United States.

Risk selection also makes evaluation of the financial impact of managed care more difficult. With their restrictions on access to specialty care, HMOs are thought to appeal to healthier patients. Therefore, some apparent cost savings may be the result of differences in the underlying demand for services between sicker FFS enrollees and healthier HMO enrollees. Evaluations of Medicare managed-care plans indicate such favorable selection is taking place. (See ProPac, 1996; Physician Payment Review Commission (PPRC), 1996.)

There is concern that the financial incentives providers face to reduce utilization in managed-care plans (especially capitation) will reduce quality by depriving some patients of necessary services. Available studies, however, indicate that HMO and FFS plans provide comparable levels of quality on process and outcome measures. A review of available data on capitation did not find evidence of degradation of quality under capitated payment, but noted that proper design of the capitation scheme (such as having sufficiently large risk pools) is important to obviate quality risks. (See Berwick, 1996.)

Concerns about access under managed care again arise from restrictions on specialty care. This would most severely affect enrollees with chronic illnesses, who are disproportionately large users of specialty care. (See Neff and Anderson, 1995.) On the other hand, managed care plans are well situated to coordinate the often fragmented care that chronically ill patients receive under FFS. A coordinated and comprehensive strategy of disease management could improve outcomes for chronically ill patients at the same time as it reduces expenditures. (See Wagner et al., 1996; Dubois, 1996.)

Even after more than a decade of experience, it is far from clear whether managed care can control a country's aggregate health care spending in the long run. MCOs have mostly enrolled under-65 workers and their dependents, whereas the heaviest users of health care services are those over 65. Medicare offers an option to enroll in HMOs, but so far only about 13 percent of Medicare beneficiaries have chosen that option, and for those who enroll it does not reduce costs for Medicare overall, because of risk selection. (See McMillan, 1993; Levit et al., 1996.)

Developing-Country Experience with Managed Care

As mentioned above, managed care has been primarily employed in high-income countries, predominantly in the United States. As a result, the literature on managed care in developing countries is very sparse. In part, this is because few developing countries have had widespread public, social, or private insurance for long enough to encounter severe medical care inflation problems. It is also because developing countries have chosen to address inflation through global budgets rather than managed care.

Still, some developing countries have adopted managed-care strategies. For example, Chile's government has strongly encouraged the growth of HMOs. (See Miranda et al., 1995.) Twenty-two percent of the population is enrolled in HMOs, which are called ISAPREs (*Institutos de Salud Previsional*). The main attraction of ISAPREs appears to be that they offer significantly greater amenities than the public system. In terms of how they work, the Chilean government takes a mandatory deduction of 7 percent of wages for health care and adds an additional 2 percent subsidy for low-income workers. Workers may choose to use the public system or to use their deduction to pay the premiums for one of the private-sector ISAPREs. However, only for better-paid workers is the deduction plus subsidy enough to cover ISAPRE premiums; thus, enrollees tend to come from the higher income strata.

Other countries allow the formation of HMOs. One of the best examples is Colombia, which, under a 1994 health reform law, allowed social insurance payroll deductions to be used for enrollment in either public- or private-sector HMOs. Workers pay 12 percent of their wages into either public or private HMOs called *Empresas de Medicina Prepagada* or EMPs. Each EMP that enrolls a patient receives a capitated payment of approximately $150 per year per patient. The exact amount of the capitated payment is adjusted by the government on the basis of age and sex. To maintain financial sustainability of the overall system, higher-paid workers cross-subsidize poorer workers: Contributions in excess of the capitated payment level go into the National Pension Fund; underfunded contributions are paid out. (See Hsiao et al., 1995.) In 1995, Ecuador tried to introduce a similar plan, but political entanglements crippled the effort and it was never implemented. Although private HMOs have joined the market, they are limited by high costs and adverse selection and remain an option for the middle and upper classes only. In South Africa some HMOs also exist and managed care is a potential option, although (as in Colombia) an unproven one, for restraining health care inflation. (See Kinghorn, 1996; Price, 1992.)

In terms of developing countries in Asia, Indonesia's state-owned oil company has considered starting an HMO, beginning in Jakarta, where the firm already owns a hospital. (See Tollman, et al., 1990.) In addition, as part of an overall health care project in Taiwan in the late 1980s that examined concerns about rising health care costs and inadequate national health insurance coverage, researchers examined the potential for introducing HMOs into the health care system. The study concluded that the current health care system was not conducive to introducing HMOs. Not insignificant among the problems were apparent cultural barriers to Chinese acceptance of HMOs. The study also found that even if other problems could be resolved, Taiwan lacked the management expertise at that time to run such an organization. (See Newhouse et al., 1988.)

Necessary Conditions for Managed Care in Developing Countries

Although the evidence on managed care in developing countries is scarce, we can draw some lessons from that evidence and from the evidence in developed countries. Successful implementation for developing countries can be defined as providing quality of care comparable to FFS plans or the public sector, at a lower cost than those systems, to a comparable enrolled population (i.e., the cost "savings" must not be based on favorable selection of enrollees). But before developing countries decide to embark on a managed-care strategy, they should carefully evaluate the experience of developed countries, to ascertain whether it meets their own criteria for success.

Several management and institutional factors must be in place if managed care plans are to be feasible. Recall that the assessment of Taiwan's potential for HMOs argued that Taiwan lacked the management expertise to run an HMO organization at that time. Thus, developing countries wishing to implement managed care must first have mechanisms to enroll patients, collect premiums, and pay claims from providers and hospitals. On the plus side, such mechanisms are required to implement social insurance, which some Asian countries have already implemented or are in the process of doing.

Second, creating managed care plans requires developing a number of management and information systems:

- To create a PPO or an IPA-model HMO, contracts must be signed with hospitals and providers. Alternatively, a group/staff model HMO would require hiring a relatively large number of physicians and perhaps purchasing or building a hospital. Forming these physician organizations and/or contracted networks would be challenging in developing countries if legal frameworks for health care contracts are not developed, or if physicians have no tradition of organizing into group practices or associations that accept reimbursement.

- Once networks are established, operating systems must be put in place: information systems are needed so that contracted providers and hospitals can report utilization of covered services and respond to utilization management mechanisms (such as preauthorization and concurrent hospital care review) that ensure that the amount of care provided does not exceed budgets, and to review claims retrospectively for legitimacy. These system requirements can be simplified if providers are reimbursed by capitation, since the risk of overutilization is transmitted to them.

- Systems to monitor quality must also be present, especially if reimbursement is by capitation and potential underprovision of necessary care is a concern. These complex management and information systems have required years to develop and refine in U.S. managed-care plans. Implementing systems of this level of sophistication is likely to be quite difficult in most developing countries.

Third, as we will discuss in Chapter 7, setting appropriate hospital and physician payment rates is challenging in any country. Rates must be set to cover legitimate costs while minimizing economic incentives to underprovide care, adopt unnecessary high technology, or engage in favorable selection. Fourth, the MOH or other government agencies must be able to adequately monitor and regulate managed-care plans. This will require regulatory authority, sufficient funding, and expertise that is not currently present in most developing-country MOHs.

Finally, managed-care plans can only be expected to reduce costs if competition for enrollees exists between plans. Otherwise, monopolistic managed-care plans could accept premiums but not take steps to correct the problems with access, quality, and efficiency that already plague existing public provision systems. The required degree of competition that MCOs require will be hardest to achieve in underserved areas with insufficient providers and facilities, such as rural areas.

Even given these considerable challenges, rapidly developing countries may consider managed care as a policy option, as the circumstances for its growth appear more fertile: health spending will grow as incomes rise, widespread social or private insurance will be developed, levels of private-sector provision of care will emerge, and professionalization and managerial capabilities in public and private sector will begin to take hold.

POLICY IMPLICATIONS

When we look across these findings, what can we say about policy focus? First, there will be a trade-off between three commonly cited objectives that improve health outcomes in a population—providing public goods, promoting equity, and insuring against catastrophic illness. Promoting health and equity, for example, focuses resources on controlling communicable diseases in primary-care settings, whereas insurance motivations for government intervention will concentrate public spending in the hospital setting—for example, on treating vascular diseases. Finding services that benefit the poor entails looking at what services they use and at the income elasticity of demand. Such services will include preventing and treating common infectious diseases at health centers in rural areas. However, protecting the poor from financial risk because of illness argues for subsidizing a network of public hospitals that already consume generous shares of the public sector's health budget. In essence, subsidies to hospitals provide catastrophic health insurance, but at the expense of subsidies to provide public goods and ameliorate equity concerns.

Second, although government decisions about financing are based on values forged in the political process, policy decisions on how revenues are raised and where resources are allocated will shape many fundamental characteristics of the health sector. User fees and other pricing mechanisms, for example, will affect utilization and where subsidies are allocated. Modifying resources through increased user fees can finance improved quality of care, but it can also reduce the access to care for the poor or the insurance value of the public delivery system. Finding the right balance between preventing diseases and treating severe illness can lead to optimal improvements in the health status of the population.

Third, to most efficiently use its public subsidies to improve health status, a government should use the following general pricing policies:

- Subsidies should be higher for those services where public care is better than private, because it leads to better health.
- Subsidies should be higher for those services where a decrease in price will lead to a large increase in utilization of clinically effective care.
- Similarly, subsidies should be for those groups (e.g., the poor, elderly, and women) where a decrease in price will lead to a large increase in utilization.
- Subsidies should be higher in areas where there is limited private care.

Fourth, although resource mobilization through user fees can cofinance curative care and private incentives that reallocate public subsidies to public health programs, there is a potential downside—decreased utilization by the poor and lower health outcomes. Dealing with this downside requires that the implications of policy changes involving user fees be considered. This argues for conducting well-designed longitudinal studies with control groups and for ensuring that user-fee policy interventions and pricing strategies are pilot-tested before being implemented at the national level.

Fifth, while social insurance (for financing) and managed care (for controlling costs) are policies that hold promise for developing countries, implementing them requires conditions and capabilities not present in all developing countries, particularly low- and middle-income ones. Before implementing these policies, countries will need to achieve a "critical mass" in terms of GDP, a formal wage sector, and urbanization—conditions that tend to be evolutionary and, hence, out of policymakers' direct control. As for capabilities, implementing the policies requires a sophisticated administrative and information resources capacity, as well as the legal and regulatory infrastructure to support the policies—capabilities within policymakers' direct control. Thus, policymakers in developing countries should take a very deliberate approach to using social insurance or managed care, developing the necessary infrastructure to take advantage of the situation when conditions are right.

CHAPTER 5: SUMMARY OF POLICY QUESTIONS, FINDINGS, AND IMPLICATIONS

ISSUES	EVIDENCE
• What are practical ways to define equity?	• There are multiple useful definitions of equity.
• How is equity measured?	• Equity can be measured with outcome, process, or structural measures, but their usefulness varies by equity type.
• How much and what kinds of inequity exist in Asia?	• Available data demonstrate that inequity remains a serious problem in most of Asia.
• What options are there to improve equity?	• Several options—ranging from financing reforms or better quality of care to national insurance—are useful for addressing inequity.
• Within these options, what are the most suitable policies and under what circumstances?	• Social insurance expansion is likely to be a better option in countries with at least a middle income; subsidies targeting the poor are better for lower-income countries.

POLICY IMPLICATIONS
• Although all governments want to help improve equity, this will always be balanced against competing needs to meet other social objectives—the priority of health equity will be subordinate to political, social, and cultural circumstances.
• Significant data gaps often prevent policymakers from addressing inequities as effectively or as cost-effectively as they might.
• Because of significant data gaps, unknown inequities exist; this means that interventions may even make inequities worse.
• To improve equity, government policy must redirect subsidies toward the financing or delivery of services to the poor.
• In the poorest countries, geographic targets, differential pricing of providers and services, and disease targeting hold the most promise to improve equity.

TOWARD BETTER EQUITY AND ACCESS: PERSISTENT POVERTY, INADEQUATE INTERVENTIONS, AND THE NEED FOR BETTER DATA AND SOLUTIONS

OVERVIEW

One of the key roles of government in the health sector we outlined in Chapter 1 is promoting equity or remedying inequities by improving access to health care. As we saw in Chapters 3 and 4, ensuring equity involves both the delivery of health care—governments need to prioritize interventions, and the financing of health care—governments need to put policies in place that enable individuals to afford those interventions.

Over the past three decades, Asian governments have made a concerted effort to improve access to health care. Many countries invested in facility infrastructure and health manpower to extend direct public provision of free or low-priced services to poor urban neighborhoods and rural areas (e.g., Indonesia, India, Papua New Guinea, the Philippines, and Sri Lanka). Some countries also expanded insurance, particularly for civil service workers and others in the formal wage sector (e.g., South Korea and Singapore) or for farmers through rural cooperatives or communes (e.g., China and Viet Nam). More recently, some governments have fostered the start-up of community financing schemes or have disseminated health cards to the poor (e.g., Thailand and Indonesia). These investments in health, combined with the development gains made possible by economic growth, as discussed in Chapter 1, have led to impressive gains in health status throughout many Asian countries.

However, such investments are not sufficient to ensure equity. Though chiefly justified on the grounds of benefiting the poor, most of the health-sector initiatives have actually ended up transferring the largest share of public subsidies to the middle class. (See Birdsall and James, 1993; van der Gaag, 1995.) For example, in many countries a substantial share of public resources support flagship government hospitals located primarily in urban settings. Even when countries support health facilities in rural areas, they are typically of low quality, lacking even the most basic equipment and drugs.

The curative services in government health facilities are often provided free or for low fees. Nevertheless, the poor tend to have lower utilization rates than the nonpoor. There are probably many reasons for this lower utilization. The poor are generally less acculturated to using health care because of lower levels of education and other factors. They often have to travel greater distances to medical facilities and have more difficulties in arranging transport, and they are less able to purchase the amenities and supplies that must be paid for outside the official fee structure. For example, in many hospitals, patients must either bring or buy on-site such basic supplies as inoculation needles, sutures, and bandages. The widespread practice of charging fees above the official fee structure further discourages the poor from using services.

Establishing national health insurance does not necessarily reduce the regressivity of public subsidies. For example, in Indonesia, civil servants have health insurance provided by a parastatal company and obtain most services from public facilities, for which the insurance firm pays a subsidized price. These insured individuals have higher use rates than the uninsured population (45 percent more outpatient visits and 65 percent more inpatient visits) at prices that are set at less than costs, so that a greater than proportional share of public subsidies accrues to civil servants. (See Gertler and Rahman, 1994.)

This is not to say that the poor have not benefited from government policies. In many cases they have, sometimes more so than the nonpoor, the above factors notwithstanding. For example, one study that estimated the distributional impact of public expenditures in Indonesia provided evidence that government health spending is associated with greater use of preventive services and better child outcomes (as reflected in shorter illness duration and greater weight for age), particularly for the poor. (See Deolalikar, 1992.)

Despite the impressive health achievements of Asian countries over the past three decades (illustrated earlier in Table 1.1), huge inequities continue to afflict vulnerable populations. As we will see, the burden of disease exacts a much heavier toll on the poor, who continue to suffer premature death and disability from communicable diseases, childbearing, and other conditions, many of which are amenable to treatment through basic medical interventions. Other vulnerable populations include children, women, ethnic minorities and indigenous populations, and rural residents. Up to half of all deaths in developing countries occur in children younger than five years. Women also bear a heavy mortality burden brought on by their lower social standing, greater financial barriers in getting access to health care, and the greater health risks imposed by childbearing. Although men's mortality is higher than women's in most developing countries, avoidable mortality tends to be higher for women. (See Murray et al., 1992a.) Rural residents generally have poorer living standards than their urban counterparts, face greater health risks because of less-developed infrastructure, and must travel greater distances to visit health providers.

Given these equity concerns, we can formulate five policy questions:

1. What are practical ways to define equity?
2. How is equity measured?
3. How much and what kinds of inequity exist in Asia?
4. What options are there to improve equity?
5. Within those options, which policies are the most suitable and under what circumstances?

The answers to these questions form the basis for the rest of this chapter.

DEFINITIONS OF EQUITY

In their cross-country comparative analysis of equity differences in 10 OECD countries, Van Doorslaer et al. distinguish between equity in finance and equity in delivery. (See Van Doorslaer et al., 1993.) Equity in finance (or equity in contribution) implies that health care is financed according to ability to pay. For example, families of unequal ability to pay would be called on to make proportionate payments for health care, payments that are not necessarily linked to the amount of care received.

Equity in delivery can have several meanings. One is that health services are distributed not according to ability to pay, but rather according to medical need as defined by the capacity to benefit from treatment. (See Culyer 1995; Wagstaff and Van Doorslaer, 1993.) Some people may have illnesses that are not amenable to treatment (e.g., terminal cancers) and would, therefore, not be defined as having a medical need. This implies equal treatment for equal need (capacity to benefit). One variant of this view holds that government efforts need only ensure physical access to facilities and removal or lowering of financial barriers. This perspective reflects the notion that "economic inequalities that stem from inequality of opportunity are more intolerable than those that emerge when opportunities are equal." (Okun, 1975, pp. 75–76.) Another view of equity in delivery does not seek to equalize treatment or opportunity per se across all groups, but instead holds that the poor and other vulnerable groups should be guaranteed an essential package of health services. The wealthy may receive better services than the poor, but as long as the poor are guaranteed a medically adequate set of services, a system can be said to be equitable.

Selecting among these alternatives requires standard-setting that is best left to individual countries, where priorities can be set to match the predominant cultural and sociopolitical values. Assessing the capacity to benefit and defining the essential package of services are concrete examples of standard-setting. These definitions must be used cautiously, however, and are less informative when assessing system performance or making cross-country comparisons.

Table 5.1 shows specific categories within each of these two dimensions of equity that we will consider in more detail.

Table 5.1

**Categories of Measures Within Equity in Finance
and Equity in Delivery**

Types of Equity	Measure Categories
Equity in finance	• Allocation and distribution of subsidies • Program coverage by population and service mix • Risk pooling
Equity in delivery	• Health status • Utilization (or expenditures) • Physical access and organization

Equity in Finance

As the table shows, one category of equity in finance has to do with the way that governments fund and allocate public subsidies. As we showed in Chapter 4, there is substantial variation across Asian countries in the way health care is funded—general taxation, social insurance contributions, private insurance premiums, and out-of-pocket payments—and in the relative importance of each source. Both the way revenue is raised and the relative importance of each source are important determinants of equity in finance.

Program coverage has to do with how different populations participate in public or private insurance plans, prepayment plans, or community financing programs. Another aspect of coverage has to do with the mix of services offered in the various programs. The service mix in some program designs can be set up to better address problems facing some groups (e.g., prenatal care for women) over others (e.g., rehabilitation for the elderly).

Finally, there is risk pooling, a mechanism for spreading or distributing risk across all the members of a group. For example, individuals who purchase insurance trade the certainty of a small financial loss (the price of the premium) for the uncertainty of ill health and a larger financial loss at some point in the future. Risk pooling can be accomplished through a number of different mechanisms: government-provided insurance, community prepayment plans, or other types of community finances.

Equity in Delivery

The strongest standard of equity in delivery is to ensure equal health status across population groups, so that the poor and other vulnerable groups do not suffer from higher mortality and morbidity than would other groups of higher social standing. According to this criterion, inequity is relatively great not only in most developing countries but also in many industrialized nations, where disparities in health status by income, gender, age, ethnicity, or geographic residence are often found. (See van der Gaag, 1995.) In the United States, for example, the infant mortality rate for African Americans is twice the rate for white Americans, and maternal mortality is nearly three times higher among African American women. (See U.S. Bureau of the Census, 1996.)

The problem with using an equity standard based on health status is that many factors outside the reach of the health sector affect health outcomes (e.g., housing, safe water, nutrition). Therefore, even if the health care system comes close to achieving equity in the delivery of services, it may not produce equal health outcomes.

Equity can also be defined based on measure of health care utilization or health care expenditures. Under this standard, the probability of obtaining health services (the contact rate), the use rates, or the expenditures are similar across population groups. In practical terms, this means that the poor have the same number of doctor visits per year as the nonpoor, after controlling for illness levels.

To some extent, though, utilization measures share a common problem with health status measures. Utilization is determined not just by the presence of health

Box 5.1: Difficulties in Achieving Equity

Clarion calls for greater equity—embodied in WHO's rallying cry "health for all by the year 2000" and adopted by governments the world over—have served as the impetus for much of the health reform fervor sweeping across Asia and the rest of the world. Despite widespread support in industrial and developing countries alike, government efforts to achieve greater equity are bedeviled not just by finite budget limitations, but by social forces as well.

First, improving equity must be balanced against multiple, legitimate health-sector goals, such as improving efficiency, improving quality, and controlling costs. Rarely will a single policy simultaneously satisfy all such objectives, thus forcing governments to make trade-offs between competing objectives.

Second, health reform takes place within a political context. As a result, entrenched interests representing a country's elite and its middle class often overwhelm those without a political voice, blocking policies that entail a significant redistribution of resources.

Third, philosophical and ideological differences often underlie much of the debate on equity. Characterized by the classic egalitarian/libertarian debate, this split produces fundamental disagreements about what constitutes equity. (See Donabedian, 1973.) In terms of health care, the egalitarian point of view argues that good health is a necessary "capability" for pursuing life's activities.

The egalitarian perspective places emphasis on equalizing health outcomes across population subgroups (i.e., the poor should have infant mortality rates as low as those of more privileged groups). (See Sen, 1985.) The libertarian point of view favors equality of opportunity, rather than equality of outcomes. Emphasis is placed on equalizing access to care (in terms of physical proximity and the lowering of financial barriers) or on equalizing the opportunity to use care. That there are differences in use rates or in health outcomes (once access is equalized) merely reflects differences in personal preferences and in the values individuals place on good health.

These ideological differences represent more than the debate between opposing philosophies. They undergird national policies that emphasize equal access (a single tier of medical care created by setting both a floor and a ceiling), regardless of income or policies that guarantee basic health services (a multitiered system that sets the floor but has no limits on the ceiling) for the poor and other marginalized populations. The two endpoints of the spectrum are represented by the social insurance systems of the OECD countries and Australia at the egalitarian end and the United States at the libertarian end, with its largely private insurance–based system augmented by public financing for the poor and the elderly. (See Peabody et al., 1996c.) No country is purely one or the other: The OECD countries allow individuals to purchase private insurance and higher-end services, while the United States provides public funding to assist the poor and the elderly. Nonetheless, the two pose a stark policy choice. (See Feachem, 1997.)

resources but by other factors that affect the demand for health care (such as illness and its determinants—nutrition, sanitation, or conditions in the environment), education levels, cultural factors (such as the perception of benefits associated with treatment), and the many other factors that affect care-seeking behavior.

Another way to define equity is by access to care. Physical access represents the opportunity for use and is simpler to define operationally. It is the presence of resources (hospitals, clinics, doctors, and other health care workers) to provide the means for getting health care. It reflects both availability (proximity, convenient hours of operation, etc.) and affordability (including both the monetary and time costs incurred in obtaining care).

How equity is ultimately defined will drive the selection of policies undertaken to improve access to health services. For example, from the 1960s through the 1980s, many Asian countries focused on the delivery side and formulated policies that largely emphasized physical access, such as meeting uniform standards of beds per 1,000 population and physicians per 1,000 population. However, once the basic infrastructure was in place, efforts to improve access turned more toward the finance side to remedy the financial and nonfinancial barriers to access, using targeted subsidies and insurance and/or prepayment schemes. Policymakers also turned toward influencing the use of services, with the emphasis on supplying preventive care, primary health services, and cost-effective curative services, redirecting patients away from hospitals and toward local health centers, and providing them with incentives to do so.

MEASURES OF EQUITY

As we discussed previously in Chapters 2 and 3, we measure health care interventions using three sets of measures: *outcome measures*, which measure how people fare and whether their health status improves; *process measures*, which reflect the practices of medicine, such as the provision of services that prevent disease or promote and prescribe actions for good health, or how medical procedures are performed; and *structural measures*, which involve what is needed to provide care, such as personnel and facilities or the organization of the health care delivery system.

Table 5.2 shows the wide range of outcome, process, and structural measures of equity across the types and categories of equity.

Outcome Measures

On the finance side, outcome measures reflect how well a program ultimately does in reaching the poor or other targeted populations (such as the sick, the elderly, or children). Benefit-incidence ratios—which show the percentage of public subsidies accruing to each income group (e.g., quintile or decile)—are an example of an outcome measure that enables policymakers to assess the distributional consequences of financing policy.

On the delivery side, outcome measures—such as mortality and morbidity rates (described in detail in Chapters 2 and 3)—are typically used to measure health status.

Process Measures

On the finance side, process measures are used to determine how a program is carried out—which of the targeted population is actually reached, who is eligible but gets excluded, etc. On the delivery side, process measures include many different measures of utilization by service provider type. Expenditure measures are sometimes used as substitutes for utilization, because they tend to be more widely available and because they aggregate all kinds of use into a common metric (money) useful for comparison purposes. Another set of process measures looks at travel times or distance. Even where medical care is free, travel costs can be a prohibitive financial barrier.

Table 5.2

Measures of Equity by Type of Equity

Equity Type	Type of Measure		
	Outcome	Process	Structural
FINANCE			
Allocation and distribution of subsidies	• Benefit-incidence ratios • Payment to share of income ratios • Concentration indices	• Tax evasion rates in informal sector	• Percentage of government expenditures for public health and primary care vs. hospital and other curative care • Progressive tax/contribution rates
Program coverage by population and service mix	• Coverage rates for primary health care services • Participation rates	• Cost of covered services	• Eligibility criteria or means testing • Sources of financing personal health care expenses
Risk pooling	• Proportion of income going to health care	• Medical loss ratios	• Size of risk pool • Rates of impoverishment due to high health care expenses
DELIVERY			
Health status	• Mortality rates • Morbidity rates • Avoidable or preventable deaths • Life expectancy • Burden of disease	• Admissions for preventable conditions (negative measures) • Successful treatment versus total treatment • Costs versus benefits	
Utilization		• Contact and visit rates, immunization rates, prenatal visits, referral rates • Forgone health care • Expenditures by type of service per capita	• Cultural relevance (e.g., language, health beliefs)
Physical access		• Distance, travel time, or travel costs to nearest medical provider	• Provider skills/training • Number of doctors/nurses/midwives; number of hospital beds, drug and equipment stocks

Structural Measures

On the financial side, structural measures are used, for example, to measure the percentage of government expenditures spent on hospitals versus primary and preventive care versus drugs, or they are used to measure eligibility criteria and means testing for program coverage and targeting accuracy. They are also used to measure whether a progressive tax or contribution rate explicitly reduces the financial burdens on the poor as a target population.

On the delivery side, structural measures are used to measure physical access in terms of the availability of facilities (physical proximity and number of hours the facility is open) and the number of personnel (doctors, nurses, and health workers). Cultural relevance, although hard to quantify, includes such elements as language compatibility and understanding of local traditions and health beliefs.

Usefulness of Measures for Policymakers

How useful are these measures for policymakers in determining whether health care interventions are effective in improving equity? Ultimately, policymakers want to be able to know how much impact interventions have, so the most useful measures are those that enable them to do this. On the finance side of equity, outcome measures, such as benefit-incidence ratios and measures of progressivity in financing, meet these criteria and are very useful policy tools. However, the answer is exactly the opposite on the delivery side of equity.

Although health outcomes—such as mortality and morbidity rates and life expectancy—are ultimately what policymakers want to improve, the problem with using health outcome measures to assess equity is that many factors affect health status besides the use of health services (e.g., nutrition, access to potable water, and tendency of the poor to minimize sickness because of different expectations about what is normal). Given this more diverse set of outcome determinants, the conditions for improving outcomes fall under multiple ministries in most countries and are outside the direct control of the MOH, whereas the conditions for ensuring utilization and access are more directly under the control of the MOH. It is therefore misleading to attribute all the variation in health outcomes to inequities in the health care system, or conversely to attribute all the gains in health outcomes to interventions designed to improve them.

In addition, even if we could directly link health interventions to their impacts on health outcomes, the impacts are not immediate. Changes in health outcomes take place over a long period of time, while interventions to affect them take place on an ongoing basis. This means that interventions must be continually evaluated to determine their effectiveness. Another disadvantage of outcome measures, particularly mortality measures, is that death is a relatively rare occurrence compared to illness.

Finally, the concept of "mutability" is important in deciding on the usefulness of equity and access measures. (See Andersen and Newman, 1973.) This means that a measure must point to policy changes that might bring about behavioral change. Enabling factors—such as how the health care system is structured or organized to promote access and utilization—are the most mutable. For example, the RAND Health Insurance Experiment demonstrated the effect of changing health insurance benefit structures on health services use. (See Manning et al., 1988.) Health beliefs have some degree of mutability, since they can sometimes be influenced to effect behavioral change or alter care-seeking patterns.

For all these reasons, the use of process and structural access measures is frequently advocated on the delivery side as the simplest and most direct approach to measuring equity. (See Birdsall and Hecht, 1995.) Unfortunately, most of the available measures are outcome measures. Although process measures (which reflect the actual treatments rendered) are more closely linked to outcomes, they require provider surveys or observational studies (or clinical data), which are not yet widely available in developing countries.

THE PERSISTENCE OF INEQUITY

Having good measures is clearly critical to determining inequities in countries and to determining the effectiveness of interventions to remedy them. When evaluating equity, it is particularly important to have good-quality, disaggregated data. To measure the effects of poverty on health, data are needed on outcomes by income class that can be used to guide policy efforts in developing countries. Unfortunately, as we discussed in Chapter 2, there is a paucity of data in this area. The major international research effort to quantify the global burden of disease through a common metric—disability-adjusted life years or DALYs—cannot yet report illness burdens by income class for a substantial number of countries. DALYs, however, are available to measure the impact of gender and age inequities.

Data that *can* support analyses linking illness burden or health-care use to income, gender, or age generally come from surveillance systems and household surveys. Unfortunately, as again shown in Chapter 2, nationally representative surveys are available in only a modicum of Asian countries. More countries collect facility-level or other administrative data. However, such data capture information only on those who use the services—they do not account for nonusers. And even for users, facility-level data only show socioeconomic status.

Beyond concerns about data availability, much of the data we do have are not as useful as they could be, because they tend to be collected on an ad hoc, rather than routine, basis. Lack of consistent data over time means that trend data are even scarcer, making it difficult to examine whether differentials in health care use and outcomes by income class are increasing or becoming smaller over time. The end result is that most of the currently available datasets are cross-sectional. Fortunately, this situation is likely to improve, since the number of countries sponsoring large-scale household surveys has grown over the last five to ten years. As these datasets become routine, they will be able to support longitudinal analyses.

Although such disaggregated sociodemographic data are sparse and, when available, generally cross-sectional, disparities in illness burden and access to health care of vulnerable groups are significant enough in Asia that they can be seen fairly easily. In the next section, we use the available datasets to briefly describe the scale and distribution of poverty in Asia. We then assess measures of health status, utilization, and access. Although we make some cross-country comparisons (addressed in significant detail in Chapter 2), our focus here is on within-country disparities across groups in Asian countries. We first look at regional disparities in health outcomes as one way to assess how well central governments have done in balancing the allocation of resources across various regions. We then look directly at the experiences of specific subgroups of the population—the poor, women, children, and rural residents—that have been the prime focus of most government interventions to improve health. Information on the scope and magnitude of existing inequities is presented to better inform the development of policies to remedy these inequities.

Poverty in Asia

The economic dynamism that has characterized much of Asia over the past two decades has helped to lift a significant portion of its population out of poverty. In only the 15 years from 1970 to 1985, poverty declined by roughly 20 percent across Asia (excluding China, for which data were not available). The decline occurred in both urban and rural areas, falling from 42 percent in 1970 to 34 percent in 1985 in urban areas; and from 61 percent to 47 percent in rural areas. (See Mills and Pernia, 1994.)

However, even with this decline, large segments of the population in Asia—330 million or one-third of the urban population and nearly 800 million or almost one-half of the rural population—still do not have the resources to maintain a minimally adequate standard of living. (See Mills and Pernia, 1994; Quibria, 1994.)

Selected country-specific data are presented in Table 5.3, which shows poverty incidence (head count index and numbers of poor persons) in urban and rural areas for two time periods, in the early 1970s and late 1980s. The head count index, one of the more commonly used poverty measures, is simply the percentage of the total population living below the country-specific poverty level. Because of differences in poverty definition and data quality, the data in Table 5.3 are not necessarily comparable across countries, but they do reveal the regional differences and temporal trends within each country.

Table 5.3 shows that poverty incidence is typically less in urban than in rural areas and that the decline in poverty has been quite significant in those countries undergoing high rates of economic growth, such as the Republic of Korea, Malaysia, and Thailand. But even in these high-growth-rate countries, substantial portions of the population remain poor. In countries with only modest economic performance (e.g., the Philippines and South Asian countries), poverty reduction has been slower.

The data in Figure 5.1 corroborate this apparent relationship. The figure shows that an individual country's rate of decline in poverty is strongly correlated with its GDP growth over time.

Within-country assessments have shown that not all groups benefit equally from economic growth. Often, benefits accrue only slowly to certain groups of the poor and to disadvantaged areas of a country. (See World Bank, 1990a.) For countries with annual per capita GDP between $150 and $1,000 (22 of 44 Asian countries discussed in Chapter 2), income differentials may even grow worse as GDP increases. (See Mills and Pernia, 1994.) In such countries, the incomes of the poorest segment of the population tend to increase more slowly than the national average. These findings have implications for designing policies to better meet the health care needs of the poor. They suggest that it is not enough to rely on economic growth to improve the living standards of the poor. Specific sectoral policies are also needed to improve access to health services for the poor.

In summary, despite the dynamic economic growth for which Asia is well known, there remain large numbers of poor people throughout Asia, with nearly 1.1 billion living below the poverty level. The large numbers of poor can easily

Table 5.3

Poverty Head-Count Ratios in Selected Asian Developing Countries

Country/Year	Total Population in Poverty		Urban Population in Poverty		Rural Population in Poverty	
	% of Population	Millions	% of Population	Millions	% of Population	Millions
Bangladesh						
1973–1974	72.7	55.7	63.2	4.4	73.7	51.3
1988–1989	47.1	48.4	33.4	6.3	43.6	42.1
India						
1972–1973	51.5	291.5	41.2	47.3	54.1	244.2
1987–1988	29.9	237.7	20.1	41.7	33.4	196.0
Indonesia						
1976	40.1	54.2	38.8	10.0	40.4	44.2
1990	15.2	27.2	16.8	9.4	14.4	17.8
Korea, Rep. of						
1970	23.4	7.5	16.2	2.1	28.3	5.4
1984	4.5	1.8	4.6	1.2	4.3	0.6
Philippines						
1971	52.2	19.7	40.6	4.9	57.7	14.8
1991	44.6	28.0	36.7	10.0	50.7	18.0
Sri Lanka						
1978–1979	22.3	3.3	19.4	.6	23.1	2.7
1986–1987	27.4	4.4	12.3	.4	31.4	4.0
Thailand						
1975–1976	31.7	13.3	17.6	1.6	35.6	11.7
1990	18.0	10.1	10.1	1.7	21.4	8.4

SOURCES: ADB Regional Technical Assistance Projects on Rural and Urban Poverty, 1992, 1994c; World Bank, 1990a; Mills and Pernia, 1994.

overwhelm the resources of developing countries. Thus, designing policy to ensure access to basic health services for the poor remains a huge challenge. The next section examines the experience of Asian countries in meeting this challenge and identifies some of the sources of continuing inequities.

The Degree of Intercountry Inequality in Asia's Health Sector

Despite Asia's impressive economic achievements and its overall progress in improving health over the past two decades, gains have not been achieved uniformly throughout the countries in the region and within the countries themselves.

Country Variation in Health Outcomes. The tremendous variation in health outcomes across countries (as discussed in Chapters 2 and 3)[1] is summarized in Table 5.4.

Table 5.4 compares three health outcomes—life expectancy, under-five child mortality rates, and adult (male versus female) mortality rates—in selected

---

[1]Despite the aforementioned problems with using health outcome measures as evidence of inequity and poor access, our description of country differences draws on these measures because they are more readily available and because ultimately they represent the outcomes of ultimate interest.

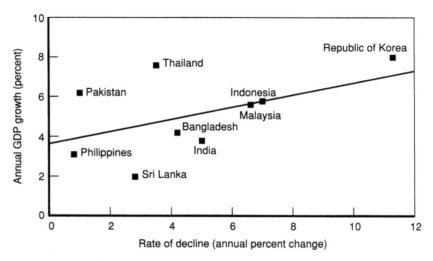

SOURCE: Mills and Pernia, 1994.

NOTES: Bangladesh, India, Malaysia, and Philippines, circa 1970–1990; Republic of Korea, 1970–mid-1980; Indonesia and Thailand, mid-1970–1990; Pakistan and Sri Lanka, 1980–mid-1980.

Figure 5.1—Poverty Incidence Decline and GDP Growth

countries in Asia with those in two developed countries, the United States and Japan. Overall, seven million children under the age of five die in Asia, mostly from preventable diseases. They represent approximately half of all under-five deaths in the world, with India alone accounting for 25 percent of them and the other developing countries accounting for another 15 percent. Even China, which is one of the best performers among the developing countries in Asia, has under-five mortality rates that are four times higher than the United States and seven times higher than Japan (the world leader). With the exception of Sri Lanka, the remainder of the Asian countries have adult mortality rates that are two to three times those of Japan.

Looking across developing Asian countries, we observe that current life expectancies vary from a low of 52 years in Lao to a high of 72 in Sri Lanka, and that mortality rates are very uneven. For example, India's under-five child mortality rate is currently more than twice as high as China's, but not as high as those of Bangladesh, Pakistan, and Lao. The adult mortality rates, while less uneven, still show significant variation.

When we look at one outcome measure, change in life expectancy (Figure 5.2), we see that enormous variation exists over time. Myanmar, China, the Republic of Korea, Malaysia, Sri Lanka, and Thailand achieved big gains in life expectancy over a 30-year period. Bangladesh, India, Lao PDR, the Philippines, and Kampuchea continue to struggle, having posted much smaller 30-year gains, so that health indicators now lag behind those of other developing countries with similar GDP levels in and outside of Asia.

Table 5.4

Mortality in Selected Countries of Asia—A Comparative Perspective

Country	Life Expectancy at Birth (1995)	Mortality Rates (Deaths/1,000)		
		Under 5 (1995)	Adult Males (1990)	Adult Females (1990)
Bangladesh	57	148	295	244
China	69	44	201	150
India	62	102	272	229
Indonesia	64	65	278	212
Pakistan	63	107	296	263
Thailand	69	43	242	163
Sri Lanka	72	20	158	92
Lao PDR	52	148	345	280
Papua New Guinea	57	84	374	327
Philippines	67	48	234	172
Japan	80	6	120	63
U.S.	76	10	157	75

SOURCES: World Bank, 1993a.; UNICEF, 1996.

Health status differentials associated with income or other measures of socioeconomic status persist in many countries in Asia and other regions of the world. A review of 14 developing countries (3 in Asia) revealed that in many of the countries infant mortality in the lowest income groups is more than twice as high as that in the highest income groups. (See also Gwatkin, 1993.)

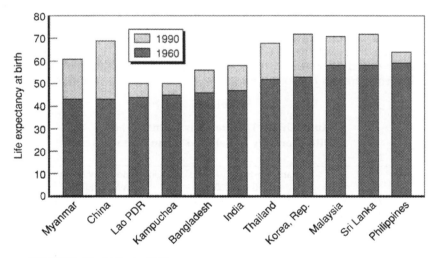

SOURCE: World Bank, 1993a.

NOTE: 1960 equals height of the dark bar; 1990 equals entire height of the bar. The gain in life expectancy (light gray portion) is the difference between the two.

Figure 5.2—Gains in Life Expectancy for Selected Asian Countries, 1960 and 1990

Table 5.5

Sex Differentials in Infant and Child Mortality in Selected Asian Countries

	Infant Mortality (0–1 yrs) (Deaths/1,000)		Child Mortality (1–4 yrs) (Deaths/1,000)	
Country	Male	Female	Male	Female
Bangladesh	107.3	93.4	46.7	62.3
India	88.6	83.9	29.4	42.0
Pakistan	102.1	85.5	22.0	36.5
Sri Lanka	39.5	24.7	10.0	10.1
Indonesia	73.5	58.8	29.9	26.5
Philippines	43.5	32.9	27.6	24.7
Thailand	45.0	31.0	11.0	11.0

SOURCES: DHS reports: Bangladesh, 1993–1994; India, 1992–1993; Pakistan, 1990–1991; Sri Lanka, 1987; Indonesia, 1994; Philippines, 1993; Thailand, 1987.

Infant and child mortality rates also vary by sex and geographic differentials. Data from the Demographic and Health Surveys (DHS) system (Table 5.5) show that despite lower *infant* mortality rates for females relative to males, females have significantly higher *child* mortality rates (ages 1–4) in Bangladesh, India, and Pakistan. (For DHS reports, see http://www2.macroint.com/DHS/.)

By location, as shown in Table 5.6, urban mortality rates are significantly lower than rural mortality rates for most developing countries in Asia, most likely reflecting the higher concentration of health services in urban areas.

Although the geographical differentials in mortality rates are likely to be driven as much by nutrition, sanitation, and behavioral factors as by differences in access to, and use of, health care services, there are known, effective health interventions—such as health services for mothers before and during birth, immunizations, oral rehydration therapy, birth spacing, and nutritional supplements—that can improve health outcomes and infant mortality in particular.

Table 5.6

Rural/Urban Differentials in Infant and Child Mortality in Selected Asian Countries

	Infant Mortality (0–1 yrs) (Deaths/1,000)		Child Mortality (1–4 yrs) (Deaths/1,000)	
Country	Rural	Urban	Rural	Urban
Bangladesh	102.6	80.9	56.4	36.3
India	94.3	59.4	40.4	20.1
Pakistan	102.2	74.6	33.0	20.6
Sri Lanka	29.9	34.7	10.3	5.6
Indonesia	75.2	43.1	33.0	16.2
Philippines	44.3	31.9	30.5	21.5
Thailand	41.0	27.0	12.0	8.0

SOURCE: DHS reports: Bangladesh, 1993–1994; India, 1992–1993; Pakistan, 1990–1991; Sri Lanka, 1987; Indonesia, 1994; Philippines, 1993; Thailand, 1987.

Persistent, Serious Inequities Within Countries by Outcome, Income, Education, Location, and Gender

There are even more dramatic differences when we look at inequities within Asian countries. Of the many dimensions that capture the breadth and depth of the problem, health outcomes and variations of these outcomes by income, education, urban versus rural, location, and gender provide the most complete picture. They also establish a basis for interventions, which is discussed in the next two sections.

Intracountry Variation in Health Outcomes. Figures 5.3 and 5.4 and Table 5.7 illustrate the wide variation in infant mortality rates across different states in India, provinces in Papua New Guinea, and provinces in Indonesia, respectively. Figure 5.3 and Table 5.7 also have data on average per-capita income and show a general relationship between infant mortality rates and per-capita income at the province (or state) level, with the exception of Kerala in India. Although the health indicator shown in the figures and table is just the IMR, the male and female 45Q15 adult mortality and the 5Q0 child mortality rates show similar patterns of variation across Indian states.[2]

The data in Figure 5.4 show the marked differences in infant mortality by province in Papua New Guinea. Although almost all provinces experienced significant

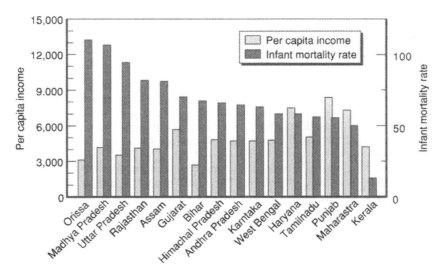

SOURCES: Cashier et al., 1995; Registrar General of India, 1993.

NOTE: Infant mortality rates per 1,000 births in 1993; per capita income in 1990 Rupees. This is a partial sample of states.

Figure 5.3—Per Capita Income and Infant Mortality Rate, Selected States in India, 1985

[2]This nomenclature denotes the probability of death over a given interval beginning at a given age. Thus 45Q15 is the probability of death between the ages of 15 and 60 and 5Q0 the probability of death before the age of 5.

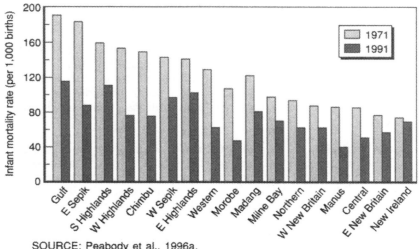

SOURCE: Peabody et al., 1996a.

NOTE: Two provinces—Enga and National Capital District—are excluded because of a lack of data in 1971.

Figure 5.4—Infant Mortality Rates, Selected Provinces in Papua New Guinea, 1971 and 1991

improvements in infant mortality over the 20-year time span, the magnitude of the gains varied substantially by province. For example, the gain in New Ireland is negligible, while the gain in East Sepik is significant.

Table 5.7 presents similar intracountry variation by province for Indonesia. Along with the IMR, it presents a number of other factors expected to influence this outcome measure, such as (1) health care use and expenditures; (2) percentage of births attended by a doctor or midwife, and percentage of health centers without a physician; (3) poverty incidence; and (4) degree of urbanization.

Figures 5.3 and 5.4 and Table 5.7 illustrate the substantial intracountry variation in one key health indicator, the IMR. The data point to disparities by region and provide some evidence that poorer provinces tend to have higher mortality rates. However, they cannot reveal the role played by poverty as distinct from the role played by greater urbanization, a better infrastructure, better sanitation, and greater availability of health services in wealthier provinces. (See Over et al., 1992.) The next section takes a closer look at health service outcomes, utilization, and access for the poor and other populations.

Impact of Public Versus Private Spending on Outcome. A few studies have tried to assess the effect of public-sector expenditures on health outcomes. They looked at the impact of publicly supported services (e.g., preventive versus curative care) on IMR after controlling for regional income level. Two longitudinal studies (without controls) covering 14 states in Malaysia over a three-year period (1986–1989) and 13 regions in the Philippines over a seven-year period (1983–1990) led to different conclusions. In Malaysia, two public health interventions (immunization and provision of safe water) led to declines in infant mortality, whereas provision

Table 5.7

Infant Mortality Rate and Indicators of Provincial Socioeconomic Status
and Health Infrastructure, Selected Indonesian Provinces

Indicators	East Java	NTB	West Kalim.	East Kalim.	West Sumatra	Nat. Average
Infant mortality rate per 1,000 births (1990)	64	149	81	58	74	71
Percentage poor (1990)	22	28	34	14	13	20
Monthly household expenditures (Rp.)	26,805	23,164	29,409	40,792	31,628	30,338
Per capita health expenditures (Rp.)	5,847	6,153	9,756	13,981	7,991	5,842
Population density	678	167	22	9	81	93
Percentage urban (1990)	28	18	23	20	49	31
Health centers with no MD (%)	4	8	5	8	7	11
Births without antenatal care (%)	12	25	20	11	3	13
Births attended by provider (%)	34	13	29	52	70	36

SOURCE: World Bank, 1995e.
NOTE: Kalim. = Kalimantan; NTB = Nusa Tenggara Barat, Rp. = rupiah

of curative services (as measured by the number of government medical personnel per capita) had no significant effect on health status. The effect in the Philippines was not as strong and the results were sensitive to different specifications of the statistical model: The data show a significant interaction between regional income and the effects of public expenditures, indicating that government provision of health services improves health status in poor areas, but providing such services in wealthier areas has no such effect on health status. Hammer (1997b) reasons that the greater substitutability of private for public services in wealthier areas explains this difference. This is plausible because greater public spending in poorer areas can increase access. And although it should be possible to empirically test the public/private substitution effect, these two studies did not include measures of the private sector supply response.

Presently, direct information on private providers is rarely included in assessments of public-sector program performance, largely because of difficulties in getting data on private providers. However, studies that have included such data show that there are substantial interdependent effects. This implies that omitting private-sector supply responses could bias evaluations of public-sector programs or policies. A possible approach for overcoming deficiencies in private-sector data is using sensitivity analyses to estimate net effects under varying assumptions about the private-sector supply response. (See Alderman and Gertler, 1989; Hammer, 1997b.)

Illness Burden for the Poor. Existing national-level datasets demonstrate the seemingly obvious: Poor health is concentrated among the poor. Researchers who have examined these data note, however, that the degree of inequality varies substantially across national settings. (See Gertler and Rahman, 1994.) For example, one counterintuitive finding is that the poor are not necessarily worse off if they live in the poorest countries. In some of the least affluent countries, the differentials in health outcomes between the poor and nonpoor are actually smaller than in countries with higher incomes. In these "poorer countries with better health," it appears that public policies aimed at improving the health status of the poor have made a difference, enabling the health outcomes of the poor to more closely approach the outcomes achieved by the wealthy. (See Griffin, 1992a.)

Box 5.2: Dual Relationship Between Income and Health

In its report on the state of health research, the World Health Organization (WHO) comments on the bidirectional relationship between poverty and health. The report asserts that three-quarters of the improvement in life expectancy over the past few decades is due to the effects of rising incomes. At the same time, it argues that the evidence also suggests that good health is a precondition for improving the economic well-being of the poor themselves and, thus, that the overall health of a country's population promotes the country's economic development. (See WHO Ad Hoc Committee, 1996.)

In terms of the first argument, the poor benefit most from investments in health because their health status tends to be worse to begin with. This is the result of suffering the long-term effects of lower nutrition, for example, and of being more exposed to unsafe water and other hazards of poor infrastructure. The poor also benefit more from investments in health because they often rely on physical health (strength and vigor) to earn a living (farming, manual labor, etc.). Serious illness in poor families leads to impoverishment partly because of the depletion of family resources to pay for medical care, but more often because of lost work days and sometimes even a permanent reduction in work capacity. For example, the WHO report notes that "the elimination of deformity in employed lepers in Tamil Nadu, India, would increase their annual earnings more than threefold." (See WHO Ad Hoc Committee, 1996.)

In terms of the second argument—that good health promotes economic development—better health might contribute in three ways. First, it leads to healthier, more productive workers who are able to participate in the labor force longer. Using the example of Tamil Nadu again, we see that treating the complications associated with leprosy—surgical and rehabilitative therapy that can correct deformities of the arms and legs or often improve sensation in the extremities—was estimated to add $130 million to India's 1985 gross national product by returning workers to payrolls and increasing family incomes. (See Htoon et al., 1993.)

Second, better health leads to increased future productivity through schooling and the acquisition of technical skills by the young. Future productivity and economic growth will depend on human capital development, which, in turn, depends on having healthy children. For example, if children are malnourished, they are at risk of dying prematurely—or, if they do not die, they are more likely to be retarded, orphaned, or handicapped. (See Summers, 1992.) A 1995 study shows that stunting associated with lack of early health interventions predicts lower future earnings. (See Strauss and Thomas, 1995.) In addition, family planning and prenatal care can reduce the costs that come from pressures on the existing infrastructure or government services generated by an expanding population.

Finally, decreasing the burden of disease—particularly preventable and infectious diseases—leads to better health, which, in turn, reduces medical expenditures and thus frees government resources to be used elsewhere. (See Gillis et al., 1983.) For example, the prevention of one case of tuberculosis—successful treatment of one smear-positive case costs less than $4 per year of life saved and is even lower when done as an outpatient—not only directly benefits the patient but indirectly benefits others, especially those in the same household, by stopping transmission. (See Murray et al., 1993.) As a result, the treatment further reduces health expenditures for expensive chemotherapy, hospitals, and other medical resources.

This finding notwithstanding, the experience across Asia shows that in most countries the poor continue to suffer higher infant and child mortality, higher adult mortality, greater incidence of disease, and lower life expectancy. Unfortunately, within-country data differentials by income are available for just a few countries. Differentials by education level are more widely available and can serve as a rough proxy for income. Before we present cross-national comparisons using the more widely available education data, we first examine some of the evidence available on income differentials.

Household survey data from rural areas of China are illustrative. A 1993 survey collected data on three standard indicators of health status—incidence of infectious disease, life expectancy, and infant mortality. The poorest respondents (lowest household expenditure quartile) had worse health on all three indicators (Figure 5.5). Compared to the wealthiest quartile, the poor had an infectious disease incidence that was three times higher, life expectancy that was 10 percent lower, and an infant mortality rate that was twice as high. Although health status improves with each jump in income from the lowest to the highest quartile, the biggest gain occurs in making the transition from the lowest quartile to the next. Given the significantly worse standing of the poorest people, health interventions targeted to this group would seemingly reap big gains.

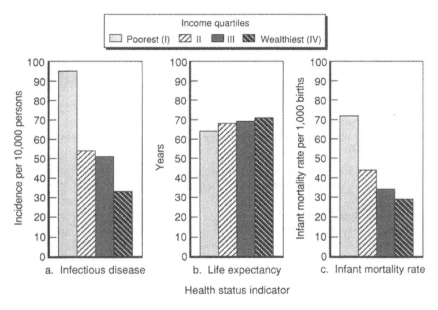

SOURCE: World Bank, 1997c.

Figure 5.5—Health Status by Income Quartile, Rural China, 1992

Other data from China provide more information on the disease burden by income group. Data on cause of death can be obtained through disease surveillance systems. Unlike household data, disease surveillance systems often cannot directly link health care indicators to income on an individual basis. Instead, disease burden (in this case, cause of death) and income are measured over an areawide basis. The income variable, therefore, represents the average income for all households in the area.

In China, a system of 47 disease surveillance points collected data on adult female mortality (45Q15) and the cause of death, grouped into the three major categories: communicable diseases, noncommunicable diseases, and injuries. Communities were ranked by average per-capita income (actually, the industrial and agricultural output per capita). The poorest women (residents of the poorest quartile of communities) had the highest mortality rates for all causes of death (Figure 5.6). The mortality rate ratio of the poorest income group to the wealthiest was 3.5 for communicable diseases, 1.3 for noncommunicable diseases, and 2.3 for injuries. (See Murray et al., 1992.) These ratios suggest that communicable diseases disproportionately affect the poor.

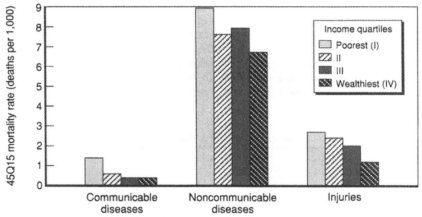

SOURCE: Murray et al., 1992b.

NOTE: The 45Q15 mortality rate is the probability of dying between the ages of 15 and 60.

Figure 5.6—Female Adult Mortality Rates by Cause of Death and Average Community Income, China, 1987–1988

A recent World Bank country assessment reports that much of China's infectious disease burden—tuberculosis, diarrheal disease, nutritional diseases including iodine deficiency disorders—is concentrated in poor and remote areas. (See World Bank, 1997c.) It notes that half the children living in households below the poverty line are stunted because of malnutrition. Other studies, such as one on agricultural workers in the Philippines document the debilitating effects of stunting on physical capacity and report that adults whose growth was stunted because of poor childhood nutrition are less productive and earn lower wages than adults of average height. (See WHO Ad Hoc Committee, 1996.)

There is still more evidence that the poor suffer a greater burden than the wealthy. As we mentioned above, DHS data do not include income or wealth information; however, we have used the data they do include to create a wealth indicator. To do this, we used a group of factors generally indicative of wealth: whether a household has running tap water, whether it has a flush toilet, whether it has electricity, and whether it has adequate flooring (i.e., wood or cement versus sawdust or dirt). Each factor of wealth was assigned an equal weight (a value of one). The factors were summed, resulting in an indicator of wealth measured from zero to four.

Figure 5.7 shows graphs for three DHS countries using this wealth indicator— Bangladesh (1993 data), Philippines (1993 data), and Kazakhstan (1995 data)— across seven health care measures: (1) percentage who never used contraception;

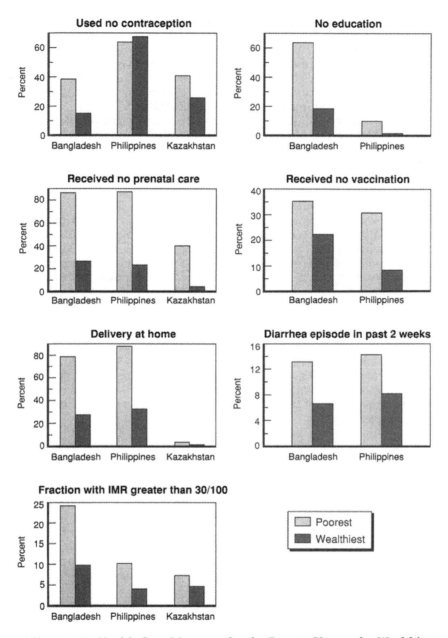

Figure 5.7—Health Care Measures for the Poorest Versus the Wealthiest, Bangladesh, Philippines, and Kazakhstan

(2) percentage of women who did not receive prenatal care from a doctor; (3) percentage of women with deliveries in home; (4) percentage with an IMR greater than 30 per 100; (5) percentage with no education; (6) percentage who did not receive vaccinations; and (7) percentage of individuals who had diarrhea episodes within the past two weeks. The graphs compare the poorest individuals

with the wealthiest (i.e., those with zero factors of wealth versus those with four factors of wealth).

The graphs in the figure show that the poor are indeed worse off than the wealthy across all seven measures. The disparate IMRs between the poor and the wealthy are indicative of the overall trend. Bangladesh is typical. Among the poor, almost a quarter of the people suffer from an IMR of 30/100 or higher. In other words, for 25 percent of poor families, it is probable that one third of their children will die within the first year of life. It is also striking that in every category examined except contraception, Kazakhstan had better results than the other two countries. Although some may claim this difference could result from data error or overreporting, the DHS data are among the highest quality available.

Illness Burden by Education Level and Residence. Because of difficulties in measuring household income or household per-capita expenditures in countries where the informal labor sector is still large, many surveys in Asia have not attempted to collect such data. To partially circumvent this problem, education level is frequently used as a proxy for income. Health measures are often reported by an education level of the household head. The exception to this are measures related to pregnancy, birth, and infant and child mortality, which are reported by the mother's education level.

Geography of residence is another disaggregation of measures of health status and health service use. It is generally divided into two (urban and rural) or three (metropolitan urban, other urban, and rural) categories. Although Asia is home to many of the world's megacities, it should be underscored that much of its population still resides in areas classified as rural. As noted earlier, poverty incidence remains much higher in rural areas (47 percent rural versus 34 percent urban on average).

Table 5.8 reports child mortality by residence and level of mother's education for a number of countries for which DHS survey data were available. The years in the first column denote the time period during which the DHS was fielded. The data reveal two patterns. First, the within-country data show the expected pattern. Mortality rates continue to be higher in rural areas and for children of less-educated mothers. This is consistent with data drawn from earlier time periods and from other countries around the world, and this pattern is observed in both high-mortality and low-mortality countries. It appears, therefore, that whether mothers get some education has a large effect on child mortality, even in countries that have managed to reduce mortality rates overall.

The second distinctive pattern is that the variation in infant and child mortality between urban and rural areas is greater in high-mortality countries than in low-mortality countries. Figure 5.8 depicts the urban-rural differentials in infant mortality by country for the seven countries shown in Table 5.8. The figure shows both the overall level of mortality in each country and the size of the urban-rural differential. Differences between urban and rural areas are pervasive in all the countries listed, except Sri Lanka.

With the DHS data, we can examine whether there are differences in the use of MCH services that might help explain the patterns in infant and child health outcomes. Table 5.9 shows the use of four measures of MCH process of care used

Table 5.8

Under-Five Child Mortality Rates by Residence and
Level of Education, Selected Asian Countries
(Deaths/1,000)

| Country/Year | Average | Place of Residence | | | Level of Mother's Education | | |
		Urban	Rural	None	Some Primary	Primary Completed	Secondary or More
Bangladesh 1993–1994	150	114	153	170	134	105	90
Pakistan 1990–1991*	120	94	132	128	107	87	50
Papua New Guinea 1991	123	63	137				
Indonesia 1991	107	84	116	131	125	102	47
Philippines 1993**	64	53	73	152	80	46	36
Thailand 1985	49	35	52	74	49	—	21
Sri Lanka 1985***	42	39/41	40/73	71	43	—	41/26

SOURCE: DHS reports: Bangladesh, 1993–1994; Pakistan, 1990–1991; Indonesia, 1994; Philippines, 1993; Thailand, 1987; Sri Lanka, 1987; Peabody et al., 1996a. (Note: Reports postdate the years of data collection.)
NOTES: Child mortality is measured over the preceding five-year period and is calculated as deaths in infants and children from birth to five years of age per 1,000 births.
*The category "primary completed" includes those who attended middle school.
**Categories in the Philippines are slightly different: Primary refers to elementary school and includes those who attended some elementary school as well as those who completed elementary school. Primary completed includes those who attended some high school. Secondary or more includes those who attended some college.
*** For Sri Lanka, urban residence is divided into metropolitan and other urban, respectively; rural residence is divided into rural and estates, respectively.

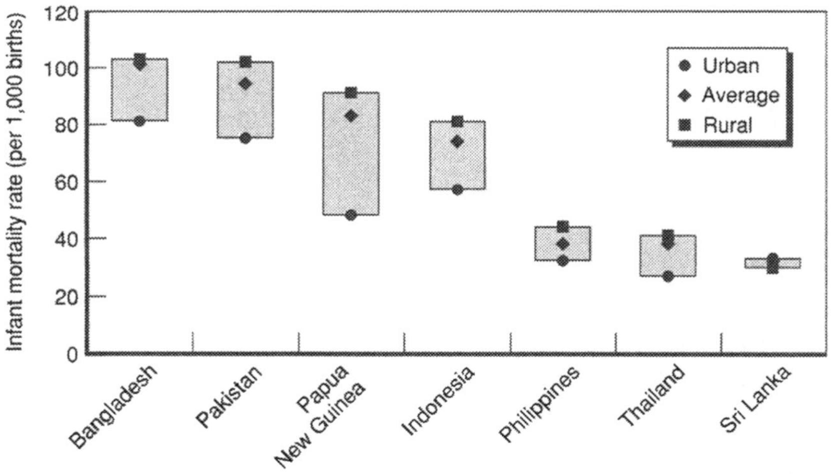

SOURCE: DHS reports: Bangladesh, 1993–1994; Indonesia, 1994; Pakistan, 1990–1991; Philippines, 1993; Sri Lanka, 1987; Thailand, 1987.

Figure 5.8—Urban-Rural Differentials in Infant Mortality Rates,
Selected Asian Countries

by mothers: (1) prenatal care; (2) deliveries in the hospital (as opposed to births at home); (3) deliveries attended by trained health personnel; and (4) full vaccination of children between 12 and 23 months of age.

Table 5.9

Use of MCH Services by Residence and Level of Education,
Selected Asian Countries (%)

Process Measures		Residence		Level of Mother's Education			
Country/Year	Average	Urban	Rural	No Education	Some Primary	Primary Completed	Secondary or More
Percentage of Births with Some Prenatal Care							
Bangladesh 1993–1994	27	56	24	18	30	27	60
Pakistan 1990–1991	30	60	17	22	41	59	85
Indonesia 1991	80	94	74	56	75	85	97
Philippines 1993	92	94	90	75	89	94	98
Thailand 1985				48	78	—	94
Sri Lanka 1985				87	96	—	98–99
Percentage of Deliveries in a Health Facility							
Bangladesh 1993–1994	4	20	2	1	2	3	16
Pakistan 1990–1991	13	33	5	7	17	43	59
Indonesia 1991	21	50	9	7	10	18	53
Philippines 1993	28	32	44	4	12	29	62
Thailand 1985							
Sri Lanka 1985							
Percentage of Deliveries Attended by a Doctor or Nurse/Midwife*							
Bangladesh 1993–1994	10	35	7	5	6	8	33
Pakistan 1990–1991	19	42	8	11	26	52	69
Indonesia 1991	32	65	18	12	20	28	70
Philippines 1993	53	53	73	9	35	60	84
Thailand 1985				44	64	94	99
Sri Lanka 1985				80	92	96	99
Vaccination Coverage of Children 12–23 Months**							
Bangladesh 1993–1994	59	70	58	52	59	67	79
Pakistan 1990–1991	35	46	30	31	39	57	52
Indonesia 1991	48	65	41	26	42	51	67
Philippines 1993	72	73	70	43	68	72	82
Thailand 1985				—	82	83	94
Sri Lanka 1985				90	87	—	95–99

SOURCE: DHS Reports: Bangladesh, 1993–1994; Pakistan, 1990–1991; Indonesia, 1994; Philippines, 1993; Thailand, 1987; Sri Lanka, 1987. (Note: Reports post date years' data were collected.)
*In Pakistan, the nurse/midwife category includes family welfare workers.
**Children who are fully vaccinated (i.e., those who have received Calmette-Guérin bacillus (BCG), measles, and three doses of DTP and polio).— = missing data.

On all four process indicators of health care use, utilization rates are substantially lower in the highest-mortality countries. Slightly less than three-fourths of the births in Bangladesh and just over two-thirds of the births in Pakistan involved no prenatal care. This problem was particularly acute in rural areas. For example, in Pakistan only one in six rural births was preceded by any prenatal care. The difference in use of prenatal care between Bangladesh and Pakistan and the other countries is quite dramatic: In the other countries four out of five women had at least some prenatal care.

The other three process measures show smaller but still quite sizable differences in use of MCH services between urban and rural areas. Even within the set of countries with lower mortality rates, these rates are associated with higher rates of MCH service use. If MCH inputs are effective in improving birth outcomes and child health, it seems possible to lower mortality rates in Bangladesh and Pakistan by providing basic MCH services targeted to rural and low-income families. Although most deliveries still occur at home or outside of formal health settings, some of these deliveries are assisted by trained health personnel (the trained attendant rates are higher than the facility delivery rates).

Mother's education levels are very strongly associated with differences in the use of the four MCH services in all the countries listed except Sri Lanka. The experience of Sri Lanka is different for two reasons: its uniformly high utilization rates across all four types of MCH services and the relative uniformity in use across all education groups. For example, although Sri Lankan women with no education were somewhat less likely to obtain prenatal care than more educated women, the vast majority (87 percent) of women with no education used such care (compared to 96–99 percent of more educated women).

Care-seeking behavior in response to illness symptoms in children showed similar patterns across the six countries. The DHS surveys collect point-prevalence data and treatment decisions for common symptoms in children—fever, cough, and rapid breathing (indicative of acute respiratory infection), and diarrhea. In general, the decision to treat (taking the child to a health facility or giving a particular remedy) showed the expected positive correlation with the mother's education (e.g., utilization rates increase as education increases) and relatively small differentials—urban populations decide to seek treatment at only slightly greater rates than rural populations.

In making urban/rural comparisons, it is important to understand that urban populations need to be differentiated even further by those who live in slums and those who do not. A 1996 publication by the Bangladesh Bureau of Statistics provides regional data that can be broken down into three geographical categories—metro nonslum, metro slum, and rural—for a number of health outcome, process, and structural measures.

Figure 5.9 shows the results for seven different measures—DTP/polio doses given to children between 1 and 2 years of age, measles vaccines given to children between 1 and 2 years of age, antenatal care for women, diarrhea incidence for boys, personnel used in delivering babies, and place of delivery for babies, and place of diarrhea treatment for boys—in the Chittagong and Dhaka regions of Bangladesh. Overall, we see that metro (urban) nonslum dwellers do better than urban slum dwellers on all the measures. This figure clearly shows that slum dwellers are more like their rural counterparts than their fellow urban residents.

The graphs also tell an interesting story when we break them down by the three types of measures. The one outcome measure is diarrheal incidence; the four process measures are for vaccination and antenatal care and the three structural measures concern place of treatment and personnel. In terms of the one outcome measure—diarrheal incidence—metro nonslum dwellers were better off than rural dwellers, but female metro slum dwellers were worse off than both. In terms of process measures, the story is similar. With the exception of DTP/polio vaccination in Dhaka, metro nonslum dwellers are significantly better off than metro slum dwellers.

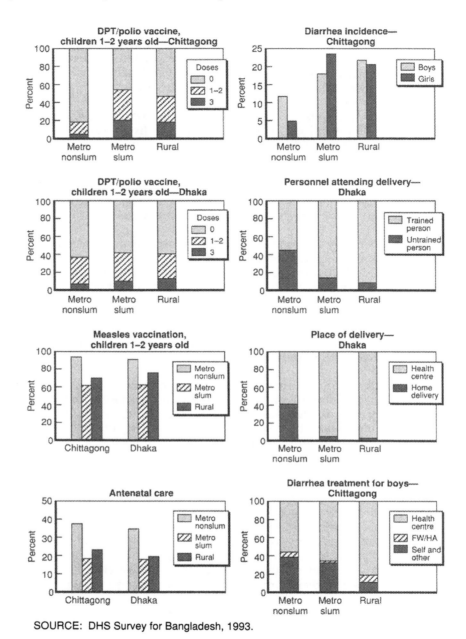

SOURCE: DHS Survey for Bangladesh, 1993.

Figure 5.9—Health Measures for Metro Nonslum, Metro Slum, and Rural Dwellers in Chittagong and Dhaka, Bangladesh

In terms of the three structural measures, the story is different: Metro nonslum dwellers fare better than metro slum dwellers, who in turn fare better than rural dwellers. These findings seem to reflect access problems to facilities in rural locations within the Dhaka region.

Access and Use of Health Services by the Poor. Utilization rates, like health status, differ dramatically by income class. Data from Indonesia are illustrative. Figure 5.10 shows that there is a steep income gradient in visit rates. Individuals in the richest quintile make 0.31 visits to health care providers per month, but individuals in the poorest quintile make only half as many visits (0.14 per month). Although the nonpoor use more of both public and private medical care services, they tend to rely more on private providers (for 55 percent of their care) as their income rises, compared to the poor, who receive somewhat less (40 percent) private care. It is remarkable, however, that even among the poorest segment of the population, a significant amount of treatment is obtained from private providers.

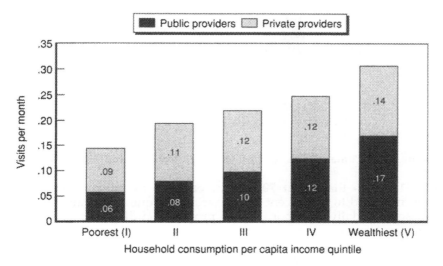

SOURCE: Biro Pusat Statistik-Republik Indonesia (BPS), 1992.

Figure 5.10—Monthly Visit Rates of Ill Persons to Providers by Income, Indonesia, 1992

Data from Viet Nam depict similar patterns. The health care reforms introduced as part of Doi Moi (a wide-ranging economic reform program), implemented in the late 1980s, expanded the role of the private market. While the public sector still provides all inpatient care, it is no longer the main provider of outpatient services or drugs. The private market includes private doctors, paramedics, pharmacies, and drug dispensaries. Recent data from the 1993 Viet Nam LSMS on utilization rates by type of provider show how privatization has affected access to medical care.

The Viet Nam LSMS collected data on contact rates—the proportion of individuals who are sick and seek care. The contact rate, although slightly lower for individuals in the poorest income quintile, is quite high overall (96 percent for the poorest quintile and 99 percent for higher quintiles, as shown in Figure 5.11).

However, the type of providers from whom treatment is sought varies widely between the poor and nonpoor. More probing shows that part of the reason contact rates are so high is the widespread practice of self-medication accomplished through contacts with private pharmacists.

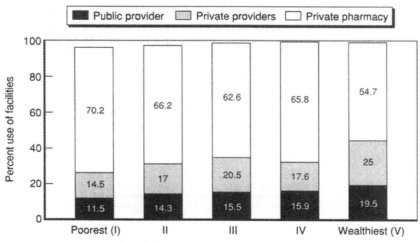

SOURCE: Gertler et al., 1997.

NOTE: Totals do not sum to 100 because some people who are ill either self-medicate or do not seek care.

Figure 5.11—Contact Rates for Ill People by Income Quintile, Viet Nam, 1993

Figure 5.11 shows that about 70 percent of those in the poorest quintile self-medicate compared to 55 percent in the wealthiest quintile. It appears that many Vietnamese, especially the poor, bypass professional diagnosis and treatment in favor of self-diagnosis and treatment (thereby avoiding payment for the professional component of a medical visit). Such a pattern of health care is potentially serious—these informal treatments could exacerbate problems of drug resistance (self-medicating individuals may take less than the full course of treatment) and adversely affect health status. It also could limit use of preventive services, since medical providers often use curative visits to deliver other services that prevent disease and promote good health.

In Viet Nam, a preference for private over public providers is exhibited by both the poor (15 percent versus 12 percent) and the wealthy (25 percent versus 20 percent). Despite this preference for private providers, it is noteworthy that the wealthy tend to use public providers 20 percent of the time whereas the poor use them 12 percent of the time.

Why is it that the nonpoor use public health facilities at much higher rates than the poor when health care is priced low enough to be affordable to everyone? One reason is that the price of obtaining care, borne by the consumer, includes not only the fee charged at the facility but also the cost of travel to the facility and the value of the time lost from work. Thus, even when the fee is zero, the cost is positive and can be quite large. When fees are zero, time prices play a stronger role in determining the choice of medical care provider. (See Dor et al., 1987.) In Indonesia, as in many Asian countries, medical care facilities are located much closer to the nonpoor.

As shown in Figure 5.12, the poor must travel about 50 percent farther than the nonpoor to reach a modern medical care provider. Therefore, despite monetary prices being close to zero, the poor pay higher real prices than the rich because of the geographic distribution of facilities. Furthermore, higher price elasticities among the poor relative to the nonpoor indicate that the poor reduce use more sharply than the rich in response to those time prices. (See Gertler and van der Gaag, 1990.)

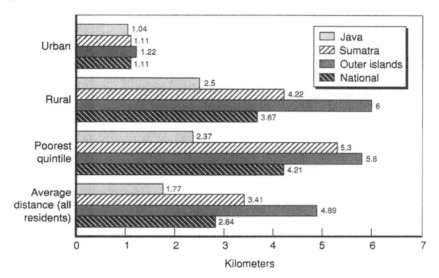

Figure 5.12—Access to Medical Care, Indonesia, 1992
(kilometer (km) to closest provider)

Gender Differentials. The problems that women face in getting access to health care reflect the larger social problems they face. These include greater difficulties in enrolling in education, lower income-earning capacity, lower decisionmaking authority in spending household resources, and all the other challenges inherent in their lower social standing in most countries. The literature on household resource allocation provides evidence that household resources are less likely to be spent on female household members. (See Thomas, 1994.) In South Asia, which has the highest prevalence of protein energy malnutrition, iron-deficiency anemia, and Vitamin A deficiency in the world, these disorders are especially severe among females and are probably a manifestation of this problem. (See Jamison et al., 1993.)

Consequently, women are more likely than men to suffer from stunting caused by protein deficiency and from anemia and iodine deficiency as well. One policy implication of this finding on household resource allocation patterns is that making cash transfers to households to alleviate poverty is probably less effective in improving the health of women and children than improving access to health services (since the cash transfers would tend to be used primarily for adult males in the household).

Women also face threats to their health from pregnancy, a high-frequency and sometimes high-risk event. Small pelvic size in stunted women, for example, increases the risk of maternal and infant mortality. Maternal malnutrition is also associated with poor maternal and infant health. Each year, some 430,000 women in developing countries die from pregnancy-related complications. (See Jamison et al., 1993.)

Given all these threats, it seems surprising that adult male mortality tends to be higher than adult female mortality. This phenomenon can be largely attributed to biological, behavioral, and genetic differences between the sexes. Table 5.10 shows gender differences in the probability of death among adults, age 15 to 60. In most countries, male mortality rates are higher. Even if the age range is restricted to the reproductive years (25Q15 or between the ages of 15 and 40), male mortality still tends to be higher. (See Murray et al., 1992.) However, studies that distinguish avoidable deaths from unavoidable show that females tend to have higher rates than males—a finding indicating that timely and effective medical intervention could reduce female mortality.

Table 5.10

**Adult Mortality Rates by Gender,
Selected Asian Countries, 1985–1990**

Country	45Q15 Mortality Rate	
	Male	Female
Bangladesh	33.7	37.9
China	16.6	14.9
India	32.8	29.4
Indonesia	28.8	23.2
Kampuchea	42.1	36.1
Laos	40.8	35.6
Malaysia	20.4	14.5
Myanmar	29.8	24.1
Nepal	29.5	35.6
Pakistan	25.2	28.0
Papua New Guinea	44.7	41.8
Philippines	28.6	22.7
Sri Lanka	22.5	12.7
Thailand	27.9	21.9
Viet Nam	23.2	17.2
Asia as a whole	23.5	20.0

SOURCE: Adapted from Feachem et al., 1993.
NOTES: Data for China are from 1986; India, 1970–83; and Sri Lanka, 1983.

A closer look at Table 5.10 shows that for three countries—Bangladesh, Nepal, and Pakistan—female mortality rates typically exceed those for males. This suggests that gender disparities in health status are significantly greater in these three countries than elsewhere in Asia. Several factors may partly explain the higher female mortality rates in these countries. First, women have a particularly difficult time attaining education. In rural areas of Pakistan, only 10 percent of females age 5 and over are literate compared to 35 percent of men. Comparable rates in urban areas are 34 and 51 percent, respectively. (See Alderman, 1992.)

Second, cultural practices restrict the ability of women to travel alone in these countries. Women who wish to seek health care must often be accompanied by a male family member, which could serve to suppress the number of visits to health providers made by women. Data presented earlier (see Table 5.9) showed that the use of MCH services was far lower for women in Bangladesh and Pakistan than it was for women in other Asian countries.

These countries also have exceptionally high levels of infant and child mortality. The higher mortality rate for adult females may put infants and children at risk. Matlab, a rural community in Bangladesh, has served as a disease surveillance site since the early 1970s. Studies in both the 1970s and in 1983–1985 found that maternal deaths were associated with higher infant and child mortality. The latter study found that a mother's death was associated with an increase in two-year mortality rates of almost 50 per thousand for sons and 144 per thousand for daughters. Although one might expect that the death of a father could lead to similarly large effects because of the expected decrease in household income, the effect is much smaller: A father's death was associated with an increase of about 6 per thousand for both sons and daughters. (See Over et al., 1992.)

Several researchers raise a note of caution about interpreting cross-sectional gender data. (See Rahman et al., 1994; Strauss et al., 1993.) These researchers argue that biological differences in the age structure between men and women and differential mortality rates by gender lead to a selection bias. First, because of higher female life expectancy, women in any survey sample are likely to be older than men and, thus, may appear to have worse health on average if the data are not adjusted by age. Second, because adult males have higher age-specific mortality rates than females in most countries, differences in the *prevalence* of ill health may affect estimates of gender differentials in the *incidence* of ill health.

For example, even if males and females have the same incidence of poor health over their lifetime, as sick men die the remaining male cohort is relatively more robust and thus may appear to be healthier in a cross-sectional survey. This effect may confound estimates of gender differences in adult ill health.[3]

Figures 5.13 and 5.14 present (unadjusted) gender differences in health status among adults 50 years of age and older (based on self-reported measures of physical functioning) for two countries, Malaysia and Bangladesh, respectively. (See Rahman et al., 1994.) Gender differences adjusted by age and controlling for socioeconomic factors are presented for Bangladesh in Figure 5.15 for a single measure of health status—the percentage of people who have difficulty with one or more functional activities.

The unadjusted figures show that women tend to fare worse than men across a variety of physical functioning measures. Correcting for mortality selection and socioeconomic differences narrows the gender gap, particularly at older ages, but the gaps persist. These gender disparities in health status could result partly from biological differences and partly from differences in behavior (e.g., nutritional differences), life experiences (e.g., pregnancy), or differential access to health services.[4] Childbearing, in fact, may be one important determinant of ill health in women, particularly in areas with high fertility and poor health infrastructure. (See Strauss et al., 1993.)

---

[3]Controlling for this "mortality selection" requires adding the individuals who have died in the interim between some reference age and the age observed in the survey sample. Survival probabilities generated from age-specific mortality rates obtained from vital registration data can be used to make this correction.

[4]The researchers dismiss reporting bias as a possible explanation given that gender differentials are observed across a wide spectrum of countries.

216 Policy and Health: Implications for Development in Asia

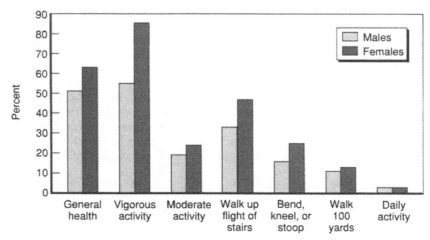

SOURCE: Rahman et al., 1994.
NOTE: The general health measure is the percentage of people who report their health as poor on a three-scale rating of good, fair, and poor. The physical function measures are the percentage of people who say their health limits each specific activity.

Figure 5.13—Percentage of Adults 50 Years of Age and Older with Poor Health and Limitations in Physical Functions by Gender, Malaysia, 1992

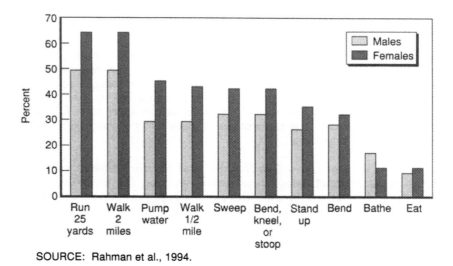

SOURCE: Rahman et al., 1994.

Figure 5.14—Percentage of Adults 60 Years of Age and Older with Limitations in Physical Functions by Gender, Matlab Surveillance Area, Rural Bangladesh, 1992

OPTIONS FOR ADDRESSING INEQUITY

As the data presented above illustrate, large disparities in outcomes, utilization, and access remain in Asia. These disparities are compounded by associations with income, education, residence, and gender. What policies are best when it comes

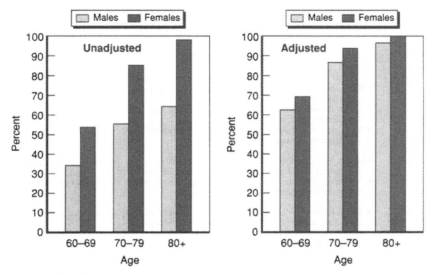

SOURCE: Rahman et al., 1994.

Figure 5.15—Proportion of Adults 60 Years and Over in Poor Health by Age, With and Without Adjustment for Mortality Selection and Socioeconomic Functions, Matlab, Rural Bangladesh, 1992

to addressing these disparities? As discussed in Chapter 1, governments have five ways to improve equity: inform, regulate, mandate, finance, or deliver. Table 5.11 lists a series of options to address inequity, organized around these five roles of government.

In terms of informing, governments can address equity issues in three ways. First, they can conduct health education and community outreach for poor, less-educated populations to teach the benefits of such practices as oral rehydration, safe birthing, breastfeeding, family planning, smoking prevention, and safe food handling. Second, since inappropriate demands and expectations by consumers often lead to the misuse of drugs (e.g., seeking antibiotics or steroids to treat a common (viral) cold or not seeking treatment for STDs, acute respiratory infection, tuberculosis, and parasitic infections), governments can train doctors and educate individuals. Finally, since much of the burden of disease stems from pregnancy-related complications and the diseases of children, governments can target health education efforts toward women.

In terms of regulating, governments can encourage more-rational use of resources and better targeting of subsidies to the poor by pricing differentially by levels of service. They can set fees low at public health centers and high at hospitals, but waive or reduce the higher hospital fees for patients referred from public health centers; they can also establish sliding fee scales based on income or proxy measures of ability to pay.

Table 5.11

Options to Address Inequity by Government Role

Government Role	Option to Address Inequity
Inform	• Conduct health education/community outreach for poor, less educated, and rural populations. • Train doctors on more-appropriate drug use and health education, so they can teach their patients. • Target health education training efforts, particularly toward women; use indigenous educators.
Regulate	• Set prices and establish referral procedures to encourage more-rational use of resources and better targeting of subsidies to the poor. • Set drug prescribing rules and establish payment systems to provide incentives for more-appropriate drug use.
Mandate	• Require new doctors to practice for a minimum time in rural areas, urban slums, or other areas with health manpower shortages. • Mandate private provision of social insurance and require businesses and other employers to participate. • Design cross-subsidies to finance enrollment of poor women and the elderly in the insurance plan.
Finance	• Establish government-sponsored health insurance and provide subsidies to enroll target populations. • Establish community financing or prepayment schemes. • If relying on user fees to increase cost recovery and generate resources, design subsidies targeted to the poor to reduce financial barriers to care. • Design subsidies that adhere to the five pricing principles identified in Chapter 4.
Deliver	• Provide preventive and primary care in government health centers and subcenters; reduce waiting times and improve quality. • Provide curative care in government hospitals with better targeting of subsidies. • Invest in categorical disease programs where benefits accrue disproportionately to poor; prioritize funding to reduce funding for diseases or services where a substantial share of benefits is captured by the nonpoor. • For villages too small to sustain health clinic staffed by doctor, encourage localities to join together to support a rotating doctor.

NOTE: The five options for public sector intervention (arranged according to degree or intrusion) are drawn from a discussion by Musgrove (1996).

Mandating options include requiring new doctors to spend some time practicing in areas with health manpower shortages and mandating private provision of social insurance and designing cross-subsidies to finance enrollment of the poor into the insurance plan.

In its financing role, governments can establish government-sponsored health insurance and provide subsidies to enroll target populations or community financing or prepayment schemes. If governments rely on user fees to increase cost recovery and generate resources to finance health care, they can design subsidies targeted to the poor to reduce financial barriers to care. And finally, given the four pricing principles elaborated in Chapter 4, governments can design higher subsidies (1) for services where public care is better than private, (2) for services for which demand is more elastic, (3) for individuals whose demand is more price-elastic, and (4) for those services and in those areas where there are limited private-sector alternatives.

On the delivery side, governments can provide preventive and primary care in government health centers and subcenters, reduce waiting times, and improve quality (through better training of doctors and health workers and acquisition and maintenance of low-tech equipment such as scales, blood pressure cuffs, sterilizers, and cold storage units); they can also maintain better stocks of drugs and supplies to dissuade patients from bypassing local public health centers in favor of more-distant, but better-equipped, hospitals.

They can continue to invest in categorical disease programs where benefits accrue disproportionately to the poor. These include diseases that have higher prevalence among the poor or treatable diseases that often go untreated because treatments are expensive (e.g., tuberculosis, leprosy, and STDs). Governments can also prioritize interventions to reduce funding for diseases or services where a substantial share of benefits is captured by the nonpoor.

Policies to improve access to health services are seldom adopted as stand-alone solutions. Because ensuring good health for poor women and other vulnerable populations is a complex social process that depends on economic development, environmental conditions, disease states, and behavioral responses on the part of providers and patients (discussed in Chapter 6), no single policy option is sufficient by itself to improve equity. Moreover, the problems that confront a country's health sector are multiple and interdependent, as illustrated by three examples of typical health-sector problems:

- The inability to maintain adequate levels and quality of inputs (staff, equipment, supplies, drugs) at government facilities and the seemingly inexorable logistical problems in deploying those resources that are available;

- The maldistribution of facilities in a country, leaving segments of the population unserved and a skewed distribution of services favoring expensive and curative treatments over simpler but effective preventive and primary health services;

- Inappropriate pricing policies and poor targeting of subsidies that (1) inhibit expansion of the private sector (e.g., free family planning commodities cause downward pressure on private-sector prices, making sustainability difficult) and (2) worsen rather than improve the equitable distribution of government resources (as when middle- to high-income groups capture most of the benefits of public subsidies).

Because of these interdependencies, acting to achieve one goal (improving equity) to the exclusion of others could exacerbate other problems. Therefore, a strategy to create a more equitable system requires an integrated package of health-sector reform that restructures incentives across all components of the health sector—financing, health manpower training and deployment, organizational structure and management, facility location and staffing, and delivery of services. In designing such an integrated package, policymakers must inevitably balance trade-offs between multiple, sometimes competing, objectives: increasing access for the poor and other vulnerable populations, improving quality, stabilizing provider income, shifting services from tertiary to primary care settings, reducing waste, and controlling expenditures.

Although this chapter has focused on financing and delivery, the bottom line is that improving equity requires more than just making improvements in how services are financed and delivered, as Table 5.11 shows. Implementing those options requires being able to change provider and individual behavior through information programs (e.g., education and training), regulation, and mandates—concerns that form the basis of Chapter 6. And carrying out any of these options also requires a strong health care management and organizational structure—concerns that we address in Chapter 7. Ultimately, improving equity requires the political will to redistribute resources from the wealthy to the poor, from men to women, and from income earners to the young and the old.

SUBSIDIES VERSUS SOCIAL INSURANCE EXPANSION

Cross-country experiences to date have led to some common policy prescriptions that remedy the structural impediments in the health sector and that improve equity. The following sector-wide strategies emerge from this book:

- Regardless of a country's financial means, prioritizing national policies based on disease burden and cost-effectiveness (DALYs, HeaLYs) is likely to improve resource allocation decisions (Chapter 3).

- Resource generation through user fees at public facilities and/or through social insurance can lead to more equitable financing of the health system (Chapter 4).

- Empowering families and providers can lead to more-participatory forms of community health planning that are likely to be more responsive to local problems and concerns (Chapter 6).

- Decentralizing public-sector health facility management, strengthening the public-sector capacity to monitor and regulate health services, and expanding the private sector and its integration into management and service delivery can improve the system's use of resources (Chapter 7).

Despite these common prescriptions for improving equity, some options are ultimately likely to be more beneficial and cost-effective than others depending on a country's or locality's circumstances. Such circumstances include the following:

- **Economic, Geographic, and Sociodemographic Characteristics**—the size of the formal versus informal sectors of the economy, the level and distribution of income across the population, the distribution of the population across urban and rural areas in a country;

- **Community Infrastructure**—a country's roads, transportation, water, sewerage, and telecommunication resources;

- **Health Infrastructure**—the number and distribution of trained providers, the quality and distribution of health facilities, the availability of drugs and medical equipment or supplies, the role of the public sector in a country versus the private sector;

- **Institutional Capacity to Administer or Monitor Programs**—a country's regulatory infrastructure, for example, and the availability and reliability of information systems for monitoring and enforcement purposes;

- **Degree of Decentralization**—how a country divides responsibilities between the central government and local levels of government.

There is a spectrum of countries in Asia, ranging from those with low capabilities within these areas to those with high capabilities, as Figure 5.16 shows. We argue that depending on where countries fall along that spectrum, various options for addressing inequities make more or less sense.

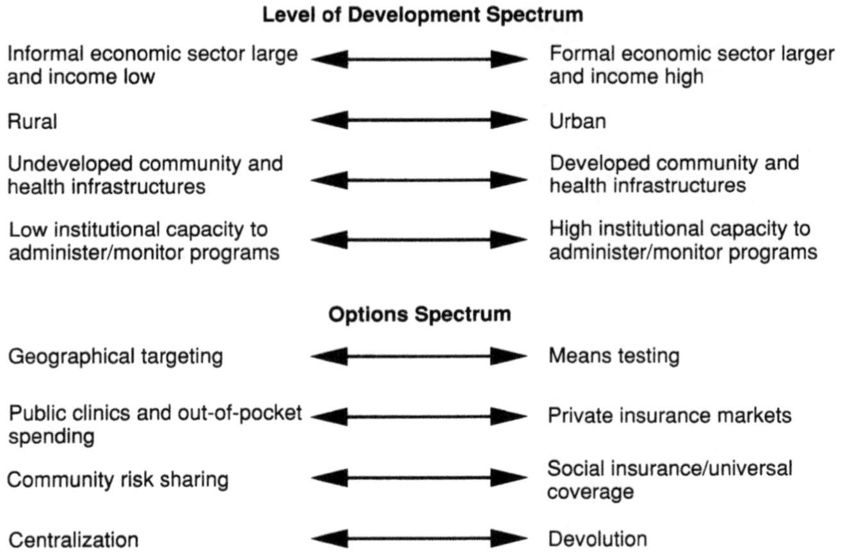

Level of Development Spectrum

Informal economic sector large and income low	Formal economic sector larger and income high
Rural	Urban
Undeveloped community and health infrastructures	Developed community and health infrastructures
Low institutional capacity to administer/monitor programs	High institutional capacity to administer/monitor programs

Options Spectrum

Geographical targeting	Means testing
Public clinics and out-of-pocket spending	Private insurance markets
Community risk sharing	Social insurance/universal coverage
Centralization	Devolution

Figure 5.16—Options for Improving Equity in Financing Depend on Level of Development

Addressing Equity at the Low End of the Spectrum—The Potential of Specific Targeting

In poor countries where average incomes are geographically segmented, governments can more effectively use their limited resources by redirecting resources to areas with the poorest populations and/or the greatest disease burden. This practice is referred to as targeting. It is the identification of those who will or will not be eligible for a social program. (See Grosh, 1996.) Targeting in the health sector generally focuses on the poor or those who are at greater risk of illness or poor access—women, children, the elderly, and rural residents. The benefit of targeting subsidies or services to the poor and other vulnerable groups is that it concentrates resources on those who need them most and shifts them away from those who don't, thus allowing governments to achieve a greater impact on vulnerable groups for a fixed budget.

Box 5.3: Geographic Targeting in Indonesia

Recognizing that much more needs to be done to help the millions still below or near the poverty line, the government of Indonesia initiated the Presidential Instruction on Poor Village Development (Inpres Desa Tertinggal, or IDT) in 1994. This is designed to deliver direct financial aid to the poor people living in the poorest one-third of Indonesia's villages. The IDT program represents a government strategy to geographically target its poverty alleviation efforts at localized pockets of poverty. How useful is the targeting approach?

Using the government's information base—SUSENAS[5]—which collects measures of both the social and economic welfare of households in Indonesia—the IDT program monitors changes in welfare status to update targeting criteria. It also uses the PODES[6]—which collects a wide range of information on the physical, social, and economic infrastructure of every village in the country—as the primary data source for the current system of identifying and ranking poor villages. (See Biro Pusat Statistik (BPS), 1994.)

Household expenditures from the 1993 SUSENAS were merged with measures of village characteristics from the PODES to determine which village characteristics were significantly correlated with village-level economic well-being for both the sample of SUSENAS villages and for all villages. Using the estimated household per-capita expenditure for all individuals within a SUSENAS village, researchers calculated two measures of village economic well-being: (1) village average per-capita expenditure, and (2) proportion of village residents below the official poverty line. Researchers created four sets of village rankings, from lowest average per-capita expenditure (or highest proportion poor) to the highest average per-capita expenditure (or lowest proportion poor).

The study finds that different sets of village characteristics are associated with village economic well-being in different regions: The village characteristics that are associated with urban village economic well-being are substantially different from those associated with rural village economic well-being. These findings indicate that targeting systems based on village characteristics should be flexible enough to permit the village criteria to vary across urban and rural areas, as well as regions.

One of the key criteria for evaluating the efficacy of a targeting mechanism is the percentage of the target population reached. While all four targeting methods are efficient, the regional-proportion-poor method is the most efficient. Nevertheless, the targeting efficiency of all methods declines dramatically as the number of villages increases. For example, targeting the first 10 percent of villages with the regional-proportion-poor method identifies 22 percent of the poor. Increasing the threshold to 30 percent of villages increases the percentage of poor identified to 56 percent. Thus, even if one were to target the poorest 30 percent of villages, one would only identify slightly more than half of the poor population.

However, targeting is not a panacea. It introduces new costs, such as the administrative costs of identifying the vulnerable groups. Other costs (which would be associated with a nontargeted benefit as well) stem from losses associated with the disincentive effects of providing the targeted benefits.

There is generally believed to be a trade-off between targeting accuracy and targeting costs: As the accuracy of targeting increases, so do the costs. (See Besley and Kanbur, 1990.) The effectiveness of targeting programs is generally assessed according to three criteria:

---

[5]*Survey Sosiala Ekonomi Nasional* (National Socio-Economic Survey).
[6]*Potensi Desa* (Census of Village Potential).

- **Undercoverage (Type I Error):** This occurs when policy fails to exempt someone from paying the fee who should be exempted. The greater the undercoverage, the fewer the number of poor protected by the price discrimination method. An extreme example of Type I error would be if facilities charged everyone the full cost of delivering the service. In that case, Type I error would be 100 percent.

- **Leakage (Type II Error):** This occurs when policy exempts someone who should not be exempted. The greater the leakage, the greater the leakage of potential revenues from the nonpoor, leaving fewer subsidies available to reach the poor. An extreme example of Type II error would be if everyone were given free care. In this case, all potential revenues would be lost and Type II error would be 100 percent.

- **Administrative Costs:** The costs of identifying the poor and implementing price discrimination (charging more to the nonpoor) can swamp all the gains from price discrimination. There are clearly diminishing returns to making price discrimination methods more precise. Administrative methods vary from inexpensive procedures, such as geographic price discrimination and targeting by age and gender, to costly procedures, such as a sliding fee system with social worker verification.

Given these assessment criteria, four common types of targeting mechanisms are available: (1) individual assessment mechanisms; (2) geographic targeting; (3) self-selection; and (4) indicator targeting. What distinguishes them is the administrative requirements used to identify individuals or groups to be targeted.

Individual Assessment Mechanisms. Individual price discrimination based on means testing is the ideal method for maximizing coverage of the poor and minimizing the revenue loss from providing subsidized care to the nonpoor. Targeting of individuals is generally the most accurate method. In addition to means tests based on household income or assets, individual applicants can be assessed according to other criteria as well (e.g., gender).

Unfortunately, experience has shown that administrative costs (partly because of lack of data) and low application rates make this method ineffective in most countries. For example, in both Indonesia and Viet Nam, the poor can get the fee waived through an affidavit of indigence. Financially indigent persons can request that their local village head or local official issue an affidavit that exempts them from paying fees for health services at all public health facilities and schools. However, few people seem to take advantage of the opportunity. (See World Bank, 1995c, 1995e.)

It is not clear why the systems are failing. Several possibilities exist: People may not know about the benefit; prices are so low that the benefit is not worth the opportunity cost of obtaining it; local officials may be charging a fee to issue the affidavit; facilities may charge a fee to accept the affidavit; or there may be a social stigma associated with receiving it.

The corollary problem of having too few data is how economic well-being can be measured in an economy where the majority of the population pay no income tax and where a good portion of economic resources are home-produced.

Without accurate, fast, and administratively simple methods of identifying poor individuals, an individual exemption mechanism may exempt too many people and, consequently, sacrifice substantial revenues. While the government may not want to use individual exemptions, doing so may be useful in certain circumstances where other methods of protecting the poor are unavailable or in cases where the poor can be easily identified.

Geographic Targeting. An alternative method of implementing a pricing policy that protects the poor is geographic targeting. This policy aims to tailor the fee structure or the provision of services to the socioeconomic composition of the population served by each facility. Facilities located where the poor live would charge zero or near-zero fees; facilities that serve primarily nonpoor households would charge larger fees. Indeed, facilities in wealthier areas could charge fees equal to or in excess of unit costs. A facility-level fee schedule that increases with the economic status of the households in the facility's service region would imply that government subsidies are pro-poor in that they are largest in the poorest areas.

Although the idea of geographic price discrimination is straightforward in principle, its implementation is quite complex. Populations within a region are not homogeneous. Every region has some households whose income is below the government's definition of poverty. In those regions where a large percentage of the population are poor, the government can keep fees low enough to protect the majority of the poor without experiencing high levels of leakage. However, in regions with a low percentage of poor, the government would have to choose between forgoing substantial revenues from those able to pay in order to protect a small number of poor or not protecting the poor to capture revenue from the nonpoor. In this case, it would be cost-effective to screen the poor at the facilities or employ an individual discrimination method.

Using geographic price discrimination in rural areas where the poor are concentrated is a promising method to protect the poor without a large sacrifice of revenues to administrative costs. Long travel times should prevent people living in wealthier areas from switching to the lower-fee facilities in poorer areas when fees in the more affluent areas are increased. However, the method has limited potential in urban areas, where the poor are intermixed with the nonpoor and most facilities are easily accessed by both poor and nonpoor.

Differential Pricing by Level of Service and Self-Selection. An alternative approach to protect the poor in urban areas is through differential pricing by level of service. The notion is to have low subsidies for services valued by the nonpoor and high subsidies for services used mostly by the poor. In particular, the government should subsidize service for which demand is income-inelastic.

In general, this would mean keeping subsidies low at hospitals and specialty clinics and high for outpatient services. If an individual first goes to the outpatient primary care clinic and requires a higher level of care at the hospital, the registration fees are waived at the hospital. In this pricing structure, fees are lower if the patient enters the system at the lowest level, and progressively higher the

> **Box 5.4: Risk-Sharing in Rural China**
>
> Starting in the late 1950s and continuing through much of the 1970s, Cooperative Medical Schemes (CMS) were introduced in the rural villages of many counties in China. Under the CMS, farmers prepaid a fixed amount into a village-managed fund. In many places, local governments also contributed. The fund covered preventive and basic health care services at the commune health station, which was staffed by a rural health worker ("barefoot doctor"), and reimbursed farmers for part of the cost of using services at higher levels of care (township and county facilities).
>
> Although problems existed (e.g., sometimes a village fund was depleted prior to year end, in which case no reimbursements were made for the remainder of the year; sometimes villages/communes mismanaged the funds; and, in some places, few preventive services were provided), the CMS succeeded in spreading risk across all the farmers within a village or commune and provided a stable source of revenue for the village health worker. Health outcomes in China improved dramatically. While this was likely largely the result of improvements brought about by rapid economic growth, the reductions in urban/rural differentials in health utilization and outcomes are believed to have resulted partly from increased access to health care in rural areas as a result of CMS.
>
> Economic reforms and the shift toward a market-oriented economy began in 1979. This led to the end of the rural communes, which led, in turn, to the dissolution of the CMS funds and the collapse of the risk-pooling mechanism. Simultaneously, government financing of township health centers and county hospitals was reduced. Whereas these facilities had formerly received nearly all their revenue from the government, now only 20–25 percent of their expenses was covered through government sources (primarily for base salaries and some new capital investments). Government funding of preventive care and immunizations was also reduced, such that nearly half the revenues for preventive services now come from patient fees. Farmers must now pay out-of-pocket for medical care, and, as a result, many forgo care they cannot afford.
>
> A recent study of 30 poor counties in China collected household data (approximately 11,000 households) in 180 villages from 1992 to 1995. Nearly one-third of these villages (30 percent) had no village doctor. Without a stable source of revenue, many rural doctors have either left the villages for employment elsewhere or have resumed farming. Moreover, more than one-fourth (28 percent) of individuals who were ill did not obtain health care for financial reasons, and one-half of those referred to a hospital did not go because of the cost. A study that compared health service use between poorer and richer households (divided into three groups) found some differentials in outpatient use and even greater differentials in inpatient use. These data suggest that health outcomes in rural areas may be stagnating, a phenomenon attributed to declines in access caused by the collapse of the CMS. Despite continuing economic growth, infant and child mortality rates have shown almost no improvement since the mid-1980s.
>
> Recently, China has initiated efforts to revive a restructured CMS system. Since 1994, it has worked with WHO and the World Bank to design and implement CMS in a small number of rural counties. In December, 1996, the government issued a call for the national expansion of CMS. In addition to expanded access and a broader-based distribution of risk, the reintroduction of CMS will coincide with better training of rural doctors, hopefully leading to better health. (See Hsiao, 1995a; Hsiao and Liu, 1996.)

further up the system the patient enters. This pricing structure provides an affordable portal of entry into the health care system through the health centers and allows those willing to pay to bypass the health center and go directly to higher levels of care. Since it is the nonpoor who are willing to pay to bypass the lower levels, they will be charged higher prices and thus receive lower subsidies. As discussed in Chapter 4 in the subsection "Adjusting Resource Allocation to Use Facilities More Effectively," this type of strategy is useful because it can also have budget implications through reduced costs. Governments have two policy levers in differential pricing and self-selection: Not only can they charge different prices, but they can also improve the quality of care. The appropriate balance will depend on the cross-price elasticity between primary and higher-level facilitation and the costs of administering disparate user fees.

Indicator Targeting. Indicators serve as proxies for determining eligibility or benefit levels for clinical, nutritional, or other social service programs. The use of indicators reduces the data-gathering burden and expense associated with individual means testing by enabling policymakers to readily identify members of a more-disadvantaged group or class. Programs can then be targeted to all members of this group. The indicator serves as a proxy that differentiates between those likely to need the benefits being offered from those less likely to need them. Although there will likely be some leakage from treating all such members identically, it makes sense to use indicator targeting if the leakage is less costly than the administrative burden of running a means-tested program.

Criteria for choosing indicators might include the following: (1) they are easily observable or not costly to measure; (2) they are not easily fungible, manipulable, or subject to fraud; and (3) they are strongly correlated to being at risk because of poor financial standing and/or greater-than-average medical need. For example, one group thought to be at great risk and, therefore, often the target for assistance is pregnant women and newborn infants. Other frequently used indicators include disease (e.g., diarrhea, acute respiratory infections, tuberculosis, or AIDS), age/gender (children, reproductive-aged women, and the elderly—all of whom are viewed as having special medical needs), occupation (farmers are viewed as being at financial risk for not being able to afford medical care; commercial sex workers are viewed as being at increased risk for contracting sexually transmitted diseases), land ownership, and ownership of particular durable goods or other assets. Geographic targeting, discussed above, is another type of indicator targeting in which a household's region or neighborhood is used as an indicator, since it is generally easier to identify low-income neighborhoods rather than individuals with low incomes. (See Besley and Kanbur, 1993.)

In addition to identifying groups to assist or subsidize, indicator targeting can also be used to identify those most able to pay the full cost of care (under a user fee policy, for example). One such group is the insured or those employed in the formal wage sector. Insurance status or employment in the formal sector are good indicators of those most able to pay, because employed or insured people tend to be wealthier than the general population and to use more medical services.

The Evidence on Targeting Effectiveness. Targeting advocates believe that by shifting from universal provision to targeted programs, governments can better reach the poor and other high-priority groups—such as women and children—within limited budgets. (See Datt and Ravallion, 1993; World Bank, 1990a.) Critics of targeting say that such programs have failed to cover many of the poor, failed to prevent leakage of benefits to the nonpoor, and even reduced the funds dedicated to the poor because of the administrative costs of screening (See Gelbach and Pritchett, 1995.) Others note that if targeting becomes more successful in shifting benefits to the poor and other marginalized groups, political support for these programs in the general population could be eroded. (See Alderman, 1991; Ravallion, 1992.)

What do empirical studies say about how well targeting programs reach the poor and other priority groups? Studies of targeting outcomes in developing countries for a broad range of social programs are reported by Grosh and Van de Walle and summarized here. (See Grosh, 1996; Van de Walle, 1995.) Recognizing that the costs and benefits of targeting depend to a great extent on program design, both authors assess the impacts of alternative design features.

Based on her analysis of 30 targeted programs in Latin America, Grosh finds that even the least-effective targeting programs have progressive incidence (that is, they benefit the poor disproportionately). The share of program benefits accruing to the lowest two income quintiles ranges from 59 to 83 percent. No one type of targeting mechanism outperformed the others (e.g., the median share of benefits going to the poorest two quintiles is 73, 72, and 71 percent for individual assessment, geographic targeting, and self-selection, respectively).

Grosh also finds that the administrative costs of targeting have tended to be overestimated. Median administrative costs for the three mechanisms is 9, 7, and 6 percent of total program costs, respectively.

Van de Walle finds a more mixed set of outcomes. Although targeted programs did benefit the poor, the evidence suggests that for some types of programs, lump-sum transfers to all households, rich and poor alike, would achieve the same incidence. (The examples concerned poverty reduction efforts rather than health programs, which can be expected to have better incidence.) One problem is that as a result of low take-up (the nonclaiming of benefits by those who are eligible), the poor do not benefit as much as intended. (See Atkinson, 1996.)

Van de Walle emphasizes the importance of considering behavioral responses to targeting. As with other social interventions, targeting may cause individuals to alter their behavior, and these behavioral responses can greatly alter administrative costs and the distribution of benefits. For example, in Sri Lanka, the provision of a benefit (food stamps) had adverse work incentives—reducing work by two to three days per month, which represented 33 percent of the subsidy's value. (See Sahn and Alderman, 1996.)

Indicator targeting, using multiple indicators, is one alternative to individual screening. Appleton and Collier recommend using gender along with other indicators such as landlessness and rural residence (e.g., the Grameen Bank credit program). (See Appleton and Collier, 1996.) Van de Walle notes that letting the poor select themselves minimizes targeting costs and results in well-targeted benefits.

Three lessons can be drawn from the above studies. First, in countries with relatively low GNP and where the majority of workers are either agrarian or work in the informal rather than the formal wage sector, governments can best improve access through direct service provision, a focus on vertical disease programs that target treatable conditions, and subsidized prices. In countries where everyone is universally poor, the government need not target its support, since all individuals are needy and stand to benefit more or less equally from government support.

Second, when the above condition is *not* met, targeted programs tend to have more progressive incidence than universal provision or across-the-board subsidization of health services. In choosing a targeting mechanism, the optimal design depends on many factors, including the characteristics of the poor—who the poor are, how many there are, and why they are poor—and country-specific circumstances such as infrastructure development and administrative capabilities. (See Van de Walle, 1995.) This means that data gaps and poor data quality can hamper efforts to relieve inequities. The careful design of programs to achieve equity goals requires a data-driven assessment of these circumstances as well as information about the likely behavioral responses of consumers and providers.

The Middle of the Spectrum—The Potential for a Two-Track Policy of Social Insurance

As discussed in Chapter 4, universal coverage for low- and middle-income countries in Asia is not a viable option for a number of reasons, including inability to pay, inability to absorb the cost inflation that is part of such coverage, and administrative infeasibility. However, in countries where universal coverage may not be feasible on a national scale (i.e., where large segments of the population reside in rural areas or participate in the informal economy), a two-track policy of social insurance in the large urban areas and community insurance or prepayment schemes in the rural areas may be feasible. For example, in China, workers in state-owned enterprises or in private companies have long been covered by government and labor insurance, whereas insurance for farmers has only recently become a policy focus with efforts under way to revive the cooperative medical systems that collapsed following the economic transformation of the past two decades.

Similarly, in Indonesia, government workers have long had government health insurance (financed by a 2 percent payroll tax), and recent efforts at insurance expansion have targeted the private sector through a law mandating employer-sponsored insurance. The formal insurance is being supplemented by a policy of community financing in rural villages (known as Dana Sehat, whereby village residents contribute to a village fund used to purchase health services) and subsidized care for the poor (known as Kartu Sehat, in which the poor are exempted from user fees at government health facilities).

The High End of the Spectrum—The Potential of Universal Coverage

For countries at the high end of the spectrum that have high per capita GDPs, real GDP growth, a high level of urbanization, and developed management and institutional infrastructures, universal coverage can be a very useful option for dealing with inequities.

More specifically, in countries where a sizable portion of the workforce is engaged in the formal wage sector, some type of social insurance is feasible. The poor can participate in such systems if cross-subsidies are built into the system, drawing funds from those who can pay to help support those who cannot pay on their own. To be workable, governments must have the regulatory capacity to collect premiums and sanction evaders. Insurance enables risk-pooling across individuals and across time, so that an individual's payments are relatively small and predictable. To improve equity, subsidies can be used to support the

Box 5.5: Achieving Equity Through Universal Coverage: The Experience of Japan

Japan's path toward universal coverage began as early as 1922, when it enacted its first health insurance law—Employees Health Insurance (EHI). The law applied to all industry employees with five or more workers and included their dependents. In 1938, the country enacted a second major health insurance law—NHI—to cover farmers and the self-employed voluntarily in a private insurance society. That law was substantially revised in 1958 to require coverage for anyone either not covered under NHI or enrolled in a voluntary society. With the inclusion of other occupational categories—civil servants, school teachers, and agricultural workers—in mutual aid associations throughout the 1950s, 99 percent of the Japanese population was covered through either EHI, NHI, one of the special occupational groups, or public assistance. Universal coverage was achieved in 1961. In the more than three and a half decades since, how has Japan's health care system fared in achieving equity?

Achieving equity in access to care was one of the key forces behind the drive for universal coverage in Japan. As such, all the plans—despite minor differences in premiums and copayment rates and in plan benefits—rely on a nationally uniform fee schedule. This means that the fees for care are uniform, regardless of who the patient is, what the physician's level of experience is, and where the care is provided. The end result is that patients are not charged extra for almost all services and doctors have no incentive to deny care for fear of not being paid. In addition, out-of-pocket copayments, beyond a given amount per month (set lower for low-income individuals), are completely reimbursed, regardless of plan.

As a wealthy nation, Japan can ensure equity by heavily subsidizing the various plans to protect the financially disadvantaged. In 1989, direct subsidies from the general budget ranged from as low as 16.4 percent for government-managed plans for small companies to as high as 50 percent for NHI health insurance for the self-employed and pensioners, with the elderly covered by a 30 percent subsidy through a pooling mechanism of national and local governments. (See Ikegami, 1991.)

The end result of such government management is that Japan has achieved a remarkably equitable health care system. In 1988, a Tokyo Metropolitan Government survey revealed that individuals' income levels had no effect on their utilization rate or on the health expenditure per person. (See Tokyo Metropolitan Government, 1989.) And in a 1985 national survey conducted by the Ministry of Health and Welfare, less than half of one percent of those people who said they were sick and did not see a doctor indicated that not having enough money was the reason. (See Japanese Ministry of Health and Welfare, 1986.) Finally, only 12 percent of the cost of health care services provided under health insurance comes from out-of-pocket expenses for copayments.

Still, although Japan's social insurance has achieved great success in providing access to care, it is also encumbered by incentives that lead to inefficiencies (e.g., overprescribing of drugs, excessively long hospital stays, and churning of outpatient visits).

enrollment of poor women or other vulnerable populations in the insurance plan (described in Chapter 4).

The experiences of Canada and England demonstrate the potential effect that a policy of universal coverage may have on improving equity. In both countries, long-standing inequities in access and utilization were reversed following the introduction of universal coverage in Canada and a national health service in England. (See Hornbrook, 1995.) Before the introduction of these national programs, people lower in socioeconomic status had worse health, were less likely to seek care, and used relatively fewer health services than others. With the introduction of universal coverage, these patterns changed—access to, and use of, health care services more closely reflected indicators of the need for care, such as health status. Nonetheless, health outcomes are still strongly related to socioeconomic status, with the poor experiencing greater morbidity and worse health outcomes. (See Cockerham, 1990.)

Within Asia, the experience of Japan and South Korea demonstrate that it is possible to move toward more-equitable systems of finance and delivery. For example, the Republic of Korea, which adopted universal coverage through national health insurance in just 12 years, mandated minimum benefits packages, along with maximum reimbursement rates to providers, in an effort to increase primary care services and participation of the poor. The resulting universal coverage has led to an expansion of clinical care, so that every urban resident and 62 percent of the rural population now live within 30 minutes travel of a facility.

Of course, equity problems still persist in South Korea despite universal coverage. High copayment rates—as much as 55 percent—disproportionately affect the elderly and the poor who live on fixed or limited incomes. Physician ratios for the rural population, where the elderly are concentrated, are well below the national average. To further improve access and improve equity, the government offers both supply-side and demand-side incentives. On the supply side, tax incentives are given to providers locating to rural areas and subsidies are provided to construct facilities. The government also continues to operate facilities in remote rural areas. On the demand side, the government subsidizes insurance premiums for the self-employed, for the poor, and for insurance societies covering the rural population. (See Peabody et al., 1994.)

POLICY IMPLICATIONS

Improving equity as a means of insuring social justice and promoting the general welfare is both a goal and an ongoing challenge for governments in Asia. While all governments want to help remove the inequities that threaten their most vulnerable populations, governments engage in a constant struggle to find the right balance between equity, efficiency, and other social objectives, which pits them in a continual search for "better ways of drawing the boundary lines between the domain of rights and the domain of dollars." (Okun, 1975, p. 120.) Where a country draws the boundaries depends on the priorities it assigns to different and sometimes competing social objectives; its own political, cultural, and ideological ecology; its level of economic development; and the state of its health care infrastructure.

A second point is that improving equity within countries is about political choices. This chapter focused on the structural barriers and best solutions, but better equity must ultimately involve a discussion of reallocating resources. What defines equity is different in each country and depends on social and cultural factors as well as political.[7] As we have seen, one useful way to begin this discussion is to distinguish between equity in finance and equity in delivery and to measure equity in terms of outcomes, process, and structure.

---

[7]The social and cultural issues are discussed in Chapter 6, while the political issues are discussed more fully in Chapter 7.

A third point, described more completely in Chapter 2, is that significant data gaps exist. The gaps hinder the ability to precisely assess inequities. In the extreme, lack of data means that inequities are undetected and untreated. Furthermore, being able to precisely identify specific inequities within a region or population is critical if policymakers are to selectively intervene with strategies that are the most effective and least costly. Without precise data, policymakers are likely to implement programs that do not reach the vulnerable populations most in need of support; they are also likely to implement programs that reach people who do not need the help, thus wasting valuable and scarce resources.

Fourth, in the absence of data and evaluation, policy may lead to interventions that actually make inequities worse. A common example seen in Asian countries is publicly supported urban hospitals that subsidize the more affluent within the cities and not the rural poor. This type of unfair subsidy may happen either because policymakers are not aware of the inequity or because, in the absence of data, decisions can be made for purely political reasons.

Fifth, to improve equity, governments should focus their policies on redirecting their subsidies toward the financing, and in some cases the delivery, of services to the poor. Subsidies can be allocated in different ways—by geographic targeting, differential pricing, and clinical targeting. The exact strategy depends on such factors as concentration of the poor, disease prevalence, and health care (e.g., prenatal) needs.

CHAPTER 6: SUMMARY OF POLICY QUESTIONS, FINDINGS, AND IMPLICATIONS

ISSUES	EVIDENCE
• What is involved in changing health behaviors?	• Changing health behaviors requires understanding the factors that affect them and designing interventions accordingly.
• How can individuals be changed/motivated to improve their health-seeking behavior?	• If designed properly, a mix of education and communication techniques can be used to change individual behavior.
• How effective have countries been in changing individuals' behavior?	• Education and communication programs have proven useful for promotive, preventive, and prescriptive interventions but should be used in concert with other programs.
• How can provider practices be changed?	• Adhering to a set of established principles increases the opportunity for changing provider behavior.
• How effective have countries been in changing provider practices?	• Despite sparse evidence, guidelines and CME show promise, but implementation difficulties abound.
• What can be done to include stakeholders and develop consensus?	• If designed properly, community participation strategies can encourage participation and build consensus.
• How effective have countries been in including stakeholders and developing consensus?	• Community participation strategies show promise, but are resource-intensive and hard to sustain.

POLICY IMPLICATIONS

- Policymakers should devote more resources than they currently do to conducting behavioral studies.

- Policymakers should carefully plan and evaluate health promotion strategies at a pilot level before implementing them on a larger scale.

- Education activities should not be used alone and should be integrated with other interventions.

- Policymakers should ensure that commissioned studies are grounded in conceptual frameworks or models about how to change behavior.

- In trying to change provider behavior, policymakers should combine, at a minimum, such approaches as education, guidelines, financial incentives, and regulatory sanctions.

GOVERNMENT AND THE IMPROVEMENT
OF HEALTH BEHAVIORS

OVERVIEW

The ultimate objective of health care services is to improve health status. In Chapter 3, we saw that choosing the right set of clinical interventions is critical to achieving better health within constrained resources. Chapters 4 and 5 discussed ensuring that all people can afford, and have access to, those interventions. In addition, ensuring that the appropriate medical infrastructure and institutions are in place is also key to achieving better health, as we will see in the next chapter.

However, none of these factors is enough to guarantee improvements in health status. Any intervention—whether clinical or enabling—will not improve the health of individuals if the individuals do not choose to take advantage of it, or if providers do not offer the intervention to their patients. For example, a government can decide to fight a measles epidemic by providing immunizations for children, by allocating public subsidies away from curative services and toward the primary preventive care services, and by geographically targeting communities most in need of measles immunization. None of these interventions, however, will improve measles immunizations for children if the parents do not choose to bring their children into the clinics that provide the service and if community health workers are not skilled.

Figure 6.1 expands the relationship presented in Figure 2.1 to show how health policy affects health status and is mediated by changing behaviors of the stakeholders. The various interests and incentives of each stakeholder must be considered before policy can be transformed into better health outcomes.

As the figure shows, individuals' (patients') attitudes, behaviors, and lifestyles are fundamentally important to their health status and to the actions they take to

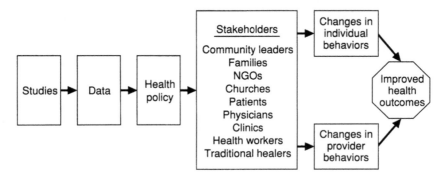

**Figure 6.1—Process to Design Changes in Health Behaviors That
Lead to Improved Health**

improve it. Just as important, providers also make choices about the care they provide their patients based on their own attitudes, behaviors, and lifestyles. In addition, the interaction between individuals and providers and the management of interests of multiple stakeholders in health systems are critical to changing health status. The bottom line is that health policy interventions must contain a component designed to change and motivate the behavior of all those involved.

Given this need to change and motivate behavior, we can formulate seven interrelated questions. We further divide them into questions of what is known about changing behaviors and how effectively change has been implemented:

1. What is involved in changing health behaviors?
2. How can individuals be changed/motivated to improve their health-seeking behavior?
3. How effective have countries been in changing individuals' behaviors?
4. How can provider practices be changed?
5. How effective have countries been in changing providers' practices?
6. What can be done to include stakeholders and develop consensus?
7. How effective have countries been in including stakeholders and developing consensus?

The answers to these questions form the basis of the remainder of this chapter.

INTERVENTIONS TO CHANGE HEALTH BEHAVIORS

What makes it so difficult to change health behaviors in a country is that so many factors—most of them not quantifiable—are involved in creating those behaviors in the first place. Figure 2.2 described these factors as cultural, social, political, and institutional. Here we look at them as they relate to individual behavior.

At the broadest level, "culture"— defined as the shared system of knowledge, values, religious beliefs, customs, and practices—shapes individuals' models of how the world works (e.g., beliefs about disease causation, prognosis, and cure). For example, ethnic groups often differ in their acceptance of specific types of service. Women from several West African ethnic groups but with similar income, education, and access to prenatal care services use services with different frequency. (See Barlow and Diop, 1995.) Similarly, families in Tamil Nadu, India, attend the medical college's outpatient clinic for simple diarrhea "dorsham," but they consult traditional healers for "dorham," which is a more serious form of diarrhea. They consider dorham a matter of ritual pollution that allopathic medicine cannot help. (See Weiss, 1988; Wouters, 1992.) Gender preferences for children, in which parents more frequently seek health care for boys than girls, also have been documented in India and Bangladesh. (See Ganatra and Hirve, 1994; Paul, 1992.)

Such cultural beliefs about disease causation, prognosis, and cure are tenacious, following people when they move from one country to another. In one study of tuberculosis among Vietnamese immigrants in New York state, researchers found that many of those they interviewed maintained strong culturally based beliefs about the disease. Nearly half of those interviewed believed tuberculosis was caused by hard manual labor or smoking, and a little less than half felt that modern medicines were not needed to treat the disease or that a physician's advice on treatment was not important. (See Carey et al., 1997.)

Beyond culturally based beliefs, an intricate web of social relationships with family, friends, and coworkers influences health-related decisions. These relationships will define both the social support that can be counted on in case of illness and the reciprocal obligations to provide support to others. For example, in a study about how to treat neonatal hypothermia in China, researchers noted that Chinese mothers are traditionally confined to bed for one month after giving birth, so that when babies become ill, they are brought to the hospital by other family members. More specifically, surveys showed that fathers brought them 82 percent of the time. Given this understanding about how families behave, researchers realized that preventive education programs needed to be directed to fathers. (See Peabody et al., 1996b.)

Political and economic systems mobilize resources to protect or restore well-being, but they also influence lifestyle choices that affect health. These systems not only shape the local communities in which individuals live, but also connect them to larger-scale national and global systems. Anti-smoking campaigns, for example, have grown from localized public health efforts to a global referendum. In more-affluent countries, voluntary (e.g., airlines) and regulatory initiatives (e.g., smoke-free workplaces) have led to decreases in smoking prevalence. These growing efforts have gradually transcended national boundaries and now form an effective counterforce against international tobacco interests.

Within the cultural, social, political, and institutional context, health care delivery can be characterized in terms of three partly overlapping approaches: popular, folk, and professional. Most illness is managed in the popular sector. This includes health-related activities by individuals, family members, or personal social networks. Serious or persistent illness may warrant recourse to the professional sector, where individuals go seeking a healing specialist (a physician) or an institution (a hospital). Care in this sector is organized and regulated with formal standards of care and training. Alternatively, care may be obtained in the folk sector from practitioners who function without formal regulation, such as traditional religious or secular healers. (See Kleinman, 1978, 1980.)

Policy development for health improvements should be conducted with an appreciation for the multiple determinants of behavior and the contextual layers into which changes will be introduced. This means recognizing the complexity and interconnections of the systems in which interventions occur and considering the wide range of effects that initiatives may have. It also means being open to questions about the cultural appropriateness of policies and being willing to investigate and make adjustments when undesired effects are encountered.

Because community, health, and other systems are complex and closely interwoven, it can be difficult to design policies that achieve intended results in one area without producing undesired side effects in other areas. For example, efforts to improve living standards by developing rural infrastructures may result in the more rapid spread of infectious diseases because of increased population mobility. Likewise, changes in the medical system may be resisted or undermined by forces intrinsic to other systems. Policies designed to protect individual

---

Box 6.1: Culture and Individual Behavior: AIDS in Thailand

The epidemic of HIV/AIDS sweeping across Asia is a major health threat in the region and has severe social consequences. Because no curative therapy exists and no affordable treatment is available in developing countries, most control efforts have focused on prevention. Therefore, understanding the social and cultural contexts of behaviors that promote transmission is especially important in designing programs to control the disease.

Thailand has been hit especially hard by HIV/AIDS. From the initial cases that appeared in 1984, the incidence has exploded in the 1990s to seroprevalence rates of 30 percent or more in high-risk groups. By 1993, an estimated 750,000 were infected. (See Weniger and Brown, 1996.) Since the majority of cases are occurring in young, economically productive people, the social impact of AIDS in Thailand has been severe. While initial cases appeared in homosexuals and IV drug users, the rapid increase in cases of late has been primarily among commercial sex workers and their customers, and from them to subsequent contacts (wives, newborns).

Several social factors have contributed to this pattern. Economic development has shifted resources and job opportunities to urban areas and stimulated migration of young people from rural areas to the cities. Migration away from villages and the adoption of less circumscribed lifestyles have reduced the influence of family and other social institutions over young people's sexual activity. Once infected through contacts in urban areas, young people frequently return to their villages and spread the disease locally.

Traditional norms of sexual behavior may also have promoted transmission. While most young women are expected to remain chaste, young men are given more license. Much early sexual activity for men takes place with commercial sex workers, typically in high-volume, low-paying brothels staffed by young women lured from rural areas by promises of jobs. Visits to brothels are also a forum for social activity and bonding among male peer groups. (See Muecke 1992; MacQueen et al., 1996.)

After initially downplaying the epidemic, the Thai government has mounted an aggressive campaign to fight the spread of HIV. Social research on factors contributing to transmission has helped enhance the effectiveness of this campaign. The major elements of the control program have included educational programs in elementary schools, workplaces, and community settings; a media campaign, primarily through televised messages; and a major effort to promote condom use in brothels, with a goal of 100 percent compliance. (See Nelsen et al., 1996.)

There is evidence that these efforts are having a significant effect on reducing the spread of HIV in Thailand. Awareness of the disease and risk factors is high. Brothel activity by Thai men is declining, while use of condoms and treatment of STDs have increased dramatically. And rates of new cases among young men seem to be declining. (See Nelsen et al., 1996.)

---

health—for example, controlling tobacco use—may be resisted by groups for whom the economic consequences are detrimental, such as farmers and small-scale retailers.

Fortunately, as mentioned earlier in Chapter 2, methods are available to generate critical information about cultural and social factors that can be used in policy development. Ethnographic research (such as the work that determined the critical role of fathers in preventing neonatal hypothermia in China) can develop information on local cultural values, decisionmaking processes, social networks, and political structures; such research uses a variety of methods—participant observation, qualitative interviewing, surveys, and social network analysis.

For example, researchers have constructed a survey to understand the separate and combined importance of cultural, infrastructure, and clinical factors in treatment-seeking behavior of women in low-income urban areas. The survey— designed to be implemented in Kampala, Uganda—explicitly includes questions intended to get at the importance of social support, social life, networks, and autonomy in why women seek treatment. (See Wallman and Baker, 1996.) Methodologies such as "focused ethnography" and "rapid ethnographic assessment" have been developed to obtain policy-relevant information on cultural factors in a timely manner. (See Manderson and Aby, 1992; Scrimshaw and Gleason, 1992; Beebe, 1995; Bennett, 1995.) Surveys and focus group interviews also can be used to inform policy development and implementation, as well as to analyze the results of policy initiatives and explore causes of any unintended outcomes. (See Khan and Manderson, 1992.)

To ensure that ethnographic studies yield valuable policy information leading to behavioral change, it is important to pursue research that will improve measurements of cultural variables. It is also important to use protocols to conduct the studies. For example, two ethnographic studies were performed in Bolivia to examine parents' understanding of ARI in children using a protocol developed by WHO. The studies concluded that prior planning—e.g., ensuring that disease control programs have the necessary resources and personnel for program activities—was necessary to translate ethnographic data into concrete program-relevant actions. (See Hudelson et al., 1995.)

Policymakers need to understand more generally how any behavior is formed and how it can be changed. Given the complexity of the factors that influence behavior, being able to conceptually model such influences is valuable. There are a number of models that seek to explain how behavior develops and how it can be changed. One such model is shown in Figure 6.2. The model, by Ajzen and Fishbein, highlights two important factors that affect individuals' actions: their underlying belief structures about what they should do (personal belief structures), and their perceptions of what others think they should do (social and cultural norms). (See Ajzen and Fishbein, 1980.) These factors lead to an intention to act and, ultimately, to a behavior. Therefore, to influence health behaviors, desired behaviors must be shown to be consistent with personal or professional beliefs, as well as with the cultural values and social norms within which they live and function.

Another model—known as the transtheoretical model (TM) of behavioral change (or the stages-of-change model)—has been used for years to help researchers design intervention components to help change health behaviors. (See Prochaska and DiClemente, 1983, 1984; Prochaska et al., 1992.) The model describes behavioral change as an incremental process that proceeds through five stages: precontemplation, contemplation, preparation, action, and maintenance.

The major value of developing and using such models is that they lend a framework and a credibility and rigor to what is essentially a qualitative process. Unlike many clinical interventions, where one can actually witness the impact of the intervention on health status, interventions that change behavior do not necessarily lead to observable changes in individuals' health status—the behavior might lead to health improvements that would not be manifested for many years

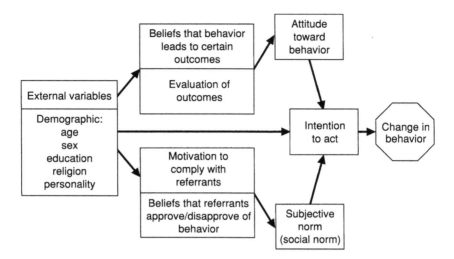

SOURCE: Based on Social Change Theory of Ajzen and Fishbein (1980).

Figure 6.2—A Model of How to Change Behavior

or even in the next generation. Or there might be no change at all if the intervention targets the wrong behavior or if other important factors harming health are also not corrected. So it is important to distinguish between the change in the behavior itself, the effects that behavior change may have on health status, and the effects of other factors.

For example, one could claim that an individual who changed behavior to practice safe sex did so as the result of a health education program designed to promote safe sex. However, it is possible that the behavior change was the result of witnessing a close friend die of AIDS and had nothing to do with the intervention. Similarly, on the provider side, one could claim that a provider changed his patient care behavior as a result of voluntary clinical guidelines or financial incentives, when in reality the change resulted from watching one of his patients die from inappropriate treatment. Being able to separate out these exogenous factors is critical in determining whether interventions to change behavior (as part of interventions to improve health status) actually work and should thus be funded by policymakers.

Beyond understanding the factors that influence behavior change, understanding the nature of how people change also has important design and evaluation implications. Knowing that change is incremental and hard to maintain, for example, means that studies evaluating behavioral change in relation to changes in health status should be longitudinally designed. In other words, even if a study shows that behavior changed and that, as a result, health status improved, the behavior change (and the positive change in health status) may dissipate over time; so a study that is not longitudinal may overrate the effectiveness of the intervention. And, of course, the converse is also true: A study design that only measures behavior change over a short time frame may show that the change did not work and did not affect health status, when, in reality, it did work (and affect health status) in the long term.

Box 6.2: Focus Group Discussions with Village Women in China

Women are central to any country's primary health-care agenda because they are responsible not only for their own health but also for that of their children. A starting point for interventions to improve health is to gain a critical understanding of women's perceptions of the health needs and problems of their families and themselves and how these issues are linked to their daily lives. Wong et al. (1995) used focus groups with rural village women in Yunnan, China, for this purpose. What they learned from the focus groups highlights the power of this ethnographic technique, when used carefully and with respect for the participants.

The focus groups were undertaken by the Women's Reproductive Health and Development Program in Yunnan as part of an effort to develop community-based mechanisms for developing and evaluating health improvement activities in poor communities. The focus groups were one element of the needs assessment. A total of 28 separate discussions were conducted over a two-week period, with 169 women participating. Discussion guides were prepared that covered women's perceptions of the most pressing health concerns and issues in their villages; of their concerns about reproductive health, including family planning; of their perceptions of work and family life in the villages; and of their roles in the home and community. The facilitators and recorders of the focus groups received training in focus group methods that consisted of role playing, testing and revising questions, and final pilot focus group discussions to check procedures. Women were selected to participate in the focus groups based on demographic criteria.

Below is an example of what the women said about their labor burdens and health:

"Ai! Who has time to think about their health? We rural women get up early when it's still dark, and don't stop working until we drop into bed at night. Working like that is already enough to make life miserable. We don't have any time to think about how to protect our health. Just give us more time to rest!"

And here is an example about what they said about women's and men's shares of work:

"Of course, men take care of the heavier tasks while women do the lighter chores. Men and women are equal, but I always have more work to do."

Finally, here is an example of what they do when they do not feel well:

"If I don't feel well, I usually don't say anything to anyone. After a while, I usually feel better. My family becomes concerned only if I can't do my work."

The focus groups clearly showed how the women's time and energy are dominated by their daily work demands and lower social position than men, affecting their health status and every aspect of their approach to seeking health care. This implies that service hours and methods for reaching village women must be compatible with their work schedules, and that they must be provided with support for their daily responsibilities so they have enough time to obtain health services.

EDUCATION AND COMMUNICATION TECHNIQUES

Individuals make three basic kinds of choices about their health. They make *promotive* choices that influence their health (e.g., eating a balanced diet or not smoking). They make *preventive* choices about seeking health care (e.g., getting immunizations, seeking prenatal care, and improving sanitation practices). And they make *prescriptive* choices about seeking treatment and following medical advice (e.g., completing a course of medication or returning for follow-up care).

Effective health promotion activities, consisting of a mix of education and communication (E&C) programs, can encourage people to make better choices in each of these areas. For example, in the promotion and prevention areas, programs often include educational activities aimed at individuals. These are combined with community or nationwide promotion initiatives to motivate people to change personal behavior. E&C programs are common for hygiene, for dietary habits, for knowing when to obtain immunizations or knowing when to seek care for, say, ARI. In the prescription area, E&C programs are often conducted individually to guide patients in managing health conditions (education on diet for people with diabetes; or instruction in taking prescribed antibiotics).

Such health promotion programs are a public good: Most educational messages benefit entire population groups, yet the suppliers have no way to obtain payment from all individuals benefited. Private providers have few financial incentives to undertake these programs. Thus, E&C programs are usually sponsored by governments and nongovernmental organizations and are viewed as a public investment in health. They are also investments in cost control, since they seek general reductions in the incidence of preventable health conditions or undesirable individual behaviors (e.g., motor vehicle injuries related to substance abuse).

While E&C programs provide potentially powerful techniques that can yield enduring new behavior patterns, many have not been shown to improve health outcomes. Thus, E&C programs need to be carefully designed to be effective. More specifically, an E&C program should consist of:

- an assessment of health education needs and priorities,
- an intervention strategy to change behaviors, and
- an evaluation of the impacts of the program.

An Assessment of Health Education Needs

Over the years, health educators have developed a number of conceptual models of the factors that contribute to human health behaviors. Three of the best-known models are shown in Table 6.1. Researchers have found that educational programs that use these or similar behavioral models to guide the choice of their intervention techniques were more effective. (See Richards, 1975; Kanaaneh, 1977; Simmons, 1978; Cox et al., 1983.)

As a result of experience with health education programs, several intervention guidelines have been identified. The guidelines are based on the principle that individuals must be responsible for their own actions, while having available support and contact continuity through education program personnel. Other principles are that interventions should have an individualized approach, a positive orientation for the message, and a focus on overcoming resistances or obstacles to achieving the behavior change. (See Simmons, 1978.)

Johanssen has identified four ways in which information programs must succeed to change individual behaviors. (See Johanssen, 1990.) Failure in any one of these elements will prevent a program from having its desired effects. First, the information transmitted must be understood by the users. Second, the information

Table 6.1

Well-Known Conceptual Models of Factors Contributing to Human Health Behaviors

Epidemiological	Health Belief	Diagnostic Systems
BASIC THEORY		
Behavior is the result of the relationship among host, agent, and environment	Internal and external forces influence an individual's movement toward a goal	Freely chosen behavior is determined mainly by personal factors, but also by situational factors
MODEL VARIABLES		
Personal Readiness (Host)	**Readiness to Undertake**	**Multiple Influences**
1. Recognition of problem	**Recommended Behavior**	1. Cultural and political
2. Acceptance of vulnerability	1. Motivations—health concern,	2. Socioeconomic
3. Predisposition to act	intent to comply	3. Demographic
4. Motivation to act	2. Value to reduce threat—	4. Social psychological
5. Ability to act	susceptibility to illness and	5. Individual status
6. Belief in desired action	extent of harm	6. Environmental
	3. Potential to reduce threat—	
Social Control (Environment)	efficacy and safety of	**Decision to Act**
1. Social pressure to act	behavior	1. Psychological readiness
2. Include in role		2. Start with trial
3. Acceptability of action	**Modifying/Enabling Factors**	3. Rejection if dissatisfied
	1. Demographics	4. Stable behavior if
Situation or Action (Agent)	2. Structural (costs, access)	satisfied
1. Effectiveness of action	3. Attitudes	
2. Pleasure of action	4. Provider interactions	**Change in Health Status**
3. Effort of action	5. Enabling (experience)	1. Influences as feedback
4. Previous experience		2. Leads to behavior
5. Favorable environment		change
EDUCATIONAL INTERVENTION		
The intervention (agent) has prominence over effects of host or environment	Base educational strategies on cues from an index of questions based on variables	Use persuasive communication to change attitude in favor of trial and adoption

SOURCE: Simmons, 1978.

must be accurate (or true) in the specific circumstances in which the user tries to apply it. Third, the person must be motivated to apply the information regularly and efficiently. Finally, the user must have the necessary resources, such as time or money, to support application of the new information. The first two factors relate to the educational, social, and cultural aspects of individuals' lives, while the last two relate to their individual health priorities and economic circumstances.

An Intervention Strategy

A key part of the intervention strategy for health promotion programs is how information is communicated. The evidence suggests that person-to-person communications are better than mass-media communications—television, printed material, telephone, and radio. For example, mass-media campaigns to improve nutritional status may be less effective than the same amount of money spent to provide nutrition education as part of home visits.

Why are person-to-person communications so effective? By participating in two-way communications with community members or patients, health workers develop relationships and are available to respond to questions and concerns. When health workers are treating children for ARI, for example, they can talk with parents and understand their concerns and level of knowledge and can teach them how to recognize and manage respiratory problems. This approach is consistent with traditions of "person-focused interest" that prevail in the cultures of most developing countries and with the existence of traditional social networks that are amenable to personal communication. (See Kanaaneh, 1977.)

Mass-media communications, by contrast, have limited use in developing countries. Many families cannot afford televisions or telephones, and high rates of illiteracy preclude the use of written materials, thus limiting the audience to the relatively small segment of urban and better-educated residents. Some remote communities distrust the urbanizing effect of audiovisual materials. (See Kanaaneh, 1977.) One Australian study evaluated 5,710 respondents after 588 health and sponsorship projects were completed between 1992 and 1994. Two-thirds were aware of the messages, 55 percent understood the messages, but only 4 percent intended to take action. "Action" was generously defined as either adopting the behavior or seeking more information. (See Hollman et al., 1996.) However, while mass-media communications have been found to be less effective than personal communication in motivating or introducing attitudinal and behavioral change, they can inform and reinforce the evolution of new attitudes. (See Richards, 1975; Simmons, 1978.) Recognition of mass media's persuasive powers, in this context, has been growing. (See Population Reports, 1986.)

As a result, mass media are being increasingly treated as components of larger systems, which are used in combination to reinforce each other. For example, a combination of radio and widely distributed flyers with color-coded pictograms was used in The Gambia to teach mothers how to mix ORS for treatment of infant diarrhea. A radio voice guided them through the information on the flyer, which they also had available for later reference. (See Population Reports, 1980.) In Bangladesh, Indonesia, and Nepal, social marketing campaigns used radio to sell brand-name contraceptives at subsidized prices through existing commercial outlets. (See Population Reports, 1985.) A variety of formats have been used for radio or television media, such as spot announcements, news broadcasts, interviews, talks, group discussions, and dramatic presentations. (See Population Reports, 1986.)

Where possible, counseling should be combined with techniques that enable people to learn by doing, with health workers providing guidance and feedback. An early example of this approach is rural nutrition rehabilitation centers in India that involve mothers directly in preparing foods to help in treating their malnourished children. (See Bengoa, 1974; Shah et al., 1975.)

An Evaluation Program

Ongoing controversy over whether and how to use E&C interventions to change individual behaviors is partly a consequence of the suboptimal evaluations that have been performed on these programs. In a review of over 65 journal articles that evaluated health education programs in developing countries, Loevinsohn found that only 21 percent were controlled studies employing sample sizes large enough to draw inferences with confidence, 33 percent looked at changes in health status, and only 33 percent looked at the ultimate changes in health behaviors. Only three of the articles had all desired methodological characteristics. (See Loevinsohn, 1990.) Similar conclusions were reached in a study of evaluations of water supply and sanitation projects, which cited such methodological limitations as a lack of adequate control groups, confounding variables, an inadequate health indicator definition, and a lack of control for seasonality effects. (See Blum and Feachem, 1983.)

Because so little is known about the effectiveness of health promotions, an evaluation component must be an integral part of the project design when a new health behavior intervention is developed. Standard prospective case studies are an appropriate starting point for designing health education evaluations. They should begin with the development of measurable hypotheses of educational impacts (outcomes) using a conceptual model of behavior. Outcomes for control groups and intervention target groups need to be compared; the outcome measures should be carefully defined; and complete and accurate data on these measures should be collected.

As we discussed in the previous section, a key design decision is how to define the effectiveness of educational inputs. Measures might be developed for changes in personal behaviors (an intermediate outcome) or changes in health status (an ultimate policy goal), or both. The ability to measure the diversity of factors that can affect behaviors and, therefore, to control for their effects in evaluating program impacts is a methodological challenge that is especially critical and difficult for educational program evaluations.

An important point to underscore is that measuring changed behaviors is not the same as distinguishing the contributions of specific interventions to those outcomes. The latter element is one of the hardest parts of evaluating health behavior interventions, because education is only one of many, often interacting, factors that contribute to behavior change. This highlights the value of having control groups whenever possible and using an underlying conceptual model of the determinants of behavior to guide the design of both the health promotion strategy itself and the evaluation of its impacts.

Therefore, the E&C programs should be designed and implemented with the following considerations in mind:

1. **The design of an educational intervention program should specify target population groups and reflect a thorough understanding of the knowledge and motivations of these groups.** This should include the individuals' level of knowledge, perceptions, and beliefs about the desired health behavior, as well as any external constraints on their ability to change behaviors.

2. **Where appropriate, educational activities should be integrated with other interventions to achieve cost-effective health improvement impacts.** In many cases, neither direct interventions nor education alone can achieve desired changes in behaviors and health status. In other cases, one or the other type of intervention may have a primary role. Determining their respective roles should be an integral part of designing an intervention program.

3. **Any new educational program should be tested before broad implementation.** This could be done using pilot projects to measure costs and effectiveness and to test the program's clinical and

administrative procedures in the field. Information from process and outcome evaluations of the pilots should be used to modify programs before full implementation and to eliminate those found not to be cost-effective.

4. **Local practitioners should be empowered to provide and coordinate treatment and education services, consistent with their skill levels.** Depending on local resources, practitioners providing health services may range from physicians to lightly trained health workers. Adequate training and authority to provide care can enhance the skills and position of practitioners, improving their responsiveness to local needs and their credibility with community members.

5. **When mass-media messages are used, they should be designed to reinforce individual-level education activities.** Mass media can be effective in broadcasting persuasive messages for changing health behaviors, often working best as a component of a combined strategy that uses direct counseling along with a mix of communication media. Messages should be relevant to the beliefs, social, and cultural orientation of the audiences. Using social marketing techniques, repeated messages should be scheduled strategically to achieve message penetration.

6. **All education programs must have evaluation components and should continue to be modified in response to evaluation feedback on their performance.** Evaluation should be an integral part of any health education intervention, whether it is a free-standing program or part of a broader intervention. A program's cost-effectiveness should be evaluated periodically, using data about program operation and behavioral and health outcomes collected on an ongoing basis.

USING EDUCATION AND COMMUNICATION PROGRAMS

As mentioned earlier, individuals make promotive, preventive, and prescriptive choices about their health. Within these three categories, governments may wish to encourage many health-related behaviors. Here, we examine examples of how Asian countries have used E&C activities, together with service delivery, to achieve health improvements for their residents. The examples chosen represent important public health issues for most Asian countries, and the experiences cited reveal the variety of approaches that can be taken, depending on a country's cultural foundation and policy priorities.

Promotive Choices

In terms of promotive choices, we look at experience with two programs: management of nutritional requirements and family planning.

Management of Nutritional Requirements. Poor economic status and inadequate knowledge of nutritional needs have contributed to malnutrition in developing countries and among the poor in developed countries. One form of malnutrition is the inability to meet energy and protein requirements for an active and healthy life. (See Pinstrup-Andersen et al., 1993.) Another is deficiencies in micronutrients, such as Vitamin A, iron, or iodine. (See Levin et al., 1993.) Determinants of protein-energy malnutrition (PEM) include access to food, sufficiency of energy and protein intake, infectious diseases, breastfeeding practices, knowledge of nutrition and behavior, access to sanitation and water, and household financial status. (See also Chapter 3.)

Programs to improve protein-energy nutritional status have used diverse combination of food supplementation, economic subsidies, and educational interventions to improve health status. As part of nutrition programs, E&C plays a supportive function within larger intervention strategies. Reviews of nutrition education programs show that well-designed and well-implemented education interventions can stimulate desired behavior changes at relatively low cost. Successful participatory models have been completed in Indonesia, the Dominican Republic, Tanzania, and India. In most cases, these programs simultaneously monitored children's growth, so that education played a dual role as an information source and a coordination role for all the intervention strategies. (See Hornic, 1988.) In China, a breastfeeding promotion program for local women increased knowledge and, after four months, was associated with more than double the breastfeeding rate of the controls (44 percent versus 21 percent).

Complementarity has been found between these diverse interventions—nutrition education and such direct interventions as food supplementation, improved household resources, and food price subsidies—leading to the conclusion that integrated strategies may yield synergies in health improvement impacts. (See Pinstrup-Andersen et al., 1993.) One study in a Bangladeshi urban slum found, however, that a combination of education and food supplementation had no greater long-term effect on children's weight gain than education alone (which also had a limited impact). Although the lack of difference between the two strategies could not be explained, the author indicated that a possible reason for the limited effect of education alone was the lack of funds to buy ingredients required for the high-energy diet. (See Fauveau et al., 1992.)

Throughout the developing world, inadequate intake or absorption of micronutrients is associated with a high incidence of both physical and mental health problems that have serious social, private, and economic costs. Information on prevalence and intervention methods is most complete for iron, iodine, and Vitamin A. Iron deficiency results in anemia, often leading to cognitive dysfunction in children and fatigue and compromised immunity in adults. Iodine deficiency has its greatest effects on the fetus, women, and children, leading to postnatal dwarfism, mental retardation in children, and increased risk of perinatal mortality. Vitamin A deficiency causes night blindness, conjunctival dryness, and increased risk of respiratory and diarrheal disease. (See also Chapter 3.) (See Levin et al., 1993.)

Similar to PEM interventions, programs to prevent micronutrient malnutrition involve a mix of direct and indirect interventions. Health education techniques are used to support fortification and ensure that individuals consume the nutrients they are provided. Communication campaigns were needed to create demand for fortified salt in India and Guatemala, and failure to support fortification interventions with education was identified as a significant reason for the failure of programs in Central and South America. (See Levin et al., 1993.) Support, counseling, and concern demonstrated by the health care provider can be important factors in patient compliance, as shown by studies of compliance with iron supplementation. (See Galloway and McGuire, 1994.) General nutrition education also contributes to micronutrient malnutrition reduction efforts. For example, a control-comparison study documented that health education increased the percentage of mothers who fed their children green leafy vegetables, which are a source of Vitamin A. (See Rahman et al., 1994.)

Little reliable information exists on the cost-effectiveness of nutrition education. Cost data are particularly difficult to get when education is an integral part of larger programs. Cost-effectiveness information, however, has been developed for two PEM education programs, one in Indonesia and the other in the Dominican Republic, that successfully used a social marketing strategy to improve the nutritional status of children. (See Pinstrup-Andersen et al., 1993.)

Policymakers can use such estimates, with comparisons to those for other interventions, to formulate nutrition intervention strategies. Given the mix of activities usually required to combat malnutrition, it is reasonable to evaluate complete programs rather than individual components.

Family Planning. Health interventions to change family planning behaviors is a unique field. At one level, lengthening birth intervals has significant benefits for the health of the mother, for the infant's birthweight, and for the health and survival rates of subsequent children. But family planning programs seek to reduce the total number of children born, generally beyond the effect that increased birth intervals would have. A short-term motivation for this agenda is to reduce the costs of education and public health investments for the new generation of children. A more long-term concern is to reduce the congestion and demand on physical resources that accompanies population growth (a goal not unanimously held by all policymakers).

Family planning programs at the government level are one component of a broader set of interventions to prevent excess fertility. Direct determinants of fertility are patterns of marriage and exposure to pregnancy, breastfeeding practices, abortions, and contraception or direct fertility regulation activities. Economic development and education are documented to be among the strongest factors in reducing fertility, leading to later marriages and preferences by women for a smaller number of children. (See Cochrane and Sai, 1993; Gertler and Molyneaux, 1994.) Family planning programs reinforce these activities by educating women on the benefits of smaller families and on methods to prevent conception and manage unwanted pregnancies and by providing contraceptive materials and services.

Over the past few decades, family planning strategies have evolved from simple distribution of contraceptive information and supplies to programs that are more integrated with development and health programs. A classic example is the Pakistan population program. For many years, its "contraception inundation" program focused on distributing supplies and had little effect on fertility rates. Policy support for integrated programs was formalized when the 1994 United Nations Conference on Population and Development endorsed the notion of sustainable development and sanctioned the need for cooperation among family planning, health services, government, and nongovernment organizations. This orientation views people, especially women, as subjects of programs rather than objects. (See Khan, 1996.)

The success of family planning programs in reducing fertility depends on creating demand for contraception and then effectively responding to that demand with supplies, education, and related medical services. Although debate continues about whether demand-creation or supply-based programs are more effective, it is more productive to view them as complementary, perhaps synergistic, activities. Education programs to stimulate demand have used combinations of mass-media campaigns, community education programs, and individual counseling. Radio campaigns, for example, have been used extensively by Asian countries, some of the earliest beginning in the 1960s in South Korea, Taiwan, Pakistan, India, and the Philippines. Bangladesh, Indonesia, Hong Kong, Sri Lanka, Nepal, and China are among others that have used radio in more recent years. Programming has ranged from family planning dramas to social marketing of contraceptives sold through commercial outlets at subsidized prices. Few programs, however, have formally evaluated their impacts on fertility. (See Population Reports, 1986.)

The contraceptive services project in Matlab, Bangladesh, is an experimental program that successfully induced and sustained fertility decline in a rural traditional population of married and fecund women. Women were visited fortnightly by project consultants, who talked with them about their contraceptive needs and encouraged them to adopt contraception. The consultants were young married women who were residents of the village. Supplies and services were made immediately available for all choices of contraceptive or sterilization methods. Following these two interventions, a rapid and sustained increase in use of contraception occurred. (See Phillips et al., 1988.) Which intervention—the demand-inducing education and promotion or the supply-subsidizing services—causes the rapid increase in contraceptive use? The authors reported that a preliminary program that simply distributed supplies had little impact on utilization.

Family planning programs in Pakistan and China offer contrasting examples of some of the policy, political, and bureaucratic issues involved in many government-operated programs. Whereas China's program has been mandatory under an aggressive national policy to reduce population growth, Pakistan's program has suffered from lack of clear policy direction since its inception in the 1960s. But the programs share implementation problems related to their design as centralized government programs that have not allowed local units to adapt intervention strategies to the needs and preferences of the communities. They also have suffered from inadequately trained personnel and supply problems. (See Khan, 1996.) The impacts of China's program on fertility reduction can be related as much to its mandatory nature as to the quality of its family planning services. In Pakistan, by contrast, there may be demand for contraception that has yet to be met by the existing program capabilities.

Preventive Choices

In terms of preventive choices, we examine the experience for two key interventions: prevention of AIDS and sanitation practices.

Prevention of AIDS. Public health strategies to prevent acquired immuno-deficiency syndrome (AIDS) highlight the close relationships among health behaviors for many health problems. Until recently, STDs were controlled primarily by early detection and treatment of disease, together with tracking exposures through sexual partners. But this approach does not work for a disease that has no effective or affordable treatment methods, of which AIDS is the paramount example. (See Cates and Hinman, 1992.) Prevention of infection by modifying health behaviors currently is the only way to limit the spread of HIV and control AIDS in developing countries. Sexual practices is one set of behaviors through which AIDS is transmitted. Another is needle-sharing by intravenous drug users (IDU), which transfers small quantities of infected blood. Mother-to-child transmission is the third form of transmission. Thus, education for AIDS control can be performed independently or integrated into family planning, maternal and child health, and drug-use prevention and treatment programs.

Government responses, however, have varied substantially, partly reflecting differences in disease epidemiologies and partly as a result of political forces derived from social and cultural traditions. For example, Thailand has responded strongly to reduce the high incidence of AIDS transmitted through sexual contacts with prostitutes (see Nelsen et al., 1996), as well as to reduce incidence related to IDU. (See Riehman, 1996.) In Indonesia, where the prevalence of both AIDS and IDU is low, intervention programs are only in early development and focus on controlling sexual transmission through commercial sex. (See Ford et al., 1994.) On the other hand, despite a growing HIV/AIDS risk, India and the Philippines were slow to initiate prevention programs, both because of cultural taboos about sexual behavior and a tendency to view AIDS as a medical problem. Interventions to prevent IDU infection already are under way, and those for sexual behaviors recently appear to be gaining momentum. (See Riehman, 1996; Asthana, 1996.)

Educational interventions to reduce both sexual and drug use transmission of HIV/AIDS often combine encouragement for discontinuing a behavior (e.g., intravenous drug use or sexual contacts with prostitutes) with education on safer practices of that behavior (e.g., sterilization of needles or use of condoms). Most programs have focused on safe practices, finding that people tend to be more willing to change a behavior than to discontinue it altogether. (See Meheus et al., 1990; Riehman, 1996.) This pragmatic approach, however, may conflict with social and cultural traditions or legal precedents, such as disapproval of sex outside of marriage or laws prohibiting use of certain drugs.

Education should also be directed toward targeting groups at high risk for HIV/AIDS, using a combination of mass media and individual counseling techniques. (See Coates and Greenblatt, 1990; Meheus et al., 1990; Maticka-Tyndale et al., 1994.) In addition, an often overlooked or underdeveloped element is support for individuals in maintaining positive behavior changes. (See Carter et al., 1990.) Finally, health education stimulates demand for condoms, screening, diagnosis, and other services. Thus, education can be successful only if supported by availability of these services.

To control its AIDS epidemic, Thailand is using multiple educational strategies focused on various target groups. These include sex practices among commercial sex workers and married women at risk of infection from their husbands, and needle-use practices of IDUs. A notable example is an initiative to educate rural, married women in the Isan region on risks from husbands who have extramarital sex with prostitutes. Focus groups and surveys found that although women had knowledge of condom use, they were not practicing it, because they trusted their husbands to protect them and were unwilling to acknowledge their husbands' behaviors. A three-part intervention strategy used meetings with village leaders, a five-part audio-drama over village loudspeakers that was advertised in advance, and village meetings to plan further strategies. (See Maticka-Tyndale et al., 1994.) Education interventions for IDUs in Bangkok helped stabilize HIV infection levels, using educational materials for drug users, counseling at drug centers, and education telling drug users to sterilize needles with bleach. (See Brown et al., 1994.) New HIV infections have declined among young men, which appears to be related to changes in their sexual behavior, especially increased use of condoms. (See Nelsen et al., 1996.)

Sanitation Practices. It is well known that adequate sanitation practices, such as access to clean water supplies and sanitary latrines, hand washing, bathing, and other personal hygiene, help prevent childhood diarrhea, other infections, and malnutrition. (See Maung et al., 1993; Esrey, 1996.) In many sanitation projects, installing water wells or latrines is a direct government intervention, but proper use and maintenance of these facilities are the responsibility of individuals and local communities. Perhaps more than in any other promotive or preventive health choice, changes in personal sanitation behaviors are encouraged almost entirely by education activities (e.g., training on the hazards of infectious disease from household debris).

Desired improvements in sanitation behaviors can be especially difficult to achieve because these problems are closely intertwined with poverty and illiteracy, which create powerful barriers to individuals' abilities to make changes, even when they want to. For example, for mothers who are living at subsistence levels, adopting new sanitation practices may be a lower priority than acquiring food and caring for their children. Mothers may also be unable to understand training materials or may not have the time to be trained.

Despite these constraints, there is documentation that individual-level educational efforts can make incremental improvements in sanitation behaviors—improvements that have helped reduce infections and malnutrition in children. In Karachi, Pakistan, for example, a control-comparison study showed that health education provided to mothers by primary-care workers resulted in decreased incidences of diarrhea, respiratory infection, and fever in children. (See Akram and Agboatwalla, 1992.) The size of decreases was not reported.

Similarly, in a randomized prospective trial in Bangladesh, educational interventions improved hand-washing practices before food preparation and reduced the amount of unsanitary debris in living areas. During the six months after the intervention, rates of diarrhea were 26 percent lower in the intervention communities than in the control communities. (See Stanton et al., 1987.)

In contrast, another project in Bangladesh was not very successful in changing sanitation behaviors. The project focused mainly on installing water wells and latrines and gave only limited training and support to community members. Few families used the latrines or built new ones when the first ones were filled. In addition, maintenance of wells declined because of lack of tools or training of community members. (See Hoque and Hoque, 1994.)

Prescriptive Choices

In terms of prescriptive choices, we examine two key interventions: use of primary-care services, and use of traditional and allopathic (disease-oriented) medicine.

Use of Primary-Care Services. Timely and appropriate use of primary-care services can go a long way toward improving health for those living in developing countries, especially in the poorest rural areas. Primary-care services aim at the cluster of diseases and health issues that have monumental consequences for morbidity and mortality—malnutrition, infectious diseases such as diarrhea and ARI, and problems of childbirth and perinatal conditions. Once individuals are reached and encouraged to use the services, an intervention often can manage more than one of these problems.

Among the factors that guide individuals' decisions about whether and where to seek services are the availability and acceptability of services and the types of providers people prefer. As shown in Table 6.2, people's perceptions of the quality of services provided by a health center or clinic are influenced by attitudes of health workers and the same factors that influence choice in developed countries: waiting times, availability of medical supplies and drugs, adequacy of clinic facilities, and relationships with physicians and health workers. (See Satia et al., 1994; Aljunid, 1995; Lyttleton, 1996.)

Underuse of primary-care services in developing countries is well documented. Studies have found, for example, underuse of services for family planning, immunizations, and treatment of fever in India (see Satia et al., 1994); for nutrition rehabilitation in Bangladesh (see Nielsen et al., 1992); for postnatal care in south India (see Bhatia and Cleland, 1995); and for ORS for child diarrhea in several sites in Africa, Asia, and Latin America (see McDivitt et al., 1994).

Table 6.2

Service Characteristics That Influence Health
Center/Clinic Demand

Service Categories	Service Characteristics
Quality of service	Good clinical care by physician Well-trained health workers Respect for patient treatment preferences Provision of patient information and education
Facilities and equipment	Clean and safe physical facilities Adequate diagnostic and treatment equipment Facilities protect patients' privacy
Service convenience	Convenient location and hours Short waiting lines Support for mothers with children Available care in emergencies

Many primary-care programs have trouble sustaining themselves because they fail to account for community perceptions about the need for these services, which, in turn, affects the demand for them. For example, in studying vaccinations in developing countries, Nichter points out that although many countries have reported significant gains in immunization rates from intensive EPI programs, the people themselves frequently do not know why they are being immunized, what antigens are incorporated, and what benefits the immunization provides. The reason is that the rush to immunize precludes the time available for communicating the value of immunization. (See Nichter, 1995.)

In poor rural areas, decisions to seek care compete with other demands of people who are struggling economically. In many countries (such as China), this is especially true for women, who are the decisionmakers about health care for their children and themselves and who not only work in the fields but are also responsible for daily maintenance of their families and home. (See Wong et al., 1995.)

During the 1980s, primary-care programs to control the health impacts of ARI were designed and tested as pilot programs in Pakistan, Nepal, Tanzania, Indonesia, the Philippines, and India. (See Douglas, 1990.) These programs consisted of immunization, health education, and simplified standard case management. This strategy offers an efficient prototype for developing countries facing economic or educational constraints. It is also being adapted to child diarrhea control programs. The educational efforts of the pilot programs, which had interventions of varying intensity, demonstrated the importance of the role of education.

Studies have documented cases where educational interventions enhanced individuals' knowledge and motivation to use services, but the evidence is less clear when evaluations of educational activities have looked at improvements in health outcomes. Some examples from controlled studies illustrate the potential for educational activities to affect the use of primary-care services. A mobile unit for cervical cancer screening increased the percentage of rural Thai women who knew about the Pap smear and, in turn, were screened at least once. (See Swaddiwudhipong et al., 1995.) In rural Nepal, expansion of the training and outreach activities of community health volunteers led to increased use of the educational and other services they provided, resulting in higher ORS use rates for child diarrhea and greater treatment rates for ARI. (See Curtale et al., 1995.) Provision of increased education on breastfeeding in a Bihar, India, hospital led to an earlier start of breastfeeding and less frequent use of prelacteal feeds. (See Prasad et al., 1995.) Unfortunately, whether these behavioral changes led to changes in health, let alone sustained improvements, was not studied.

The use of prescription drugs, other pharmaceuticals, and injections is another major primary-care issue. In many places in Asia, these methods are the first choice for treating health problems. In addition, because private pharmacies are an important source of health care in many countries, the information they provide influences customers' use of drugs and decisions on when to seek other medical care. Thailand villagers, for example, often choose to purchase packages of pills from local drugstores or to obtain injections from "injection doctors," who typically do not have medical training. (See Lyttleton, 1996.) Hong Kong Chinese tonics are commonly used for self-medication, even though patients do not perceive them to be as effective as Western medicines and do not have knowledge of side effects. (See Lam et al., 1994.)

Two controlled studies in Kenya and Indonesia tested the effects of training pharmacy attendants on treating children's diarrhea and educating customers. The studies found that, compared with the controls, the trained personnel sold more ORS and discussed dehydration more with customers. One is left to wonder, however, whether this led to better health. (See Ross-Degnan et al., 1996.)

Use of Traditional and Allopathic Medicine. Consumers' decisions about providers, including their choices between using traditional and newer Western treatment methods, can have substantial impacts on their own health status and outcomes, as well as on resource allocation for their countries. As governments in developing countries expand their health care systems, they are often confronted by competing and fragmented groups of health care providers. A strategy that many countries have pursued is to integrate traditional medicine and Western medicine into a unified system of health care delivery, allowing traditional providers to focus on primary care while allocating Western technological resources to expand secondary- and tertiary-care facilities.

Worldwide, patients favor Western medicine for acute diseases but find the approaches of traditional medicine particularly appealing for treating psychiatric and chronic diseases. For example, in mainland China, where Western and traditional medicine treatments are often available side by side in the same health centers, the queues for Western medicine are longer in the acute care arena, while traditional medicine has longer queues for chronic conditions. (See Edwards, 1986.) In addition, there are numerous examples of the popularity of traditional medicine in treating psychiatric illness. (See Suryani and Jensen, 1992; Razali, 1995.) These include the use of Dervish healers by Arabs for treating psychiatric illness. (See Al-Krenawi et al., 1996.)

Traditional medicine can improve patients' decisions by fostering patient empowerment, and it can increase cost-effectiveness (as discussed in Chapter 3) by encouraging self-care when appropriate. Because traditional medicine is likely to be more culturally suitable and appropriate, especially in rural areas, it can result in changes in behavior, greater community involvement, and integration of health care into community social structures and support systems. Use of traditional medicine practitioners can also mitigate culture shock, which often leads to noncompliance with appropriate and effective Western medicine approaches. The result can be substantially greater patient compliance.

There are many examples of the successful use of traditional medicine providers in the developing world. The most notable example is the use of Chinese providers in primary care. (See Roemer, 1991.) Ayurveda still plays a prominent (although informal) role in India's health care system, covering innumerable localities, villages, and towns. (See Khare et al., 1996.) Other examples include the extensive use of medicinal plants by Salvadoran health promoters (*promotores*) and several medicinal plant projects in Nicaragua that enjoyed community participation and popular support. (See Barrett, 1994.) In Mexico, traditional birth attendants play an important role in providing prenatal and obstetrical care. (See Comey et al., 1996.)

Box 6.3: Integration of Traditional and Allopathic Medicine

Incorporating traditional medical providers into the health care policy debate has the potential to broaden the base of support for health care reform, avoid duplication, and improve resource allocation. Integrating traditional medicine and Western medicine allows traditional providers to focus on primary care, while resources allocated to technology can be used to expand specialty-care services, rather than duplicating primary-care capability.

A common problem in health care delivery in developing countries is poor coordination between primary and specialty care. This has already occurred in several Asian countries, notably South Korea and Taiwan, where community-based primary-care providers, hospital-based primary-care providers, and hospital-based specialists continue to provide overlapping care at substantial expense. (See Peabody et al., 1995c; Peabody et al., 1994.) The potential for duplication and disintegration is even greater between traditional medicine and Western medicine because of their conflicting paradigms of health and illness. Governments will need to work hard to overcome these differences, and the best way to start is by engaging both groups in the health care political process.

The WHO's 1978 Alma Ata declaration stressed community-based health care as a means of involving the community in health care planning and delivery. (See WHO, 1978.) A corollary benefit of such an approach, which relies heavily on indigenous or traditional medicine providers, is greater emphasis on prevention and primary care. Another advantage is the role such a strategy plays in fostering a socially responsible, ecologically sustainable, and economically viable world order. (See Barrett, 1996.) Implementation of WHO's policy of community-based health care has been slow and sporadic. Notable successes, however, include the use of traditional providers of primary care, such as the curanderos in Latin America; medicinal plant projects in China; and the roles of traditional birth attendants in providing prenatal and obstetrical care in Bangladesh.

Advantages of integrating traditional medicine into the actual health care delivery system include improving access to primary care and greater efficiency in allocation of limited health care resources. By providing a legitimate role for each party in the health care system, governments can foster cooperation, integration of care, and health improvements. Guidelines can be universally developed and applied to primary-care health services, whether they are provided by traditional or Western medicine–trained providers. These guidelines could include appropriate referral to suitable community (often traditional medicine) providers for primary care and to Western-trained providers for secondary and tertiary care. Finally, the dissemination of standards and practices, which is critical to effective health care delivery, can be accomplished much more easily in an integrated system.

In developing an integrated system, it is important to focus on the similarities between traditional and Western medicine in terms of the basic functions of primary care, rather than looking at the technical differences. Traditional medicine providers will be effective in the areas of health education, prevention, and promotion. Educational outreach should guide patients in their provider choices, including indications for when they can benefit from traditional medicine and when they should seek the technological prescriptive capabilities of Western medicine.

In fact, there is evidence that developing countries are beginning to consider integrating traditional and Western medicine systems. For example, in South Africa, a new insurance program now gives patients a choice of going to traditional healers—referred to as *inyangas* (spiritual herbalists)—or Western doctors. This willingness to formalize integration is driven by the realization that traditional healers have strengths, particularly in rural areas where conventional health care is scarce or expensive.

In summary, experiences with health promotion and education around the world yield a paradox with respect to the impacts of educational strategies and the attitudes of policymakers and analysts about the roles of these activities. Given that educational programs vary widely in their effects on health status, it is difficult to say how successful they are. Yet the absence of educational components in health promotion, prevention, and prescription interventions has occasionally been documented as a reason for the failure of some interventions to change health behaviors or outcomes. Similarly, while some advocates of health education may claim it is the backbone of all effective programs, doubters may fail to recognize the detailed elements of what comprises effective educational interventions.

Clearly, some of the limited understanding of health promotion interventions results from poor design and execution of the interventions themselves or a poorly designed evaluation component. In health promotion, inadequate intervention and evaluation design often make it difficult to attribute the absence of impacts to one or more multiple determinants. A number of studies conclude by speculating on various factors that might be contributing to unexpected results—many of which could have been addressed during the initial study design. Yet there appears to be a learning curve, and the accumulated experience discussed above is improving the quality of interventions. Nevertheless, governments should be cautious in starting a health promotion education program or in using education as a component of broader health or development projects.

INCREASING THE OPPORTUNITY FOR CHANGING PROVIDER BEHAVIOR

Even if individuals can be motivated to change their behaviors to seek appropriate health care, problems with how providers practice medicine still hinder the ability of governments to improve health status. Poor-quality care is particularly acute in government clinics, health centers, and hospitals, which are key providers in many communities in Asia. The problem may be worse in rural locations, which tend to have the greatest need for health status improvement. Often working under severe budget limitations, facilities struggle to supply adequately trained personnel and sufficient materials, equipment, and drugs to serve local health needs. (See Bennett et al., 1994b; Aljunid, 1995; Berg, 1995.)

Poor-quality care in government health facilities is well documented. In Papua New Guinea and Tanzania, community satisfaction was higher for primary-care services provided by church dispensaries than those provided by government facilities. These studies cited greater availability of drugs and more positive attitudes by health workers. (See Gilson et al., 1994; Peabody et al., 1996a.) Complaints about public facilities in Mali included long waiting times, shortage of drugs, inadequacy of care, and poor attitudes of nurses and physicians. (See Ainsworth, 1983.) Evaluations of India's primary-care program also have highlighted poor utilization, accusations of negligence by medical officers and workers, and low participation in outreach programs. (See Kamat, 1995.)

Because improving health status is a public policy priority for developing Asian countries, countries have focused on primary health care services. Changing provider behaviors is an important part of ensuring quality health care services. This can be done through a variety of programs: the provision and financing of training programs, mandating and regulation through testing and licensure, development and dissemination of clinical standards, external monitoring of provider performance, and research to support development of new treatment technologies. (See World Bank, 1992c; Aljunid, 1995.)

Here, our focus is on directly improving the quality of a provider's care. This is distinct from the indirect influences that come through the funding role (see Chapter 4, where we discuss ways of using funding to change provider behavior) and the mandating or regulation role (which is the subject of Chapter 7). Here, we focus on ways to voluntarily change the way doctors provide care. Available techniques for changing practitioners' behaviors in this way include education and training activities, persuasion to encourage voluntary behavior changes, and participation strategies.

Many approaches have been tried in more-developed countries. The hope is that changing providers' behaviors (i.e., the way they practice) will lead either to better health outcomes or to the same outcomes with fewer inputs (resources). Some approaches are uniquely suited to wealthier countries; physician profiling and utilization review are examples.[1] Other strategies, such as implicit or explicit chart reviews, are effective but only useful under well specified clinical and organizational conditions.

Another approach to evaluating the quality of care is to use *clinical vignettes*— open-ended clinical cases that, once they have been validated, can measure how physicians would provide clinical care for a patient. For a given case, physicians are asked about (1) taking a history, (2) doing a physical examination, (3) what laboratory or other tests they would perform, (4) their diagnosis, and (5) their treatment plan.

These five steps form the basis for evaluating clinical medicine. The "correct" responses are based on outcomes research that link process to outcomes. Vignettes control for differences in case mix variation, and—since they are also relatively inexpensive—they can be given to a large number of providers in a wide variety of settings to generate average quality scores among doctors. Another strength of vignettes is that they can be used to assess the effectiveness of policies. For example, when payment mechanisms or licensing requirements are introduced, vignettes can be used to measure changes in provider behavior. And since the criteria for measuring quality are based on outcomes research, inferences can be made about provider practices and the health outcomes of the population.

---

[1]Provider or physician profiling generally involves measuring and aggregating provider decisions or practices, such as prescriptions, and then comparing the provider with his or her colleagues. Those who prescribe "too much" or operate "too infrequently" are made aware that they are at variance from the group norm of their colleagues. Utilization review involves evaluation by a (typically) expert panel before a test or procedure is allowed to be done and generally focuses on reducing the number of unnecessary tests.

Vignettes have been developed and validated in parallel research that compares them with chart abstraction for standardized patients having nine common health conditions that are best treated in a primary care setting: coronary artery disease, hypertension, chronic obstructive pulmonary disease, diabetes, prenatal care, tuberculosis, contraception, and low back pain for adult patients, and diarrhea and cough with fever for children. (See Peabody, et al., 1998b.) The approach is currently being applied in the Republic of Macedonia as part of a facility survey. (See Peabody et al., 1998c.)

In both developed and developing countries, care management strategies have been used for some time and show promise for expansion in less affluent settings. Care management or clinical practice guidelines (CPGs) are a series of steps the provider follows before being directed to the next set of diagnostic studies or interventions. The belief is that by following these steps, the patient will get better care and resources will be better used.

In this chapter we emphasize guidelines for several reasons. First, CPGs can be introduced that apply to clinical functions performed by all clinical personnel. Second, although discussions of these issues in developing countries often focus on public practitioners, the methods can be used in both private and public settings. Third, CPGs are usually developed by working in cooperation with providers to specify the best clinical methods.

As was true with programs intended to modify individuals' behavior, any program that relies on voluntary compliance must be able to motivate practitioners. That is, practitioners must believe that they will get something of value out of changing to new clinical techniques. Health care professionals, like their patients, conduct their activities within the same multilayered context of cultural, social, economic, political, and health systems discussed earlier. However, unlike their patients, their role as medical professionals carries with it intrinsic responsibilities. To motivate behavioral change, these need to be considered, along with other contextual factors, in designing interventions to influence provider behavior.

A second factor to consider is the social position of medical professionals, which is generally one of prestige and privilege. Physicians frequently have attained the elite levels of society because of the social or educational barriers they must overcome to achieve their positions. On one hand, the differences in status and power may foster patient confidence in the practitioner's abilities and enhance the practitioner's authority and influence over patient behavior. On the other, class differences may result in gaps in communication and understanding between providers and patients. At the same time, the high status of practitioners may make them less amenable to interventions intended to influence their behavior.

A third influence on physicians' attitudes and practice is their link to the global system of biomedicine through their long and intensive training. This biomedical heritage is oriented toward the developed countries of the West. It emphasizes a scientific approach to disease, high technology, curative therapy rather than prevention, hospital-based tertiary care, and distrust for non-biomedical alternatives. (See Peabody, et al., 1992.) Unfortunately, the values this system instills may be less appropriate in developing countries or in regions with different cultural values.

Nonetheless, efforts to influence provider behavior locally may be resisted when perceived as conflicting with values intrinsic to this global biomedical system. For example, when researchers designed a series of self-instruction modules to help doctors in China treat neonatal hypothermia, they carefully translated the English text of the modules—which contained a review of pathophysiology, diagnosis, treatment, and relevant preventive measures—into the local language. However, despite promotion by the Bureau of Public Health, the program did not initially fare well. It was not until the original English text was added on the page facing the translated text that local physicians valued the instruction as "advanced and suitably sophisticated." (See Peabody et al., 1996b.)

Educational interventions may have a greater chance of succeeding with practitioners than with other groups, especially if interventions address the professional needs of practitioners, such as the knowledge needed to treat particular problems and to facilitate professional advancement. Competence, knowledge, and skill, for example, are qualities highly valued in the culture of biomedicine and are a means of advancement within the field. Changes induced in practice patterns may be sustained over the long term if they are accompanied by changes in systems of care that support the new patterns. For example, record-keeping systems may be changed to incorporate clinical reminders that reinforce changes in practice.

Intervention activities, such as using guidelines, must also work within the network of formal and informal alliances that medical practitioners develop through their personal interactions, culture of professionalism, and common interests. A sense of shared clinical standards may either lead them to participate in desired changes or spur them to act together in resisting changes they see as threatening to their professional interests. An important example is opposition to other groups of practitioners, such as traditional healers or paraprofessionals, whom physicians often view as encroaching on their domain. Thus, integrating other types of practitioners into health development programs can be met with resistance if cooperation and involvement by biomedical professionals are not actively sought in the planning and implementation process.

Given these needs, how should policymakers design interventions to get providers to improve their practices? First, because interventions may be designed to change the distribution of behaviors in different ways, there is a need to understand what the interventions are really trying to accomplish. Figure 6.3 reveals two distribution curves showing how interventions can affect the distribution of behaviors. The distribution on the left is representative of all provider behavior where the average practice clusters around the middle (x). The better practitioners are to the right, the less competent ones, to the left. One type of intervention (A)—such as physician profiling or utilization review—tries to identify all low-end performers and improve their performance. This shifts the average performance slightly toward the better practitioners $(x \rightarrow y)$. By contrast, intervention (B)—such as CPGs—tries to shift the average performance of all practitioners to the right $(x \rightarrow z)$.

Models of introducing and diffusing newer practices stress the influences of interactions between characteristics of the receiver (the practitioner), the source,

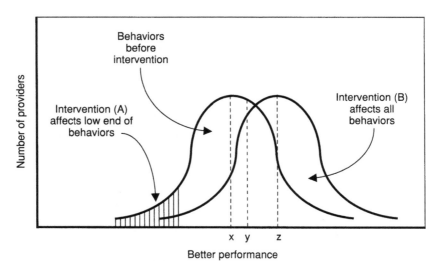

**Figure 6.3—How Interventions Can Affect Distributions
of Provider Behaviors**

the message, and the channel used to provide the information. The process of
change has been characterized as involving three stages. (See Lomas, 1991.)

- Predisposing or priming activities to trigger consideration of change;
- Enabling strategies to motivate and facilitate change;
- Reinforcing activities to sustain change.

Consensus recommendations are the basic instruments used in all stages of the
diffusion of new clinical practices. Initially, they serve as sources of information
that stimulate practitioners to consider change. In the remaining two stages,
individual practitioners may use the recommendations as goals as they modify
their behaviors, or other parties may use them as yardsticks to monitor progress
in changing practices and provide feedback to practitioners.

CPGs—increasingly used in industrialized countries confronting escalating health
care expenditures—tend to emphasize appropriateness of care and seek to achieve
more cost-effective levels of care. These interventions are designed to improve the
performance of all providers. Guidelines are commonly used today for treating
coronary disease, drug therapy decisions, cancer prevention and management,
patient monitoring during anesthesia, use of Caesarean sections, performance of
coronary artery bypass grafts, management of hypertension, management of
lower back pain, and liver transplantation. Governments and professional
organizations in many countries are not only developing but also disseminating
CPGs on a national level. At the same time, local hospitals, health plans, or other
organizations are developing their own guidelines or adapting national or
professional guidelines to their particular situation. (See Lomas, 1991; Mittman et
al., 1992.)

Unlike guidelines in developed countries, guidelines for developing countries—
such as those published by the WHO—emphasize techniques to improve the
quality of preventive and primary-care services. Guidelines serve as both clinical

standards and educational guides for health workers in developing countries. Using expert panels to develop consensus recommendations, WHO has already produced guidelines for the case management of ARIs in children, prevention and treatment of complications of abortion, essential elements of obstetrical care, thermal control of the newborn, cholera control, prevention and management of diarrhea, and treatment of tuberculosis.

Since many guidelines (such as the WHO guidelines) already exist and the issue is how to enhance their impacts on health status and treatment services, our focus here is on information dissemination and changing provider practices. Active interventions, in addition to passive information dissemination, will be necessary to bring about desired changes in provider behaviors. Insurers in industrialized countries, for example, are increasingly using a mix of education, persuasion, financial incentives or penalties, and contractual requirements or sanctions to reduce costs that result from inappropriate care.

In terms of information dissemination, four types of social influence techniques have been shown to be useful for persuading physicians and other practitioners to voluntarily change their clinical behaviors. (See Mittman et al., 1992.) The first is the use of *opinion leaders* to transmit norms or model appropriate behaviors. These leaders are respected individuals who know the targeted practitioners and whose views are valued.

Two other techniques are specific applications of small-group discussion— essentially processes of social norm development—that have been found to change individuals' attitudes and behaviors to match more closely those of group members, while also providing continuing clinical education. (See Mittman, 1994.) One is *study groups* that examine specific quality and effectiveness issues. Another is *participatory development* or *review of guidelines* to develop consensus among practitioners on acceptable clinical practices. Such methods offer considerable potential for modifying the behaviors of practitioners who work in group practices, medical clinics, managed-care plans, multidisciplinary teams, or other types of small groups.

A fourth technique is *continuous quality improvement* (CQI), which uses a range of industrial quality management principles and methods for improving the quality of services and products. (See Imai, 1986.) CQI has three key features: (1) the process consists of repeated sequences of activities; (2) small teams of workers are given the authority to carry out CQI for their services or production processes; and (3) the teams use scientific methods and data to inform their actions. In each cycle, a team identifies an issue and establishes a quality improvement goal. Then, the team designs and implements quality improvement actions and monitors progress toward its goal. By repeating this process, the team achieves a series of incremental improvements in its functions.

Although CQI has been successful in transforming many industries, it is complex to initiate and its introduction can have profound impacts on an organization's culture and operation. It is an appealing strategy for health care because, when successfully implemented, it can bring about permanent improvements in the attitudes and practices of clinical personnel. However, the leadership of a provider organization or health plan needs to be fully committed to CQI and must be prepared to manage the change process actively.

**Box 6.4: WHO Guidelines for Case Management of
Acute Respiratory Infection in Children**

ARIs are one of the most common causes of death in children in developing countries. Almost all ARI deaths are due to acute lower respiratory infection, mostly pneumonia, so the most important objective of ARI case management in children is to recognize and treat pneumonia. The case management guidelines in the World Health Organization (WHO) manual are appropriate for developing countries or areas with limited resources and an infant mortality of greater than 40 deaths per 1,000 live births. (See WHO, 1990a.) They are designed for use with children age 5 years or younger and in hospitals where X-ray and laboratory facilities are limited and diagnosis relies on clinical examination.

For example, Table 6.4.1 summarizes WHO guidelines for pneumonia management at small hospitals for the child age 2 months through 5 years with cough or difficulty breathing, who do not have stridor, severe undernutrition, or signs suggesting meningitis.

Table 6.4.1
WHO Guidelines for Pneumonia Management at Small Hospitals

Clinical Signs	Classify Diagnosis As:	Summary of Treatment Instructions
• Central cyanosis OR • Inability to drink	Very severe pneumonia	Admit Give oxygen Give an antibiotic: chloramphenicol Treat fever or wheezing, if present Give supportive care Reassess twice daily
• Chest indrawing AND • No central cyanosis AND • Ability to drink	Severe pneumonia; if child is wheezing, assess further before classifying	Admit[a] Give an antibiotic: benzylpenicillin Treat fever or wheezing, if present Give supportive care Reassess daily
• No chest indrawing AND • Fast breathing[b]	Pneumonia	Advise mother to give home care Give an antibiotic (at home): cotrimoxazole, amoxycillin, ampicillin, or procaine penicillin Treat fever or wheezing, if present Advise the mother to return in 2 days for reassessment, or earlier if the child is getting worse
• No chest indrawing AND • No fast breathing	No pneumonia: Cough or cold	If coughing more than 30 days, assess for causes of chronic cough Assess and treat ear problem or sore throat, if present Assess and treat other problems Advise mother to give home care Treat fever or wheezing, if present

[a]If oxygen supply is ample, also give oxygen to a child with restlessness (if oxygen improves the condition), severe chest indrawing, or breathing rate of 70 breaths per minute or more.

[b]Fast breathing is: 50 breaths per minute or more in a child age 2 months up to 12 months; 40 breaths per minute or more in a child age 12 months up to 5 years.

As with evaluating the ability to change individual behavior, it is important to distinguish between the change in the behavior itself and any effects that behavior change may have on health status. Thus, evaluations should measure impacts at several points in the change process: credibility of the guidelines developed, effectiveness of guideline dissemination in providing new information, changes in clinical practice in response to the new information, and impacts on outcomes and costs.

In summary, then, a number of factors are essential for successfully developing and implementing CPGs, which focus on primary-care practice issues.

1. **The chosen intervention to be developed should address high-prevalence conditions and be relevant and useful to health practitioners.** Practitioners will be more willing to participate in designing and changing behavior if they feel the intervention is addressing an important clinical quality issue.

2. **Practitioners should be involved in the development of interventions.** Physicians involved in the development process will gain a sense of ownership and be more likely to contribute to implementation than physicians who have not been similarly involved.

3. **The intervention should be responsive to the cultural context in which health services are being provided—whether it be clinical guidelines, chart abstraction, utilization review, or something else.** Given the diverse histories of cultures and traditional medicines in Asian countries, efforts to change provider behavior can be expected to differ across countries and communities within countries. This process is an opportunity to integrate the roles of allopathic and traditional medicine.

4. **There should be linkages among physicians and other health workers responsible for patient care.** Physicians often object initially to the idea of simplified guidelines and expanded roles for lower-level health workers, reflecting concerns for the integrity of clinical care. Physicians should be involved not only in development, but also in the design and execution of the supervisory system, thus supporting health workers in the functions they perform and ensuring physician supervision and coordination of care.

5. **Regular feedback should be provided to practitioners on their performance.** This step is critical for successfully using any practice standard. The most effective (and least threatening) feedback mechanism is a small-group process where practitioners can interact and work together in problem-solving activities.

6. **Stronger incentives or sanctions should be considered if voluntary participation is not effective.** In many cases, voluntary methods may not fully achieve desired changes in practitioner behaviors. Governments then may turn to additional incentives such as bonus payments or sanctions such as penalties for inappropriate service use.

IMPLEMENTING CLINICAL PRACTICE GUIDELINES AND CONTINUING MEDICAL EDUCATION

The most suitable approaches for changing provider behavior in developing Asian countries—and certainly the ones with the best data—are CPGs and continuing medical education (CME). The expansion of guidelines in developed countries, as well as lessons learned from using both CPGs and CME, shows promise in helping to upgrade clinical practices. Unfortunately, the evidence in developing countries—in Asia or elsewhere—is fairly sparse.

CME has the potential to ameliorate inadequacies of clinical care found in many settings. Self-instructional continuing education programs in neonatal care, for example, were tested for workers at four county hospitals in China to correct shortcomings in neonatal care education and practice. Although these programs were uncontrolled interventions, they increased workers' cognitive knowledge, improved essential clinical practices, and elevated the availability of essential supplies in those facilities. All the hospitals reported improvements in management of hypothermia and fewer transfers of babies to the provincial hospital. (See Hesketh et al., 1994.)

In more-developed countries, CME does not consistently improve provider practices. A meta-analysis of CME studies between 1975 and 1991 found only 50 randomized controlled trials (out of 777 published papers) that looked at changing provider behavior. Of the 50, only 18 evaluated the impact of CME on health outcomes. Perhaps even more disappointing is that only 8 studies demonstrated improvements in health status, despite the acknowledged bias toward publishing positive results. The researchers found that preventive and prescribing practices were easier to change than case management and patient counseling behaviors, probably because the latter were too complex unless they were matched with more-complex (multiple) and more-intensive strategies to change behavior. (See Davis et al., 1992.)

A study in India corroborates these disappointing results in a developing country. It found that practice changes stimulated by CME may be short-lived. Using a before-and-after design, the study evaluated how mothers' breastfeeding practices were affected by training of physicians and midwives in the benefits and feasibility of breastfeeding. Although training strengthened interventions by the practitioners, greatly improving breastfeeding practices in the short term, the impact of training fell off within six months. (See Prasad and Costello, 1995.)

CME may be especially important for drug retailers in Asia. These private practitioners often are people's first or only source of health care outside the home, and there are typically few controls on their drug distribution practices. The Nepal Ministry of Health operates a 45-hour course for private drug retailers that covers practical training, pharmacology, ethics, and legal issues. Although the program is operationally successful, its impact on prescribing patterns has not been evaluated. (See Kafle et al., 1992.) Also in Nepal, a study of a supplemental drug supply system found that, with adequate supplies of essential drugs, state health posts tended to overprescribe drugs—leading to questions about the efficacy of the MOH's CME program. (See Chalker, 1995.)

Clinical practice guidelines offer another approach to changing provider behavior. In many cases, guidelines have simply reflected local practice standards or the standards of the expert panels that developed them; in contrast, national or international guidelines are generally based more on clinical evidence.

A variety of dissemination techniques for CPGs have been used, including journal publications, distribution of booklets, press conferences, and other communications media (recently including the Internet). Despite these dissemination channels, awareness of guidelines and consensus statements disseminated in developed countries has been found to vary from a low of 20 percent to a high of 90 percent, depending on the type of guidelines or medical specialty. (See Lomas, 1991.)

Substantial work also remains to be done in disseminating guidelines in developing countries. Many private practitioners are not using such key guidelines as protocols for treating tuberculosis, use of antibiotics, and choices of prescription drugs. (See Aljunid, 1995.) Private doctors in Bombay, for example, were found to prescribe three times more expensive drugs than the national standard when treating tuberculosis, and they also used unnecessary drugs. (See Uplekar and Shepard, 1991.) In Tanzania, church dispensaries distributed antibiotics, chloroquine, and injections in higher proportion than government units, also dispensing mostly nonessential drugs. (See Gilson et al., 1993.)

In addition, although disseminating guidelines broadly in the clinical community improves knowledge, it does not necessarily stimulate changes in practices. National practice guidelines in more-developed countries have so far had little impact on physician behaviors. (See Kosecoff et al., 1987; Lomas, 1991.) For example, a study surveying nearly 1,800 U.S. physicians on how they would treat a patient with tuberculosis discovered that, even though the physicians practiced in specialties and lived in regions where tuberculosis cases were likely to be found, only 59 percent described a treatment regimen that conformed to national-level recommendations. In fact, among those physicians specializing in lung disease, only 71 percent prescribed the recommended regimen. (See Sumartojo, 1993.)

One reason for this problem is that passive dissemination methods are generally used. These introduce little incentive for physicians to translate new knowledge into new behaviors. In addition, physicians may not be accepting guidelines because they perceive the guidelines as constraints to their autonomy and to patients' choice, or as inappropriate substitutes for clinical judgment. Other barriers that have been identified include ingrained habits, malpractice concerns, conflicts with payment incentives, and organizational constraints. (See Mitmann et al., 1992.)

On the other hand, CPGs introduced in the context of rigorous evaluations have been found to improve clinical practice. (See Grimshaw and Russell, 1993.) For example, the guidelines in a program that successfully lowered Caesarean-section rates were accompanied by active education (an enabling strategy), combined with review of individual physicians' rates (a feedback mechanism). (See Myers and Gleicher, 1988.)

Few examples of the use of practice guidelines for physicians are documented for developing countries, but those that do exist indicate the potential that such activities offer. Two initiatives, one in Viet Nam and the other in Morocco, demonstrate educational impacts in cancer treatment. (See Love, 1994.) In Viet Nam, physicians participated in clinical trials in breast cancer therapy, including literature reviews, trial designs, writing of protocols, and other related activities. Through these efforts, physicians reported their clinical knowledge increased and they changed their practice approaches. In Morocco, a new clinical guidelines program began with developing guidelines for treating the most common cancers, using a multidisciplinary approach. Although the eventual impacts of these programs on clinical care are not yet known, both processes engaged and educated the learners.

An experimentally designed project in Nepal demonstrates that CME and CPGs together can be effectively used for lower-level primary health care health workers in rural areas. The study found that use of primary-care services for children improved when the functions, training, and supervisory support of community health volunteers were expanded to enable them to provide both curative and educational services. This study changed a situation where the community staff had been equipped only to provide educational services and where the rural mothers were not using their services because they preferred curative treatment to education. Among the primary-care improvements achieved were increased immunization coverage, greater use of oral rehydration therapy for diarrhea, greater use of mebendazole for intestinal helminths, and better treatment of ARI. (See Curtale et al., 1995.)

In the developing word, tensions also are encountered in changing the behaviors of traditional (or indigenous) practitioners. To do so successfully, guidelines need to be established that reflect the available evidence about the indications and efficacy of traditional treatment while retaining sensitivity to the cultural and spiritual aspects of the practitioners' services and their community roles. Special attention, by both traditional and allopathic providers, must be paid to the roles played by both groups of practitioners.

What is the best way to proceed? Given the widespread need for improved primary-care services in many Asian communities, an initial focus should be placed on mobilizing the medical community to implement existing WHO guidelines for primary health care. At the same time, work can proceed on identifying other clinical priorities for which guidelines or continuing education should be developed or adapted from existing sources.

The primary-care guidelines developed should embrace practices by all levels of practitioners involved—physicians, nurses, paid health workers with limited training, and community volunteer workers. As discussed above, several projects have shown the potential for nonphysician health workers to improve health status in a community—if they are properly trained, have guidelines to follow, and are supervised appropriately. In poor communities with poor health status and serious malnutrition but few resources to apply to the problems, such workers provide most of the primary care. These pragmatic strategies can be strengthened by providing simplified guidelines that improve the practices of community health workers. Although simplified guidelines may be considered a "second best" solution, they can help save lives by accommodating the needs and capabilities of lower-level health workers and the roles of traditional healers.

COMMUNITY PARTICIPATION STRATEGIES

In determining and implementing health policies, governments clearly must consider not only the individual attitudes and behaviors of patients and providers but also the effects that interactions among them can have on health status and the delivery of health care. Two forms of interactions stand out: the dynamics of provider-patient relationships, and the management of interests of multiple stakeholders in health systems.

Managing Provider-Patient Relationships

Provider-patient relationships are critical in shaping the delivery of health services. Because patients have incomplete knowledge about their health status and appropriate treatment technologies, they regularly rely on their doctors to present options and make or recommend health care choices.

However, practitioners often have conflicting interests, with the result that they may not always act in the best interest of their patients. For example, there will be an incentive for a fee-for-service practitioner to overtreat if patients have incomplete information on what is or is not appropriate care. Not only are information (and often decisions) on medical treatment practices and technology the domain of clinical practitioners, there are often honest disagreements among practitioners about the appropriate uses of treatment methods. As a result, patients (and insurers) face large costs and substantial uncertainty in monitoring the performance of providers. This strongly influences the structuring of economic and organizational relationships. (See Dranove and White, 1987.)

Residents of Asian countries are served by a heterogeneous group of practitioners, many of whom split their time between the public and private sectors. (See Aljunid, 1995.) For example, only about 15 percent of health workers in Indonesia work full-time in private institutions, and more than 67 percent of public-sector physicians in northern Thailand report also having private practices. (See Gish et al., 1988; Smith, 1982.) These practitioners have a major financial incentive to treat patients in their private practices, where they can earn more by providing more services and charging higher rates. Thus, they may have conflicting obligations to their public employers and patients, both of whom are relying on their professional judgments.

Conflicts also center on the quality of care provided by private practitioners. Such problems can arise when providers' obligations cannot be monitored effectively by the government or by their patients because they have incomplete information. In India, for example, private physicians have been found to prescribe more drugs and injections compared to public doctors. (See Greenhalgh, 1987; Uplekar and Shepard, 1991.) Poor integration of private practitioners into health care systems and inadequate participation in CME activities contribute to quality problems. But people in developing countries often believe that private providers render higher quality care than public facilities. (See Aljunid, 1995.) With little objective information available on the quality of clinical care, it is not clear where the truth lies.

Box 6.5: Provider-Patient Interactions and Compliance

One of the biggest challenges in prescriptive health care services is incomplete patient compliance with treatment protocols (e.g., taking drugs as prescribed, following nutritional supplement instructions, or returning for follow-up physician visits). The nature of relationships between patients and their physicians or other health care practitioners has been consistently documented to be an important factor in increasing compliance, especially the establishment of trust and demonstration of concern by the practitioner. Table 6.3.1 summarizes some guidelines that have proven effective in improving communication and patient compliance.

Table 6.5.1
Methods for Improving Communication and Patient Compliance

Methods	Description
Avoid information overload.	Concentrate on a few essential points, repeating for emphasis.
Slow down!	Speak at a pace that patients can understand, avoiding tones or body language that appear hurried.
Verify that the patient understands.	Ask patients to confirm the instructions in their own words, and what the next steps will be.
Be a good listener.	Pay attention to what patients say in both words and body language.
Use "show me" methods.	Give demonstrations, such as how to use a thermometer, and ask patients to show you the method.
Simplify written instructions.	Use a conversational style, keep sentences short, and use short words and lots of white space.
Simplify oral instructions.	Speak to patients as if explaining a medical condition to a family member; do not patronize.
Tell stories.	Story-format education has been shown to increase compliance.

The governments of many Asian countries serve as agents for their residents in providing both preventive health and medical treatment services. In rural communities, as well as urban areas with high rates of poverty, most individuals and families depend on government public health departments, clinics, and hospitals for their health-status and health-care needs. The success of the public organizations in responding to these needs depends on the availability of trained health workers and the adequacy of supplies and equipment; it also depends on how public personnel and health workers manage their multiple roles as agents for patients and for their government employers.

Managing the Interests of Multiple Stakeholders. A diversity of stakeholders in health systems generate other, often complex, patterns of relationships that must be recognized by government policymakers. Among these stakeholders are patients, clinical practitioners, health care organizations, and governments themselves. Stakeholders often have differing perspectives about health needs and priorities, and their views also are influenced by such macro issues as the burden of disease (Chapter 3), the constraints of the health financing system (Chapter 4), and inequities in access to care (Chapter 5). Governments have the opportunity and responsibility to encourage various groups to participate in developing and implementing health policies. From a pluralistic perspective, effective policy should accommodate these views as much as possible, seeking consensus among different, often competing, agendas. A sense of ownership among stakeholders is vital for the sustainability of programs and policies, as we discuss in more detail in Chapter 7.

Managing Stakeholders Using Participatory Strategies

Many health policymakers and planners argue, with justification, that health promotion, preventive health, and service delivery programs will not be successful unless their design and execution reflect the priorities and preferences of all the involved stakeholders—that is, all those with a stake in the outcome of a particular activity, in this case some form of health program. Inevitably, stakeholders have differing beliefs and priorities, which may conflict as they seek to gain their own benefits from a program.

No effort to change the behaviors of stakeholders occurs in isolation. Each individual or provider is influenced by his or her personal preferences and values, which, in turn, reflect the norms of the culture and community. In addition, as difficult as it is to achieve sustainable changes in individual behaviors, the challenge becomes more complex when these changes interact with the differing priorities and behaviors of various stakeholders in local health care markets. For example, patients may want health practitioners to be responsive to their need for information or their desire for privacy. Yet practitioners may prefer to render services rapidly to increase revenue, and this comes at the cost of time spent with patients providing information and education.

The many health practitioners serving a community have the power to influence the success or failure of a health intervention. These include allopathic practitioners working in public and private settings, traditional midwives, and other traditional healers. Allopathic practitioners may include physicians, nurses, or health workers. The variety of stakeholders poses several challenges for a health program. First, households in a community may use different types of practitioners, depending on the health condition being treated. (See Aljunid, 1995.) Second, practitioners may view the health program—or each other—as competition. Third, many of these individuals have a high status in the community social structure, although the nature of their status may vary. For example, traditional healers may be revered within the local religious tradition, whereas an allopathic physician may derive status from his or her educational level. Non-degreed health workers, on the other hand, may be awarded status if they are perceived as being formally trained and providing leadership, or they may be viewed as just another community member.

Another stakeholder group of particular concern is people in poverty, who often are target populations for health programs. Whether in rural areas of developing countries or in depressed neighborhoods in more-developed countries, the poor share a set of living conditions, personal status, and values that exclude them from opportunities available to more affluent persons. They face poor sanitation, malnutrition, disease, and ignorance. The burden of disease falls on small children and their mothers, with high morbidity and mortality rates for infants and children. (See Kanaaneh, 1977.) Working with these stakeholders to improve their health status requires sensitivity to the limits of their education, literacy, and knowledge of health practices, as well as understanding that they may view improvement in health status as less important than such basic needs as food or work.

Most health-related programs in rural Asian communities target women as a primary client because they are the foundation of the family, managing the family's daily activities and having primary responsibility for the health and well-being of the children. At the same time, women have lower social status than men with respect to family and community decisionmaking, and their own physical, social, and health needs often are the last to be addressed. Both field projects and studies have shown, however, that women can make substantial contributions to improving the health status of their communities when educated and empowered to make health-related decisions. (See Behrman and Wolfe, 1989; Caldwell, 1993; Aljunid, 1995; Manderson et al., 1995.)

How, then, should health programs or activities be designed to be responsive to—or successfully balance—such a diversity of stakeholder interests? Well-designed community participation strategies are one way to engage all the stakeholders. Local health or development programs typically start by identifying local community leaders, interest groups, and individuals who are key stakeholders and then develop community participation strategies to involve them in the program design and execution.

Three Basic Models of Community Participation

Programs that use community participation activities may be categorized by three basic models: community development, health education, or customer service. These models differ in the amount of active participation they require on the part of the leadership or individual members of a local community. The community development model requires the strongest local initiative and involvement; the customer service model requires the least. When evaluating community participation strategies, it should be kept in mind that no one approach is universally better than others. It should also be clear that compelling evidence substantiating these approaches needs to be developed.

Community Development Models—programs to establish or improve local community systems or infrastructures, such as water supply systems or drainage programs for malaria control—tend to incorporate broad, local participation. Such projects affect virtually all members of a community and typically require both local leadership and direct involvement by community members for successful implementation and sustainability. Community involvement in designing, developing, and operating a new system improves the likelihood that the system will be responsive to the local culture and priorities. Many of these projects also create jobs during both the development phase and ongoing operation of a new system, which not only is a form of participation but also contributes to the local economy. Such involvement should encourage community members to use the system after it is in operation and also to modify related health behaviors.

Health Education Models—programs to modify individual health-related behaviors, such as family planning programs or home care by families for ARI—tend to use a variety of health education and training techniques. These programs are critical to improving health status and survival in rural areas of developing countries, where preventive health programs and primary care are public health priorities. For these programs to succeed, they must gain acceptance by both the individuals or groups who are the target audiences and the communities in which they live. (See Kanaaneh, 1977.) Programs have used a wide variety of participation techniques, ranging from community needs assessments during program design through full sponsorship of a program by the local target population.

Customer Service Models—programs for direct delivery of health care services, such as primary-care clinics or dental services—tend to use more passive participation methods than the other two models. The goal is to encourage local community members to use available health services, including appropriate follow-up care. To be accepted, program providers should be viewed as both clinically competent and responsive to individual needs and values. A variety of customer service techniques can be used to ensure that services are responsive to clients. These include, for example, convenient hours of service, short waits to see a health worker, assistance to mothers of young patients in the supervision of other children, taking time to explain a medical problem and how it is treated, and asking patients how satisfied they are with services they received and what other services they wish to have. In many communities, outreach activities also may be necessary to educate individuals and community leaders on health care issues and the importance of obtaining needed care.

Key Design Issues for Community Health Programs

Regardless of which model policymakers use, several design issues appear to be important for any local health-related program initiated by an external organization (government or private). The critical success factors for execution of a community participation strategy are as follows:

1. **The program should address the health-related needs of the community.** Identification of these needs should involve not only analyses of morbidity and mortality statistics, but also qualitative information-gathering techniques, such as focus groups or interviews with community leaders and members. This process enables program personnel to become familiar with the social norms and structure of the community as they ascertain the perceptions of community members about their health status and health-related needs.

2. **The services provided by the program should be viewed as a priority by the community.** Health-related needs identified as important by the government are not necessarily the same as local priorities. Health issues compete with other priorities, especially in a poor community whose members are concerned about such basic needs as food, water, jobs, or education. Alternatively, it may be possible to elevate health issues to a higher priority by first helping a community address the concerns they view as more important and then working on the health issues.

3. **The program should be implemented to generate a sense of community ownership.** The program should demonstrate respect for the social structure and leadership of a community, sensitivity to current social and health-related values, and flexibility in working with traditional treatment methods and practitioners. Emphasis should be placed on achieving a sense of trust and partnership between a community and the external program sponsor. Program survival itself will ultimately depend on local investment of time and energy and perhaps financial investment by community members.

4. **There should be a clearly defined program leader.** The leader or leadership should be committed to investing the time and effort needed to work with the local community. This individual should have clear authority, be provided with sufficient resources to operate the program, and have the flexibility to modify program design in response to community preferences. Often, NGOs are ideally suited to this task.

5. **Government expectations for the roles of local community leadership and members in a program should be realistic.** The more extensive the behavioral changes that a program is intended to stimulate, the more important it is to have local community leadership, ownership, and participation. Volunteer contributions by community members (time or materials) should be used appropriately—not as a substitute for paid health workers or material resources the government rightfully should be providing.

6. **Adequate program organizational structure and operating procedures should be established to ensure sustainable operation over time.** The early successes of many of the primary-care programs sponsored by NGOs and other organizations are often difficult to sustain. A frequent reason is the dependence of programs on individual charismatic leaders from the outside, who, by virtue of their experience and personalities, work effectively with local communities to establish needed programs. An important, and often more difficult, task for these leaders is to create a formal program structure and train other personnel to carry on its operation—in essence, to make themselves replaceable. This may include preparation for transfer of full program control to the community as the external organization departs.

PROBLEMS WITH COMMUNITY PARTICIPATION

A variety of community-based programs have arisen throughout the Asian region, many of them in response to the Declaration of Alma Ata on Primary Health Care that defines community involvement as an integral part of primary health care. (WHO, 1978.) Most of the programs are free-standing, small-scale efforts in rural communities, which are sponsored by NGOs. Typically, the programs address such basic public health issues as infectious disease prevention, health education to encourage appropriate health behaviors, preventive health services, and primary-care treatment services.

Box 6.6: Community Participation in Primary Care in Zambia

A five-year project to improve the health status of people in the Samfya District of Luapula Province, Zambia, set out to construct three health centers, implement a primary health care strategy to enhance the health of women and children, and facilitate women's control over resources and their participation in community decisionmaking. (See Manderson et al., 1995.) Development strategies included the expansion of community infrastructure, such as new water wells and grinding mills; training of community health workers and traditional birth attendants; improved delivery of health interventions; sanitation; HIV/AIDS education; nutrition; malaria prevention; and promotion of income-generation activities.

In the first three years (1990–1993), the project trained 57 community health workers, 48 women in development (WID) leaders, and 63 headmen and chiefs (primary health care orientation). Mobile health teams and improved access to health centers reduced the time and workload for women in obtaining access to immunization. The project achieved increased attendance rates at clinics, producing over 90 percent immunization coverage of children in some communities and 76 percent coverage for maternal tetanus toxoid immunization. Distances to services such as grinding mills, health centers, water wells, and stores were greatly reduced for many households.

However, not all components were equally successful. People in some communities still have to travel more than 10 kilometers to a grinding mill and many over 6 kilometers to a health center. Also, while most women were motivated to use contraceptives, their husbands prevented them from doing so. Many men stated that women should not stop producing children "until God stops them producing."

The effect of the project on men is also important. Men felt unempowered because they were unable to gain access to loans and other benefits from the project, and some resented the favored status given to women. Many felt that the business activities and agricultural support should have been theirs. These feelings impeded implementation, leading to overt opposition, lack of assistance for women who started to learn traditional male tasks, and efforts to subvert the process or divert assistance back to men. Women were also under pressure to get personal loans to support men's activities.

Despite some resistance from men, women's groups flourished from the inception of the project. But women's workloads changed little, and in some cases the workload increased because of their involvement in income-generating activities. This may indicate a need for a more "gender sensitive" approach rather than a strict focus on WID. This approach would take into account the sexual division of labor and allocation of power in the development of projects.

Although the project was designed for the community, ownership was incomplete. Most viewed it as an NGO or government project, looking to these institutions to provide nearly all the input and giving little support to community health workers and traditional birth attendants. In addition, the evaluation team expressed concerns about the dependency on project staff and services, which had political overtones. In community meetings, people presented the evaluation team with a request list for additional resources, including a bank, glass windows for houses, another road, and health centers. Project staff in the areas tended to perpetuate this lack of community involvement. The evaluation report noted that "old patterns of thought and behavior change slowly."

The Asian experience with community participatory strategies can be grouped in terms of the three models discussed above: community development, health education, and customer service.

Asian Experience with Community Development Participatory Programs

In this category, malaria control programs offer some of the best examples of both the value and difficulties of full community participation. Since malaria control encompasses a spectrum of actions for both prevention and treatment, effective community programs will impose substantial changes on the social fabric of local communities. This makes it important to involve local community leadership and members to achieve the breadth of activities necessary to reduce the incidence of malaria and effectively treat those cases that occur.

The experience of a South India program exemplifies the challenges. (See Manderson et al., 1992.) The first efforts of the Vector Control Research Centre failed when it did not work through the official village committee. Personnel were viewed as trying to disrupt the village, because they first approached the lower-status groups in a stratified community. After months of other cooperative efforts with the village committee, growing acceptance permitted them to work with the village leadership in designing and conducting a multifaceted program to control mosquito breeding, including activities that generated income for the community. Some malaria control programs in other Asian countries have followed similar strategies. Others have focused on malaria prevention practices by community households using active local involvement.

A literacy training project for women in Indonesia demonstrates how enhancement of basic reading skills, with initiative by the individuals involved, can expand into a full empowerment process. A local women's group contracted with an NGO for a literacy program that used a teaching method that involved participants and focused on local issues. As their reading skills grew, the women decided to pursue access to clean water as the next priority for their community. With assistance from a local NGO, they organized the community to dig three wells. The success of these women was reflected in enhanced positions in the home, improved understanding of legal documents, ability to manage household finances, and greater independence. (See Manderson et al., 1995.)

Asian Experience with Health Education Participatory Programs

In this category, communities have turned either to encouraging local personnel to take up roles as medical providers or to motivating segments of the local population.

In rural China, two important forces resulted in a dearth of technically qualified health care providers. The local "barefoot doctors," with often only four to six weeks of schooling, were not trained to give sophisticated care, and the better-qualified five-year students were moving to the city to seek better pay. In Hanzhong and Ankang Community Colleges, local leaders contracted with the national government to train three-year physicians. Admission criteria were that students come from the local community, have adequate scholastic aptitude, and have strong family ties to the rural area. The curriculum was community based as well. Using medical principles, "cases" were developed for teaching. The case-based learning reflected the local population, local medical technology, and available financial resources. The combination of a three-year degree, local recruitment and training, and community-based learning resulted in a high retention of graduates. (See University of New Mexico/WHO, 1991.)

Efforts in several Asian countries to improve women's compliance with iron supplementation provide good examples of motivating segments of the local population. These programs have demonstrated the importance of active and empathetic involvement by health practitioners. High compliance levels in Thailand, Burma, and Hong Kong were attributed to highly motivated program participants and practitioners, supported by ongoing communications about the importance of taking iron pills. (See Galloway and McGuire, 1994.) The patient's perception about the concern of the provider has been found to be important. (See Woolley et al., 1978.)

Recognizing the diversity of cultures, educational status, and languages used by Asian populations, a variety of projects are using medical anthropological techniques to improve the content and language of needs assessment and communications methods for health education programs. For example, the WHO program for ARI uses a case management approach for diagnosing and treating ARI in which health workers and caretakers in the family perform complementary roles. An ethnographic study manual has been developed for use by health workers as they work with family members. (See Pelto, 1996.)

Similarly, standard needs assessment protocols are being developed in India to better understand women's reproductive health beliefs and knowledge, as well as their care-seeking decisions and behaviors. These protocols are being used by numerous NGOs across the country to provide reproductive health services for poor women in their service areas. (See Gittelsohn and Bentley, 1996.)

Asian Experience with Customer Service Participatory Programs

The implementation of an MCH project in Lao PDR by an NGO exemplifies the mix of techniques that can be used to ensure that a service delivery program is responsive to its clients. (See Manderson et al., 1995.) The project trained over 300 health workers, constructed a new village dispensary in the local area and a maternal and child health center at the district hospital to increase access to services, provided courses for village health volunteers and traditional birth attendants, negotiated free government transport to a referral center for emergency cases, and organized a local women's union that has been involved at all levels of the project. Utilization of health services and women's use of antenatal services has risen, and there has been a 50 percent increase in deliveries at the provincial hospital.

A health card system initiated by the Ministry of Public Health in Thailand uses a unique customer service approach to increasing health care coverage to rural households. (See Thailand Ministry of Public Health, 1997.) A household can purchase a health card for less than the average household spends for private health care. During the term of the health card, the purchaser is entitled to unlimited visits for preventive services, as well as a specified number of treatment services. The program encourages use of preventive care, increases use of local public health centers, reduces waiting time for hospital referrals, and protects rural households against catastrophic health care costs. It has been received enthusiastically in the villages where the cards are offered—from 55 to 100 percent of villagers have purchased cards.

Although the examples of community participation strategies described here were some of the more successful efforts, they all faced challenges in achieving sustainable preventive health or primary-care delivery programs. The wide diversity of local programs reflects the need to be responsive to the unique situation in each community. Thus far, there has been limited success in generalizing such programs to multiple locations. (See Manderson et al., 1995.)

In addition, programs with active community involvement usually are extremely resource-intensive, with program personnel investing extensive time in talking, training, and working with community leaders and members, thus allowing working relationships to grow as the community learns to trust and accept the external initiative.

Despite the challenges, there is consensus that community participation is essential to successfully develop and operate preventive health and primary health care programs. In some cases, however, governments have used community participation strategies to simply shift costs from the government to the local community. This is an inappropriate use of community participation, which is likely to fail because of lack of local support or resources.

Local involvement is especially important for government programs to improve health status in the poorest communities of developing countries, both rural and urban. Not only do these programs face daunting tasks of working with people to develop new health and hygiene behaviors—essentially requiring them to change the way they live—but they also typically have limited resources with which to work. Community participation in these programs, if well executed, offers hope for achieving and sustaining improvements, as community members experience both the benefits of the changes and enhanced self-confidence because they helped bring about those improvements.

POLICY IMPLICATIONS

What should policymakers focus on if they want to change behaviors? First, given how critical changing and motivating individual and provider behaviors are to implementing clinical and enabling interventions, policymakers should devote more resources to behavioral studies than they currently do. There is a paucity of well-designed studies of interventions to change behaviors. Finding the best ways to encourage health-seeking behaviors among individuals and to get providers to effectively deliver the interventions increases the likelihood that those interventions will improve health outcomes in the short and long term across a country's population.

Second, health promotion strategies generally are unproven; thus, policymakers should carefully plan and evaluate such strategies at the pilot level before they are implemented on a larger scale. Such evaluations need to account both for whether the intervention changed behavior and for whether the changed behavior improved health outcomes. Moreover, when policymakers do implement health promotion strategies on a larger scale, they should insist on longitudinal designs so they can clearly understand whether short-term behavioral changes (and, thus, changes to health outcomes) are sustainable over time and, conversely, whether the lack of such changes in the short term really reflects a failure of the long-term strategy.

Third, educational activities need to be integrated with other interventions to achieve improvements in health status. Although education may have a primary role, neither direct intervention nor education by itself can achieve the optimal change in behavior.

Fourth, commissioned behavioral studies should be grounded in conceptual frameworks or models about how to change behavior. There are a number of such models, several of which were mentioned above. Although supported by limited data, these frameworks can help design interventions that can lead to healthier behaviors and better practices by ensuring that important causative factors are not overlooked. Models also help in the evaluation of the effectiveness of the interventions. Along these lines, policymakers using published information from behavioral studies should critique published evaluations for their relevance to the cultural, social, and political context of each country or region.

Finally, in trying to change provider behavior, policymakers should combine, at a minimum, education, guidelines, financial incentives, and regulatory sanctions. As the models indicate, changing behavior is a complex process and under-standing how to change provider behavior is limited. Thus, it makes sense to try multiple approaches, both voluntary and, if necessary, compulsory, to effect that change.

CHAPTER 7: SUMMARY OF POLICY QUESTIONS, FINDINGS, AND IMPLICATIONS

ISSUES	EVIDENCE
• How can the objectives of the health sector be better understood?	• Understanding and informing the political process are important to enhancing MOH performance.
• How can the Ministry of Health (MOH) translate policy into programs and determine if it accomplishes its objectives?	• A formalized management system to operationalize health-sector objectives is needed.
• How should the MOH organize to carry out the policy plans?	• Organizing around programs and devolving programs to local communities, when appropriate, make sense.
• When should the MOH oversee and coordinate rather than participate directly?	• Private provision of services makes sense only when it will increase efficiency or advance another health system objective.
• What are the key infrastructure elements the MOH needs to manage?	• Managing medical technology and developing human capital are key elements of the health infrastructure the MOH should manage.
• What are the policy options for paying providers and hospitals?	• Payment mechanisms must be tailored to national circumstances and social objectives.

POLICY IMPLICATIONS

• The planning process needs to transform the political goals into operational programs that can be conducted within budget constraints and assessed by objective, measurable criteria.

• The collection and analysis of information should be tailored to the needs of managers at all levels of the MOH, rather than to the needs of statistical reporting.

• The delegation of responsibility for the provision of health care services should occur only after ensuring that local capabilities are in place and that the central government's goals for equity and efficiency are likely to be met.

• The provision of hospital services should not be delegated to the private sector unless an effective system for regulating institutional providers is in place.

• The private practice of medicine needs to be integrated into the planning and regulatory activities of the MOH.

• All regulatory systems should contain enforcement mechanisms that reward conforming behavior and that credibly punish violations.

IMPLEMENTING POLICY OBJECTIVES: THE ROLE AND RESPONSIBILITIES OF THE MINISTRY OF HEALTH

OVERVIEW

We argued in Chapter 1 that when governments pursue health-sector activities, their efforts are driven from the top down by a set of broad health-sector objectives. Governments seek to improve health status, ensure equity, and insure against catastrophic illness. Establishing and prioritizing those objectives is challenging enough, but governments have the much harder problem of managing the health-sector operations that derive from those objectives. Translating those objectives into operational programs is a difficult management task.

Just exactly how hard it is to manage health-sector activities is illustrated by the difficulties China has had during its reform efforts. A decade ago, Chinese macro health policy shifted health care financing and delivery activities toward a free market system. All levels of health facilities were encouraged to rely on user fees to support their operations. For political reasons, China continued its system of administered prices so that public hospitals continued to be run by the government. The government hospitals were only funded for basic wages and capital. User fees were intended to cover all other hospital costs. The government then set prices of many basic services at less than or equal to cost, while allowing higher prices to be charged for certain imported drugs and new high-technology procedures. Thus, hospitals and providers were able to make a profit on these services, which they could use to subsidize basic services and to award wage bonuses. But the combination of pricing policy and hospital administration rules increased utilization of high-technology services rather than decreasing it. And while cross-subsidizing basic services is potentially beneficial, it also contributed to the rising cost of care—something the government had hoped would not happen when it raised the prices for those services. (See Hsiao, 1995a.)

Based on the kinds of management problems and uncertainty that plagued China's reform efforts, we formulate six policy questions that policymakers must answer as they undertake health-sector activities:

1. How can the objectives of the health sector be better understood?
2. How can the MOH translate policy into programs and determine if it accomplishes its objectives?
3. How should the MOH organize to carry out policy plans?
4. When should the MOH oversee and coordinate rather than participate directly?
5. What are the key infrastructure elements the MOH needs to manage?
6. What are the policy options for paying providers and hospitals?

The answers to these questions form the basis of this chapter.

Unfortunately, researchers are at a significant data disadvantage in this area, even more so than they are in evaluating the behavioral interventions discussed in Chapter 6. Data that help in the implementation of effective management are difficult to obtain. The MOH, as the interface between politics and the institutions that deliver health care, is affected by the political, cultural, social, and institutional environment (as shown earlier in Figure 2.2). These factors are difficult to characterize and are hard to measure precisely. For example, stakeholder incentives, which are certain to influence policy implementation, rest on such questions as local ownership, leadership ability, and clarity of objectives. These factors are also hard to control for in a study. The result is that much of the information on management and other aspects of policy implementation comes from observational data, retrospective assessments, or case studies that are often qualitative and hard to generalize, instead of from controlled clinical trials. (See Table 2.11.)

It is ironic that the critical step of taking information from a limited and controlled experimental setting to a much broader level of policy implementation—a step that involves enormous amounts of a nation's public resources—has so little high-quality empirical evidence. While some rigorous studies are available, they are rare, and much more research is needed in the areas covered in this chapter. Although the evidence for management interventions may not be of high quality and is frequently observational, it can still be useful for policymakers, especially since management decisions cannot wait for more-rigorous studies to be conducted.

UNDERSTANDING AND INFORMING THE POLITICAL PROCESS

Not only is the MOH faced with the formidable task of translating policy[1] into programs, but it must also consider the politics that generate the policy in the first place. Developing countries increasingly have access to capital and human resources, but, as in more developed countries, sensible and effective policy is limited by political realities. The political process, for instance, is often conflicted or uncertain, and the MOH may be faced with multiple expectations generated by a variety of constituencies allied to support a specific policy. Similarly, political leaders may produce a policy that the MOH does not feel it has the resources to accomplish or that interferes with other objectives.

If MOH staff can better understand the political context that generates health policy, they can increase the likelihood that the information they provide to decisionmakers will be more relevant and that the information will address the conflicting objectives. A better understanding of the political process should also improve decisionmakers' assessment of how effective the MOH is at managing its tasks. This interface between politics and the MOH's institutional roles and responsibilities is an area where political scientists have investigated and developed some preliminary models that may help the MOH and that may lead to better MOH performance.

---

[1]To limit the discussion, policies are defined as statements developed by governments to guide activities designed to accomplish a set of objectives.

The Politics of Policymaking. To begin, we look at three reasons why the political debate is often so contentious. First, as we discussed in Chapter 1, the debate reflects different values about health. Some policymakers may value the most health for the least cost, others may want to guarantee minimum access to every citizen, while others believe that government should protect overall welfare by guaranteeing coverage for catastrophic illness. Second, policy debates are among different stakeholders. The competition over resources is about redistribution and "who gets what." Building a public hospital, for example, is not just about protecting social welfare; it is about "whose" social welfare. If policymakers choose to locate the new hospital in a metropolitan area, the choice will favor those in the city, redistributing resources away from the rural poor. Third, policy generates a political response—a positive one from the recipients and a negative one from the nonrecipients—that comes back and affects the political process that created the policy in the first place. (See Peltzman, 1976.) The MOH will have to consider all these perspectives as it carries out its responsibilities.

Policy Development. Another framework that may be useful to the MOH is considering how policy is made. Two descriptions of policy formulation are the rational process and the incrementalist process. Early on, policymaking was described as a rational process in which a problem is identified and further characterized by information and data; a policy is selected from a set of options and compared with other options based on such values as costs, benefits, and consequences; and the policy activities are put in place and evaluated for effectiveness. This model is orderly, scientific, and, as Walt (1994) points out, it assumes that policymakers behave rationally and (we add) have access to low-cost information.

Health policy objectives, however, are often not specified and are implied only by the set of activities chosen by the political process. There may be a practical reason for this. If the objectives were explicitly stated, it might focus political opposition and make policymakers more vulnerable to criticism. These observations have contributed to the articulation of the incrementalist process of policymaking. In this process, policymakers tend to choose options that are only marginally different from the status quo, for several reasons. First, policy cannot always characterize the problem or identify optimal policies. Second, rationally bound policymakers choose only the most visible solutions and identify the most obvious consequences. Third, experience shows that policy choices do not completely solve the identified problem. Therefore, policy is by definition remedial and in constant need of reform as new strategies are developed and misdirections corrected. It is not surprising that this process has been identified by many as "muddling through." (See Lindblom, 1977.)

In the incrementalist model, the policy process is inherently conservative, both technically and politically. The inherent belief is that eventually this process will get it right, but this belief is subject to how fast options are initiated and implemented and ignores the consequences of delays and gross misjudgments. While the rational process has the advantage of being able to perform "radical surgery" and introduce a more normative element to the debate about what health reforms ought to be, the incremental process is far more grounded in the realities of a local environment and considers the very practical insight that the

---

Box 7.1: The Importance of Political Leadership in Social Security Reform in Ecuador

In June 1994, Ecuadorian President Sixto Duran Ballen assembled the Presidential Commission of Reform of the Social Security as a body of the National Counsel for Modernization (CONAM) to develop alternative health and pension fund systems. As some international observers stated, most of the conditions were ripe for successful health-sector reform. There was a general consensus that the Social Security system (plagued, for example, by low coverage and a focus on medium- and high- as opposed to low-income groups) needed to be reformed, and the issue was brought to the political forefront by the president in forming the Commission. In addition, international organizations were in place to provide the economic resources and technical assistance to initiate reform. Still, the reform process failed in Ecuador because an important element was missing—appropriate mechanisms for informing the people and establishing consensus were not implemented.

The Commission's proposal in February 1995 was a technical document, developed by national and international consultants but lacking any kind of social or political support. Key social groups—retirees, social security workers, physicians working in the public and private sectors, political parties, unions, and the Indians, who up to then were covered by the "Seguro Social Campesino" (Rural Social Security)—had never been systematically consulted.

Because the reform required eliminating the monopoly of the public sector as a provider of health insurance, the Constitution had to be amended. In April 1995, the CONAM president started lobbying the country, with mixed results. In general, entrepreneurs defended the reform, while workers in the public health sector, the unions, and the Indians were suspicious. In many cases, reactions showed that the main points of the reform were not understood, partly because the CONAM had not communicated them and partly because the leaders of the extreme leftist party—the Popular Democratic Movement, or MPD—manipulated and distorted the message. For example, the Indians held a national strike demanding that Rural Social Security not be eliminated, whereas one of the main goals of the reform was actually to reinforce it. The CONAM failed to establish channels to negotiate changes to the original reform and limited itself to defending the reform passively, thus leading to confrontation rather than negotiation.

Negotiations between the Congress and the Presidential Commission were conducted in vain, partly because of the CONAM president's rigidity. Without this consensus, Congress rejected amendments needed for the reform. As a last resort and ultimate attempt to save the reform, Duran Ballen established a referendum in November 1995.

Although the CONAM changed its attitude and aggressively tried to generate a social base to support the reform, it was already too late. The window of opportunity for policy change had closed: The government's credibility was eroded by both a harsh economic crisis and by the accusation that the vice-president had engaged in corrupt activities. As a result, the Ecuadorian people voted in favor of the status quo and against the reform.

The mistakes committed in the political arena have had a significant cost, which is now being paid by all those who have seen their access to a basic service postponed.

---

politics of skillful policymaking is as much a part of successful policy as a rational technical solution.

The attempts of the Clinton Administration to reform health care in the United States during its two terms reflect the differences between the two models of policy development. In its first term, the Administration took a more rationalist approach to reforming health care. Feeling it had a mandate for radical change, the Administration tried to overhaul the entire system. Unfortunately, its efforts ran up against a political wall. Many of the key players in the debate, particularly in Congress, felt the Administration had excluded them; and in fact, very little consensus-building took place. The end result was that the Administration was accused of behaving in an authoritarian manner and the entire attempt to change the U.S. health care system failed badly.

When the Administration decided to return to reforming health care in its second term, it took a decidedly incrementalist approach. Instead of trying to change the whole health care system, the Administration chose to "fix" pieces of the system (such as the lack of adequate insurance coverage for children) around which it felt it could build a consensus. The Administration now picks and chooses its battles; as a result, it has been much more successful but reform has been incremental.

The implication of these two approaches is that, without crisis or forceful impetus for change, policymaking is likely to be incremental. Data presented by the MOH, for example, may not compel policymakers to change their strategies quickly and much-needed reform can lag behind technical developments.

Identifying Issues. Finally, there is the issue of how objectives in the health sector are defined. All stakeholders are interested in understanding which issues gain ascendancy and become part of the policy debate and which issues will be ignored. On many occasions, MOH officials must feel that the number of problems they need to address is overwhelming. From that inexhaustible list, some issues end up as the minister's priority, while others do not. Similarly, the minister may want to understand "why" he faces one particular issue, such as leprosy control, while the assistant secretary for evaluation and monitoring may want to know "why" staffing for his monitoring and evaluation division has not become a reorganization priority.

Many frameworks exist for thinking about how issues are identified and gain ascendancy, but the simplicity of Hall's model has much to recommend it. (See Hall et al., 1975.) In this framework, an issue needs to be legitimate, to have feasible solutions, and to have public support. Legitimacy refers to issues that most people feel are appropriate government concerns, such as licensing practitioners. But which issues are legitimate varies considerably from country to country. For example, while most Asian countries are involved in family planning, in China, this involvement extends to a one-child policy that is accepted by most urban residents.

If an issue is considered the legitimate responsibility of government, policymakers turn to the question of feasibility. Technical feasibility might entail, for example, whether there is the expertise to design integrated hospital financial records or train staff to work in a remote clinic. Financial feasibility deals with budget constraints and depends on choosing between several policy options simultaneously.

Even when an issue is legitimate and has feasible solutions, it must still attract support. In health, public support, more often than not, refers to the support of (or lack of opposition to) medical reforms. For example, pharmaceutical reforms carried out in Bangladesh in the 1980s rode the crest of populist political support and were coupled with external support from the WHO and local NGOs. These reforms were countered by strong opposition from the Bangladesh Medical Association and from diplomatic representatives of developed countries.

Informing the Political Process

Policies are ultimately implemented by institutions within the government. In the health sector in Asia, the institution generally responsible for setting much of the health policy and implementing policy activities is the MOH. Many researchers point out that the MOH is rarely a powerful ministry. The Ministry of Finance or the Ministry of Planning are often the most powerful institutions involved in setting health policy. Such ministries can even set health policy by establishing budget allocations and, in effect, prioritizing activities by establishing the budget. This is made worse when there is little technical input from the MOH. Other institutions also actively contribute to health policy, such as the Ministries of Education, Agriculture, and Public Works, although the specific organizations vary considerably throughout Asia. In Viet Nam, for instance, budget contractions led to "default policymaking." Because of a general overall economic decline, falling local community budgets for rural commune health clinics were not offset by central-level funding. Without MOH replenishment, the budget shortfalls effectively cut off support for the commune clinics and shifted the focus of primary care to district-level facilities.

The MOH always exists in a political environment. To improve health, the MOH not only needs to understand the political processes and policies but must also respond to the varying political forces. If, for example, it is charged with limiting the spread of HIV and chooses to use research-supported needle-exchange programs, it must contend with legitimate concerns that drug addiction rates could escalate. In this example, it is not enough for the MOH to simply assert that needle-exchange programs reduce HIV and save lives; it must also show that deaths from drug addiction will not also rise. By broadening the analysis, the MOH informs the decisionmaking process and gives policymakers more choices and options. Thus, as part of its technical role, the MOH is responsible for informing the political process.

The remainder of this chapter focuses on how the MOH, operating within the political milieu, can effectively implement health-sector objectives through its policies.

MANAGING HEALTH SECTOR OBJECTIVES

As the China example at the beginning of this chapter illustrated, the consequences of management and policy decisions are complicated. Because it is so complicated, rational planning alone is not sufficient to ensure that programs achieve their goals. Program activities and their results must be continually evaluated to determine how to improve them, and the results of the evaluations must be fed into some form of planning and evaluation process. The result of the planning process is a statement of the agreed-upon goals, objectives, priorities, and broad strategies for reaching these goals. Unfortunately, the planning process often stops at this stage of broad generalities and the plans are not translated into action. This step requires that specific programs be laid out in detail and that budgets be determined for each program.

Planning, Programming, and Budgeting System (PPBS)

Although there are a number of possible management structures that can operationalize planning, we focus our discussion on the Planning, Programming, and Budgeting System (PPBS), because it shows the place of planning and evaluation within a more complete management structure. PPBS is also useful because the concepts that it contains underlie most current planning systems, although their names differ. For example, the concepts are the basis of planning systems used recently in Papua New Guinea. Alternative systems and concepts, described by several authors, can also be used and are useful planning aids. (See Stanton and Wouters, 1992; Walt and Gilson, 1994.) Although the implementation of a full-scale performance budget has sometimes been criticized for being more trouble than it is worth, the concepts endure and remain the basis for most analytical budgeting systems.[2]

PPBS is a management system for developing and implementing long-range plans, as well as short-range plans consistent with those long-range plans. Figure 7.1 is a schematic of the PPBS process, reproduced to show the logical relationship among the major phases of the Planning, Programming, and Budgeting System process. PPBS is divided into the three phases for which the system is named. While PPBS can be carried out with a variety of steps, each phase is aimed at producing specific decisions required to manage government activities. Below, we describe the steps in PPBS that can be applied to planning health care in developing countries.

The Planning Phase. During the planning phase, government leaders determine goals, objectives, priorities, and broad program outlines. This phase is akin to the development of the five-year plan in Asian countries such as Papua New Guinea. Here, leaders need to consider the constraints that limit goals, such as hard-to-change legal mandates or political groups that would lose power or wealth. They then need to develop and set forth a statement of the government's goals for the health care sector so that the plan can be reviewed by stakeholders.

Decisions about the government's broad strategies to achieve its goals are also made during the planning phase. By strategies, we mean classes of activities—for example, public/private mix of primary health care clinics, regulation of insurance practices, or changing legislation. These are what Frenk calls "systemic policy levers." (See Frenk, 1993.)

Ideally, decisionmakers are presented with analyses of outcomes associated with alternative strategies for achieving each objective. The analyses must explain the trade-offs among the various objectives—for example, user fees might increase efficiency by reducing unnecessary services but could harm equity by reducing the access of the poor to health care, as illustrated for Indonesia in Chapter 4. (More-complete examples of the expected outcomes from various strategies are found in Chapters 3 through 6.)

During planning, these known arguments would be particularized to the circumstances of the planning environment in various ways. Interactions among the different strategies are analyzed. The analysis also involves forecasting likely changes in the environment and examining constraints that limit program

---

[2]Dean (1989) reported case-study evaluations of program budgeting in India, Malaysia, Philippines, Singapore, and Sri Lanka. However, these programs were implemented nationally, not within a specific ministry.

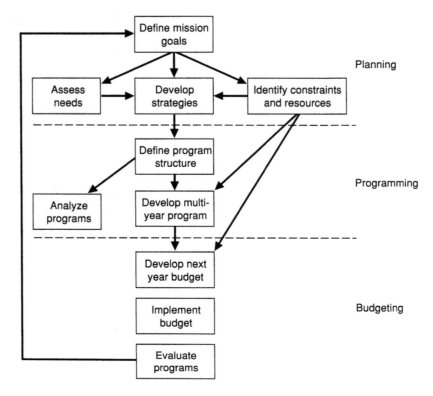

SOURCE: Adapted from McKinney, 1995.

Figure 7.1—The Three Phases of the PPBS

operations (e.g., the availability of trained personnel). Any assumptions made in the analysis, such as the level of resources or spending efficiently, must be made explicit.

The Programming Phase. During the programming phase, operational plans for implementing the chosen planning strategies are designed. This phase, akin to the annual implementation plan in Papua New Guinea, involves analyzing alternative methods for achieving objectives. Measurable criteria are chosen for each objective. Cost-benefit analyses can be used to help choose specific programs that are feasible, adequate, and more cost-effective than alternative programs. Note that the cost-benefit analyses must consider all effects of project implementation—including, for example, nonhealth effects, changes in demand for health care, or provider responses. For each program, specific multiyear goals, timetables, and budgeting guidelines must be developed. Equity considerations can be addressed here too, when choices are made about how resources and/or facilities are geographically allocated. This phase incorporates the results of evaluations of ongoing programs to look for ways to improve efficiency or equity by changing organizational, financial, or regulatory procedures.

The Budgeting Phase. Once goals and programs have been identified and multiyear plans established for each one, operational plans for the near term must be developed. The near-term plans serve as the basis for budgets developed during the budgeting year. Quantitative performance indicators should also be chosen to measure effectiveness and efficiency against those plans. In this way, the program budgeting process explicitly allocates resources to produce *outputs* that meet national health goals and objectives. This allows government leaders and other concerned citizens to review how much the budget reflects the agreed-upon goals and objectives of the health care sector. In contrast, the traditional line-item budget process only specifies various categories of *inputs* (such as personnel and supplies) and does not explicitly link them to performance.

The budgeting phase is often described by four steps.[3] The first step is to define performance indicators for major programs identified in the programming phase. For a hospital, these measures might include patient days of care provided; for a series of clinics, the fraction of expectant mothers receiving prenatal care; for a drug procurement program, the availability levels for essential drugs. The measures themselves will be produced by the information system (discussed below). The staff managing each program should be involved in developing the indicators that will measure it, since they will be held accountable for performance on those indicators.

Once performance indicators have been defined, baseline or current performance on each measure must be assessed. Target levels for each indicator should be set for the coming year and for the multiyear planning horizon. For example, a 5 percent increase in the rate of measles immunization could be targeted in the first year, with a goal of a 20 percent increase at the end of five years. Providing comparisons of baseline performance to states, regions, and districts can help managers in those jurisdictions set realistic targets for their own performance.

The second step is for each program to draft operational plans to achieve targeted performance levels. This requires defining such inputs as the personnel, supplies, facilities improvements or maintenance, and transportation needed to accomplish specific tasks; assigning management responsibility for those tasks; and establishing a timeline on which they are to be accomplished. For example, upgrading the vaccination cold chain in rural regions would require such resources as new freezers in some clinics and transport to deliver them, plus maintenance personnel and supplies to repair existing nonfunctional freezers. Of course, improving performance is not necessarily the goal for all programs; for some programs, maintaining current acceptable performance levels may be the goal.

The third step is actual budget preparation. This includes estimating costs, iterating to reconcile planned expenditures with expected available funds, and submitting the complete budget to the Ministry of Finance. Cost estimates must be developed for each task in the operational plans. This requires information on the unit costs of each input item, such as equipment repair or vehicles. Experience has

---

[3]This discussion draws primarily from the literature on well-established budgeting and government financial management practices in industrialized countries. (See Babunakis, 1976; McKinney, 1995a; Steiss, 1989.) The literature on health care budgeting in developing countries is limited. Most of the available literature on budgeting in developing countries discusses activities at the Ministry of Finance level, rather than within individual ministries. (See United Nations, 1991b; Caiden, 1980; Joseph, 1982.)

Box 7.2: Planning, Programming, and Budgeting in Papua New Guinea

The process of developing and implementing the recently completed 1996–2000 National Health Plan (NHP) in Papua New Guinea illustrates the application of planning, programming, and budgeting principles. Previous health plans had set goals that were inadequately tied to available resources, and recent fiscal strains have reduced government resources even further. The latest five-year health plan was therefore drafted to allocate resources where they could most effectively improve the health status of the nation's population.

The goal of the 1996–2000 NHP is *to improve the health status of the people of Papua New Guinea.* It establishes five policy priorities aimed at achieving that goal:

1.   Increase services to the rural majority;
2.   Expand promotion and preventive health services;
3.   Reorganize and restructure the national health system;
4.   Develop staff professional, technical, and managerial skills;
5.   Upgrade and maintain investment in health infrastructure.

These priorities were then used to guide the development of strategies and objectives for major program areas over the period of the plan. For example, major objectives of Family Health Services are to increase immunization coverage and reduce maternal mortality. The NHP specifies target levels for such measures as coverage rates for major vaccines, antenatal care, and supervised deliveries.

Figure 7.2.1 shows how these long-term national targets form the basis for annual implementation plans and budgets at the province and district level. The first step in this annual exercise is to use data from the existing health information system (HIS) to assess the burden of disease in each province. Since the most severe health problems differ across provinces, this allows tailoring of activities to meet local health needs.

Next, each province sets improvement targets for individual program activities, based on NHP policy priorities and budget ceilings from the MOH. Specific plans for achieving these targets are then written, specifying the resources necessary to carry out those plans. For

---

shown that during the first years of using a program budgeting system, staff on each program will have to spend a great deal of time developing reliable unit cost data.

The fourth step in the program budget process is to evaluate actual spending and performance against target levels of performance indicators. In this way, programs can be held accountable for the resources they receive. Specifically, operational efficiency can be assessed by computing variances between planned and actual performance.[4] For example, if increased spending on antibiotics did not decrease pneumonia mortality as much as expected, it would be considered an unfavorable variance. Corrective actions should be developed in the case of unfavorable variances; these corrections then become inputs to developing operational plans and budgets as the budget cycle starts again.

The detailed work of budgeting accomplished in these four steps may show that the resource allocation assumptions of the programming phase were not adequate to support existing programming decisions. Small modifications can be accommodated by making modest changes in scale or by stretching out

---

[4]Operational efficiency contrasts with *allocative* efficiency, which is addressed primarily in the decisions on budget ceilings for programs and prioritization of activities within programs.

example, to reduce maternal deaths, increases in health patrols to remote villages may be planned, which require resources such as supplies and transport.

The budgets for each province are then based on these annual implementation plans. Standard reporting categories for cost line items (such as personnel and supplies) are being promulgated so that budgets for all provinces can be aggregated by the MOH on both a program and a line-item basis.

The final step in the process is monitoring the actual performance against the targets in the annual implementation plans, and spending compared to budgets. These performance assessments then become inputs to the next year's planning process.

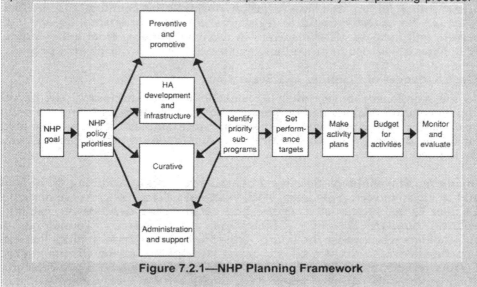

Figure 7.2.1—NHP Planning Framework

timetables. Larger changes require revisiting the analyses in the programming phase.

The planning, programming, and budgeting phases are logically sequential. When the government first intends widespread reform of the health care sector, the steps must be carried out in this order. Clearly, it is not feasible to analyze programs until objectives and goals have been clarified. Moreover, an infinite number of draft budgets would need to be analyzed unless program choices have first been made.

However, after the initial cycle, the PPBS phases are implemented simultaneously, each phase dealing with different time periods. The planning phase should cover a period long enough to make substantial progress in attaining systemwide goals and objectives—say, five to ten years. The budgeting phase covers the current year and one or two future years to provide input into the programming phase. The programming phase covers the first future year and enough additional future years (typically, three years) to allow adequate resource mobilization and efficient implementation of program changes.

Both legislators and high-level government executives use the analyses that occur during the planning phase, because planning issues usually require joint action by

288 Policy and Health: Implications for Development in Asia

both. For example, should hospitals be funded by the central government (as is now done in many developing countries), or should local governments also fund hospitals (as is done in China)? In contrast, the details of the programming and budget phases are rarely helpful with the questions that legislators need to resolve. (See Dean, 1989.) The questions addressed in these phases are likely to be largely, or even solely, the province of the executive. For example, maternal and child health services can be provided in separate clinics (as in China) or within general-purpose public health care clinics (as in the Philippines and elsewhere). This decision hinges on understanding local circumstances and capacity and is better suited for an executive decision during programming and budgeting. Although not directly useful to legislators, a careful programming and budget process will increase MOH's success in receiving funding from either legislators or donors; it will also improve the way the MOH carries out its own policies.

The Challenges of Planning and Evaluation

As we mentioned above, involving stakeholders is a necessary part of policy implementation. Making assumptions explicit, vetting trade-offs between program goals, and coordinating with other sectors are examples of where stakeholders, including donors, need to be included. But involving these parties presents challenges.

Involving Stakeholders. Successful planning requires considering both political and technical factors. (See Green, 1995; Walt and Gilson, 1994.) As we discussed in Chapter 6, the success of even the best reform plan depends on gaining the political support of some stakeholders and effectively countering other stakeholders who oppose the reform. The surest way to develop plans that can be implemented is to involve all important stakeholders in the planning process. Further, efficiency can be enhanced if plans of related agencies are coordinated. The identity of the stakeholders and the details of their involvement will depend on the political, legislative, and administrative structure of the country and on how much agreement there is on basic goals.

Who are the important stakeholders in any reform effort? They include representatives of all involved branches of government, such as the finance or taxation departments and legislators with substantial influence on revenue, spending, or legal mandates for the health sector. Routine consultations with these individuals when plans and programs are being developed will increase the likelihood that the final plan and its implementation will be accepted. It may even increase the resources available for health.

Identifying additional stakeholders depends on the particular government strategies being planned or programmed. Plans for important changes in regulation might be improved after consulting with representatives of the regulated providers—especially those who can be trusted both to have the public good as a primary goal and to understand the likely behavior of providers in the face of the regulations. If the government plans to increase NGO activity, it will need to discuss with existing NGOs the feasibility of its plan and the support (financial or other) that the NGOs might need.

All organizations that provide related services should be consulted about plans to open or close facilities or to expand or decrease the amount of services provided.

Organizations that might be concerned with such plans include NGOs, local governments, the social health insurance agency, other parts of the central government, or even drug or medical supply wholesalers. Coordinating changing levels of service will allow much more efficient use of remaining services and should avoid the duplication of facilities that so often occurs. For example, in China, many national programs are organized vertically and planning is often not integrated across programs. Consequently, there has been duplication of facilities or excess capacity, resulting in inefficiency and waste. In urban areas, the overlap involves Ministry of Public Health (MOPH) facilities, state-owned enterprises, and traditional medicine; in rural areas, the overlap is among maternal and child health centers, family planning services, township health centers, and epidemic prevention stations. (See World Bank, 1997c.) As experience in many developed and developing countries attests, it is often politically difficult to close unneeded facilities after they have been opened. Consequently, careful, comprehensive planning before opening facilities is especially important.

Of course, in considering all the important stakeholders, one often overlooked group is critical—the local population where a program is being implemented. These individuals are the end-users in the health care planning and evaluation process. As we showed in Chapter 6, community participation programs are essential if health care programs are to be successfully implemented.

Plans will more likely be implemented if one understands the position of those who might lose from the implementation. Thus, it might be useful to vet a proposed plan with organizations representing those who are likely to oppose it (e.g., civil service unions on plans for privatization, professional provider organizations on new regulations). It might be possible to negotiate with them to obtain their acquiescence to the plan; at the least, one would be prepared for public discussion of their arguments.

Involving Donors. Resources provided by donors also need to be considered in developing a country's health plan. But the need for donor involvement in planning is broader than this. Discussing the entire strategic plan with the donors might result in a better fit between donor activities and the country's needs. Green argues that donors are having an increasingly damaging effect on the planning process. (See Green, 1995.) They develop large sectoral projects that have miniplans of their own, making wider plans inoperable. In addition, they may impose conditionality, may attract the best technical planners (thus leaving none for the strategic plan), and may overemphasize operational planning (i.e., programming) while underemphasizing strategic planning.

Donors often call their projects "pilot projects" without addressing how the project might be replicated or extended if successful. Often, the level of investment is infeasible for locals. In a paper prepared for the 1996 ADB conference on health-sector priorities, one policymaker noted that "most developing countries are unable to cope with the operating and maintenance costs arising from investments made by outside agencies in health development projects." (See Ali, 1996.) Even when they do consider sustainability, donors sometimes emphasize financial sustainability rather than organizational or political sustainability.

Donor assistance has its own political constraints. Not only do donors need to show results to sustain their funding or lending, they also have their own agenda, often closely linked to national perspectives. When the project objectives conflict with national policy or when political intrusion is excessive, recipients have declined the aid (and will continue to do so). For example, food aid in African countries has been used for political leverage, and in Viet Nam development aid was refused because it was linked to human rights issues. (See Harris, 1991.)

By negotiating with donors over mutually acceptable objectives, methods, and resources, policymakers can help the donor aid support the country's plan rather than subvert it. (See Wang'ombe, 1995.) Donors need to recognize that short-term project interests may not be compatible with long-term sector development. They pursue their own need to demonstrate short-term identifiable gains to their sponsors and not necessarily the recipient country's need for long-term development. (See Foltz, 1994.) For example, the organization of the donor's project can be shaped to be implemented by a reformed MOH, thereby supporting reform rather than competing with it. (See Foster et al., 1994.) Guldner argues that in Viet Nam the absence of Vietnamese personnel in donor projects hindered their long-term effectiveness. (See Guldner, 1995.) Involving local personnel more heavily spreads innovative methods and concepts of public health and finance that donors bring. It might even be possible to replace program implementation units with more general implementation units. Evaluation of programs, if done by donors, could become a model for evaluation by the recipient country.

Greater coordination across donors could also reduce duplication and waste. A number of donors are currently implementing health management development projects in support of the civil service reform process in Laos. Interviews with Laotian officials, reported by Holland and colleagues, suggest that lack of donor coordination is contributing to a fragmented approach to health management reform. (See Holland and Phimphachanh, 1995.) Similarly, Guldner reports that the vertical organization of donor-funded national disease control programs has caused duplication of work and inconvenienced the served population in Viet Nam. In contrast, the Bangladesh Population and Health Consortium is an example of a coordinated donor process. Members of the consortium include the government of Bangladesh, the ADB, the World Bank, the WHO, UNICEF, and 10 bilateral agencies. The members collectively support the Fourth Population and Health Project, a $605 million project. During project formulation, several workshops were held in Dhaka and a conference was held in Geneva where agreement was reached on strategies and approaches to improving the health sector.

The Challenges of Programming and Budgeting

When implementing a program budgeting system, policymakers must bear several technical and accountability challenges in mind.

Technical Challenges. The greatest technical challenge in preparing program budgets is estimating the allocation of shared resources to the different programs.[5]

---

[5]Public agencies in industrialized countries also face this problem, since they, too, provide a broad mix of services in varying quantities and generally do not receive payment for those services at the time of provision. Private firms also have complex cost accounting methods. They, however, can

For example, regional managers may supervise several programs, drugs used in health facilities may be supplied from a central government purchase program, and rural health clinics may provide services that support several disease-specific programs. One solution to this problem is to define inputs, such as management and drug procurement, as separate programs. Performance indicators could then be used to measure how well the resource inputs support the needs of those other programs. Defining resource inputs as programs minimizes the sharing of resources (such as between hospitals and primary-care clinics), but managers must ensure proper coordination between programs.

Another technical challenge in preparing budgets is the constraint of essentially fixed costs. The most important of these fixed costs is personnel, who are often protected by civil service regulations. When government budgets are cut in times of austerity, personnel may remain on the payroll but not be supplied with the drugs or equipment maintenance necessary to provide care for patients. Program budgets force managers to confront these problems by estimating costs for all inputs needed to achieve performance targets. However, changes in the allocation between fixed and variable costs may have to be phased in over more than one budget year.

Yet another technical challenge is to ensure that capital costs are treated separately from recurring costs, because supplies and maintenance for facilities and equipment become recurring fixed costs in later years' budgets. Decisions about acquiring new assets at the program level should, however, be based on *life-cycle costs*, rather than just the cost of the initial capital investment. Life-cycle costing takes into account both initial capital expenditures and the recurring costs in each subsequent year. The recurring costs are usually discounted to reflect the lesser value of future expenditures.

Challenges of Accountability and Political Transparency. Beyond these three technical challenges, there are the additional challenges of accountability and political transparency. Adherence to accounting standards is essential for this task if budgets are to be used to hold programs accountable. Program budgeting, while helping with accountability, also increases the complexity of accounting, since each expenditure must be categorized both by line item and by program. Each program's budget submission must be broken down by the categories used in the overall government budget, such as salaries, housing, and supplies, so that the MOH can aggregate program budgets for its budget submission to the Ministry of Finance. In addition, the allocation of spending to different programs must be performed consistently at all administrative levels. For example, if a district receives personnel funds from several programs, it must report those funds against each program according to guidelines specified by the MOH.

Carrying out this "matrix" approach to accounting calls for using computers, which can reconcile line-item and program-expenditure categories quickly and accurately. Computers are already used extensively for budgeting by Ministries of Finance in developing countries. (See Davies et al., 1993; United Nations, 1991b.) The increase in power and decline in price of microcomputers makes their use

---

allocate the costs of overhead and shared resources to the products they sell, since all revenue received by a firm comes in return for selling its products. (See Horngren, 1982). The accuracy of these methods has been improved in recent years with the advent of activity-based costing. (See Cooper and Kaplan, 1988.)

feasible in health care budgeting by developing countries. For example, budget submissions from programs, regions, and districts could be prepared on preformatted, MOH-supplied spreadsheets and then submitted in electronic form to the MOH. However, for such a system to function effectively, adequate provisions must be made for developing programming expertise, training users, and maintaining hardware.

Another fundamental accounting discipline is accurately recording actual spending and comparing it to budgeted amounts. In addition to monitoring total spending by a program, budgeters must also record expenditures by line item[6] to determine whether the funds allocated by the MOH were expended in the planned manner. This is a powerful tool for enforcing accountability of managers at all levels.

Auditing is an important way to check that financial accounting is being performed accurately. (See McKinney, 1995b; United Nations, 1990.) In addition, nonfinancial performance audits can be done and are facilitated by the performance indicators included in operational plans for each program. (See Dean, 1989.) Effective auditing depends on the presence of good accounting records and the independence of the auditing body, such as an Inspector General's office or private firms contracted to perform audits. Audits must also be timely, which is often not the case in developing countries. (See Wallis, 1989; Esman, 1991.) However, even though effective auditing is a great challenge, its benefits can be great. In particular, it is one of the strongest tools for preventing corruption in countries where many public servants are unfortunately tempted to convert public resources to their private gain.

Beyond accounting and auditing issues, there is the political challenge of implementing program budgets and audits. Implementation should be phased in over a period of years, for several reasons. (See Babunakis, 1976.) It can take several budget cycles for managers and budget analysts to become proficient at accurately estimating costs and effectively using actual performance data as a management tool. Training and outside technical support may also be required to build the managerial and analytical expertise called for by program budgeting, where it is lacking in developing countries. The experience with program budgets in the United States indicates that political reaction can be strong when performance trade-offs are made explicit by a program budgeting exercise. The MOH must prepare in advance to defend budget choices against vigorous challenges. (See Golembiewski and Rabin, 1983; Wildavsky, 1984.) Even though program budgeting has long been advocated for developing countries (e.g., see WHO, 1983), implementations of program budgeting at the national level have often proved disappointing. Expectations may be overly optimistic, or the system is imposed on all ministries at once, or perhaps the system is insensitive to the information needs of legislators. (See Dean, 1989.) Finally, program budgeting, as presented here, does not replace traditional budget submissions to legislatures; instead, it provides the MOH with a management tool for systematically planning and measuring performance in the face of resource constraints.

---

[6]Computers can also be useful in recording and submitting this accounting data efficiently to the MOH.

Despite all these challenges, program budgets, if successfully implemented, promise numerous benefits, including more realistic planning in the face of resource constraints and greater accountability for performance. These factors improve the MOH's ability to attract funds from the central government and from donor agencies. As donors place more explicit conditions on their aid, they may be more likely to fund initiatives supported by effective budgeting and accounting systems. (See Foster et al., 1994.)

Unfortunately, given the value program budgets have, few Asian developing countries are reported to have comprehensive programming and budgeting systems in place. Papua New Guinea has implemented such a system as part of its most recent five-year plan. And to address highly fragmented health-sector funding sources and an overly centralized process, Indonesia has implemented an Integrated Health Plan and Budget (IHPB) process. (See World Bank, 1989c.) The IHPB is prepared by local governments and aggregated up through intervening administrative levels to the MOH. It also serves as the basis for performance measurement and resulting modifications to future years' plans. In India, the portion of health-sector financing contained in the national development budget is allocated to the vertical programs in the development plan. However, recurrent expenditures, mostly financed by the states, are budgeted by line item only, not by program. (See World Bank, 1992c.) In Pakistan, the development budget specifies resources by program on a "zero-based" principle and separates capital from recurring expenditures, but recurring expenditures are budgeted based on historical expenditures. (See World Bank, 1993 l.) Nepal has experienced difficulties in coordinating funding in the presence of multiple donor–sponsored vertical projects, as well as in making sufficient provision for recurring expenses. (See Henderson, 1995.)

Managing Information Resources

Effective policy analysis, planning, budgeting, management, and performance measurement all depend on accurate, detailed, and timely health information. Earlier chapters (especially Chapter 2) have discussed methods for evaluating such information. This section briefly reviews the types of systems that governments use to collect and analyze health information—routine reporting and surveillance systems, national or local population surveys, and information systems that support individual programs and facilities—and draws lessons from experience with computerized information systems.[7]

Routine Reporting and Surveillance Systems. Many countries collect data through routine reports from health facilities on morbidity, mortality, and service utilization. All facilities in a country may be required to report data on some conditions, particularly communicable diseases. China's National Disease Reporting System (NDRS), for example, reports 35 communicable diseases on a national basis. (See Chunming, 1992.)

Sentinel sites are another common method for collecting data on specific diseases. Such sites are often large facilities, such as hospitals, that provide services to a large enough population to capture significant numbers of patients with the target

---

[7]Advanced medical information systems, such as image processing and diagnostic systems, are being developed in some developing countries (Wang, 1993), but their policy significance is likely to be small in the near future.

diseases and that have the resources for detailed ongoing data collection. For example, in Bangladesh the Dhaka Medical College Hospital and several hospitals to which it transfers patients serve as sentinel sites for infectious disease monitoring; in Bombay, India, the Kasturba Infectious Disease Hospital is a sentinel site. (See Woodall, 1988.)

Countries with networks of public clinics and hospitals can use routine reporting from those facilities to collect a broad range of health information. The Philippines' Field Health Services Information System (FHSIS) collects data from all public health care facilities on mortality and service utilization for several major programs, including maternal health, child health, and infectious diseases. (See Robey and Lee, 1990.) Thailand and Papua New Guinea also have comprehensive facility-based health information systems. (See Wilson and Smith, 1991; Campos-Outcault, 1991.)

But facilities and sentinel sites may not be representative of the health status of the population as a whole, and no purely facility-based system can collect data on persons who do not use the facilities. (See Cibulskis and Izard, 1996.) China has addressed the problem of representation by establishing a network of 145 Disease Surveillance Points (DSPs). Household-level data and utilization data are collected from a stratified random sample. The network covers a combined population of 10 million (1 percent) and provides a representative sample of the nation's population. (See Chunming, 1992.)

National and Local Population Surveys. National population surveys collect truly representative data on the demographic and health status and service utilization patterns. While costly to carry out, these surveys provide valuable detailed information for program design, planning, and evaluation. The simplest demographic survey is a national census. The World Bank's Living Standards Measurement Survey (LSMS) is a more detailed survey that has collected data about health, education, nutrition, and economic status in a number of countries. (See World Bank, 1993a.) Demographic and Health Surveys (DHS) fielded in over 40 countries provide data about fertility and a range of other household characteristics. (See World Bank, 1993a; Wilkinson et al., 1993.) In addition to producing high-quality data, surveys such as the LSMS and DHS—supported by donor funding —produce results that allow planners to compare their country's performance to that of other nations.

Countries may also choose to fund focused surveys to answer questions of interest to policymakers. For example, the National Epidemiology Board of Thailand has commissioned studies to examine defined questions about environmental health, infectious disease, and chronic disease, the results of which have influenced policy decisions. (See Walsh and Simonet, 1995b.)

Rapid assessment methods have also been used to produce data on local populations quickly and inexpensively. These data can then be used by local health managers in planning and evaluating their activities. For example, sample surveys conducted in 113 villages in Gujarat state, India, produced profiles of variations in coverage rates that served as the basis for plans to target areas with the greatest unmet needs. (See Satia et al., 1994.) In Karachi, Pakistan, rapid survey methods are the basis for planning in primary health care systems that serve residents of squatter settlements. (See Husein et al., 1993.)

One study describes five uses of rapid assessment in tropical disease research: prevalence estimation, cause of death estimation, identification of high-risk groups in the population, understanding local conditions as an input to design of interventions, and ongoing monitoring and surveillance. (See Vlassoff and Tanner, 1992.)

Another study used rapid assessment to evaluate the impact of management interventions in the Kabarole district, a rural area of Western Uganda. Baseline data collected from randomly selected facilities and households were used to design a program of management interventions, such as training for health workers and managers, a supportive supervision system, minimum infrastructure standards, and increased community participation. (See Kipp et al., 1994.) Two years later, the same instruments were used to assess the same households and facilities, which showed an average of 19 percent improvement on 10 aggregate performance indicators. The authors attribute the improvement largely to the interventions, since most other factors (such as salary payment regularity and equipment maintenance) had not changed.

Yet another study describes the use of rapid household surveys to evaluate the effectiveness of a diarrhea control program in Kenya. (See Oyoo et al., 1991.) The survey found that less than half of caretakers could properly prepare oral rehydration solution, an insight not obtained from previous larger-scale surveys. These data were fed back quickly to program staff.

Finally, several researchers developed a simple Health Risk Index (HRI) incorporating such factors as adult literacy, housing quality, and tobacco/alcohol use and applied it to 600 families in a Madras, India, urban squatter settlement. (See Srilatha and Aitken, 1991.) They found the index to be a good predictor of illness and age 0–60 mortality. The HRI was then used to identify high-risk families and measure their coverage by primary-care services. The HRI is suggested as a practical tool to help health workers target their services.

Program and Facility Information Systems. More selective information systems have been deployed in support of primary health care programs, disease-specific programs, and hospitals. Several successful primary health care programs have successfully used information systems to improve population-based health services. The aforementioned Karachi primary-care information system is used to manage outreach activities by communities, as well as services provided at facilities. This information system is credited for a significant role in the 49 percent decrease in infant mortality over the first 3–5 years of the program. (See Husein et al., 1993.) An outreach program in Punjab state, India, produced comparable improvements in child health status, and the monitoring system used was cited as the most cost-effective tool for identifying health problems. (See Taylor, 1992.) A microcomputer-based information system at a primary health care center in Rajasthan state, India, helped to significantly reduce dropout rates from the immunization program. (See Singh et al., 1992.)

Traditional disease-specific programs are also supported by dedicated information systems. These show that information systems are not a panacea. An analysis of maternal and child health and family planning program information systems in 27 African, 5 Asian, and 8 Latin and Caribbean countries indicated that those systems generally did not produce the desired benefits. (See Keller, 1991.) Most systems did not provide basic output indicators (e.g., new family planning users, cost of services), and those that did were not used in management decisions.

Because of the low cost of computer hardware, computerized hospital information systems (HISs) are practical in most developing countries. Potentially large cost savings may be realized by producing better data for management purposes, so long as staff are available to enter and analyze the data. (See Song and Luo, 1995; Wang et al, 1993.) These systems can also provide data electronically to the MOH or regional health authorities. Private provider organizations and health insurance plans might also be required to submit to the MOH data derived from their management information systems as a condition of reimbursement. (See Paterson et al., 1997.)

Lessons from Developing Country Experience with Computerized Informa-tion Systems. More and more information systems in developing countries are fully or partially computerized. Computerization promises to reduce the burden of data collection on health workers, which can occupy nearly half of their working time. (See Wilson and Smith, 1991; Moidu et al., 1992.) Small-scale implementations of the computer technology discussed above have yielded promising results. For example, using a computerized information system in a health center in South Korea to collect, process, and retrieve routine health and administrative data cut the time needed by more than a factor of six, thereby increasing staff productivity. (See Chae et al., 1994.) In addition, some developing countries, such as India and China, have established communication networks to further leverage their investments in computers. (See Indrayan, 1995; Wang et al., 1993.)

There have been a number of studies on using microcomputers to collect health information in developing countries, as opposed to using computers only to perform data analyses. (See Snow et al., 1992.) Computers were used to manage collection of malaria morbidity data in The Gambia; to monitor child welfare, family planning services, and antenatal care among the population served by a hospital in Kenya; and to collect data in the field in Cape Verde, Senegal, Ivory Coast, and The Gambia. Use of microcomputers in these cases reduced error rates and speeded data collection.

However, the experience of using computerized information systems on a large scale has often proved disappointing. (See Cibulskis and Izard, 1996.) Several factors are cited for these difficulties:

- The necessary amounts of user training, equipment maintenance, and data administration (e.g., for backing up data) are difficult to sustain. (See Cibulskis and Izard, 1996.)

- Efforts must be made to make data useful to workers and managers who collect them, rather than just creating systems for reporting data to the MOH. (See Moidu et al., 1992; Sharma, 1992.)

- Although computerization can improve the capabilities and efficiency of an information system, those benefits often fail to be realized because data in the system are not tailored to decisionmakers, not collected and processed accurately, or not incorporated into planning, management, and decisionmaking. (See Finau, 1994; Sandiford et al., 1992; de Kadt, 1989; Keller, 1991.)[8]

To date, there is no compelling evidence that computer systems have been helpful in improving health status. Worse, there is the potential that large investments in hardware and software will divert resources from effective and much needed health programs.

ORGANIZING AROUND PROGRAMS WITH DEVOLUTION TO LOCAL COMMUNITIES

Implementing health-sector objectives requires using a formalized planning, programming, and budgeting system to ensure that the objectives match the programs and that the programs themselves can be monitored. But effective implementation also depends on how the MOH itself is organized.

The Organization of the MOH

Given the diversity of health-sector organizations, market structures, and political systems in developing countries, no single blueprint can be offered for organizing the MOH. Detailed descriptions of organization and management problems in developing-country health systems exist, but research on the effectiveness of different methods for addressing those problems is quite limited. Most available research evaluates the impact of policy changes such as devolution or imposition of user fees; studies of the changes in the MOH needed to successfully execute those policy changes have either not been done or have not yet appeared in the literature. The larger public administration literature offers little specific guidance for the organization and management of the MOH. (See Esman, 1991.)

Despite these limitations, the industrialized-country management literature points to two general recommendations. (See Levine and Luck, 1994.) The first is to reorganize the MOH to eliminate features that clearly hinder reform efforts. For example, if authority is devolved to states or regions, control over staffing levels and hiring policies should also be devolved to the extent that civil service laws allow. If a department is set up in the MOH to manage a particular program, that department should also receive authority over the necessary resources, such as staff, budget, and regulatory power.

The second general recommendation is to organize divisions of the MOH around the programs that form the basis for planning and budgeting, rather than having one program be the joint responsibility of several divisions. In particular, existing disease-specific vertical programs may need to be reorganized in favor of programs for publicly provided primary health care or for regulation and financing of private provisions. (See Kutzin, 1994). Where programs provide support for one another, clear performance standards should be established and monitored. For example, hospitals can be measured on how quickly they schedule referrals from rural health centers. Instances of duplication or conflict between programs should also be eliminated. For example, in China, many

---

[8]Useful guidelines for the development of effective health management information systems are contained in United Nations (1985a).

villages have competing but underutilized clinics for family planning and for maternal and child health, a result of poor coordination between the ministries that operate them. (See Hsiao, 1995a.)

Problems of Centralized Provision of Care. Unfortunately, these general recommendations offer little guidance in addressing a bigger challenge that the MOH faces. How should the MOH manage publicly provided health care delivery? While not all countries in Asia provide health care directly, many still do and could do a better job. The public provision of care is inherently bureaucratic and, hence, is subject to problems of "government failure." (See Wolf, 1986.) A familiar litany of problems has been documented, both in general discussions of developing country health systems (see Musgrove, 1996; Barnum et al., 1995; Kutzin and Barnum, 1992) and in Asian countries, including India (see World Bank, 1992c), Indonesia (see World Bank, 1989c, 1994i), Pakistan (see World Bank, 1993 l), Papua New Guinea (see Peabody et al., 1996d), Sri Lanka (see World Bank, 1988d), and Viet Nam. (See Ensor, 1995.) These problems include:

- Poor customer service, low morale, and high absenteeism in government-operated primary-care clinics;

- Insufficient drug supplies and poor maintenance practices in those clinics, leaving staff unable to provide essential services;

- Patients bypassing primary-care clinics as a result of the above problems and going directly to higher-cost hospitals;

- Waste of resources in hospitals;

- At a national level, overspending on salaries relative to drugs, maintenance, and other nonpersonnel inputs, as well as devoting too large a share of health spending to curative (versus preventive and promotive) services and urban (versus rural) facilities.

These problems are not due just to a lack of resources. Management shortcomings include:

- Limited delegation of authority;

- Lack of training among MOH staff in managing, planning, and using quantitative data;

- Lack of management training among physicians who manage facilities;

- Defective incentive structures, such as low salaries that encourage public-sector physicians to divert patients to their parallel private practices; and

- The difficulties of enforcing accountability under civil service regulations.

Excessive centralization, as mentioned above, is one of the key problems in large bureaucratic organizations with dispersed operations. This is illustrated by the hospital sector in the newly independent republics of central Asia and Mongolia. Hospitals in the Kyrgyz Republic are rigidly divided into departments based on medical specialty, with each department having a separate nursing and physician staff. The small scale of departmental operations creates substantial diseconomies. Personnel are allocated centrally to each hospital, and salaries and utility costs eat up all funds, leaving little or no funds for drugs, hospital supplies, or laboratory costs. The absence of supplies means that few patients enter the hospital, thereby exacerbating the underutilization of personnel. Since salaries are determined centrally, physicians and hospital managers have no incentive to improve care.

The former socialist economies are not the only examples of the cost of centralized decisionmaking. In India, for example, service provision targets are the basis of most primary health care planning. National targets are set, then allocated to the states, then to districts, and then to primary health centers. These targets are based on population norms and form the basis for planning supplies and monitoring the performance of workers and centers. Despite the use of population as the basis of resource allocation, poorer areas are ill served because actual services provided vary considerably. The system does not cater to local socioeconomic and geographical variations, nor does it involve and motivate local staff. (See Satia et al., 1994.)

The Potential of Devolution

Given the problems of centralized organization, devolving some of the centralized responsibilities to local levels—transferring management control of local operations, whether public health services or the provision of curative care, to a local organization—can improve technical efficiency. Decentralized programs can be designed with the knowledge of the local culture and circumstances. They can also be allocatively efficient, because resources can be devoted to the most-needed local services. With decentralization, fiscal responsibility for services rests with local managers who have incentives to improve efficiency because they can use the savings for other local purposes. Local managers also have more opportunities to reduce costs. They can tailor staff and procedures to local resources and circumstances, rather than relying on centrally determined procedures. Information can be used without delay, rather than after permission is received from central agencies. As discussed in Chapter 6, decentralization is one of a variety of strategies that may be used to increase community participation in local decisions.

Another possible benefit of devolution, at least in a large country, is that local governments can experiment with alternative ways of doing things. Some of these ways may turn out to be superior and can then be adopted in other regions. This appears to be the case in China, where rural experiments in community financing and urban experiments in insurance reform appear to have resulted in some particularly useful models for dissemination. The World Bank reports a recent study showing that some poor villages in China that used community financing delivered services more efficiently than villages that did not: They had greater use of lower-level facilities, a lower proportion of income from drug sales in township health centers and county hospitals, and lower fees for primary-care services—and they had better outcomes as measured by lower morbidity rates. (See World Bank, 1997c.)

Despite the fact that centralized organizations have acknowledged problems managing a geographically dispersed health care sector and the inherent attractiveness of devolution, there is little proof that devolution actually improves efficiency. One reason may be the difficulties in assessing the impact of devolution. Short-term implementation problems also plague most large-scale changes; these problems are difficult to separate from devolution policy. Devolution seldom occurs, for example, without simultaneous changes in training, supplies, or levels of resources.

Nevertheless, there are examples where devolution, with or without community participation, has resulted in improvements in efficiency. One study reports that communities in Indonesia were able to mobilize resources and train and supervise health workers to achieve important improvements in infant and maternal mortality. (See Kutzin, 1994.) In Nigeria, the local government in the Oji river area recognized that by leasing and borrowing vehicles for short periods of time, it could conduct immunization campaigns in outlying areas without the expense of purchasing additional vehicles. (See World Bank, 1994e.)

Problems with Devolution. When devolution does not work, there seem to be a number of possible reasons why. One of the most frequently encountered problems is an increased disparity across regions in government expenditures for health services. This appears to occur in proportion to the extent to which the central government relinquishes control over the geographic distribution of expenditures.

For example, in Laos, the devolution of governmental functions that began in 1985 included all financial responsibility for health services. All planning and budgeting functions, except for donor programs, were devolved to provincial and district levels. (See Holland and Phimphachanh, 1995.) The provinces were responsible for the local generation, collection, and allocation of revenue. However, no effective mechanism had been established by which the wealthier provinces could be taxed and the surplus used to subsidize poorer provinces. As a result, disparities between provinces increased. Those that were poor were unable to meet the costs of public services, while rich provinces could make and retain profits. The government of Laos is currently recentralizing budgetary and financial decisionmaking. However, early central allocations still show large disparities across regions in per-capita health expenditures.

Similar increased regional disparities arose among rural areas with the devolution of health care finance in China and other countries. (See Smith, 1993.) Existing inequities across provinces were heightened by the devolution of health responsibilities to the provinces in Papua New Guinea. (See Thomason, 1994.) In Viet Nam, communes support their own health care needs; consequently, the wealthier communes have more staff and services. (See Nguyen et al., 1995.) In China, public health workers have been diverted from needed work (immunizations and disease surveillance) to work for which fees can be more easily charged (water and food testing). In many parts of that country, the Epidemic Prevention Service now charges for immunizations and tuberculosis treatment. This has reduced coverage and—in the case of tuberculosis treatment—

has led to medically inappropriate, but profitable, patterns of care. (See World Bank, 1997c.)

Many other problems with devolution arise from tensions between the goals of the central government and the goals of local government. For example, local governments, even those with sufficient resources, may not want to budget adequately for health services. Public demand may be stronger for curative health services than for public health services, which require longer time periods to show effects. This public demand may sway local government officials. Lack of local support may be especially high for programs with effects that spill over to other areas, such as communicable disease prevention. For example, a case study from India describes the problem of implementing HIV/AIDS education and condom use at the local level because of conservative sociopolitical views and an emphasis on medical aspects of the disease. (See Asthana, 1996.)

Tension between the goals of the central government and those of local governments can arise over the distribution of health care resources within the local area. Local governments may be substantially under the control of local elites who arrange to obtain the lion's share of resources for themselves. (See Collins et al., 1994.)

When the devolution involves either the loss of civil service jobs or the transfer of power away from persons who hold it, there is likely to be resistance to the devolution. Such problems, identified in a cross-sectional survey and routinely collected health information, delayed the implementation of Papua New Guinea's devolution for seven years. Devolution did not advance until political intervention ensured restructuring of the Department of Health and professional support was gained. (See Campos-Outcalt et al., 1995.)

Finally, lack of skilled personnel, lack of information, or the loss of economies of scale may counteract efficiency gains from devolution. There are examples in the literature where local surpluses and shortages of supplies existed simultaneously without the knowledge of local officials at either site. In Viet Nam, communes in Do Luong district faced a shortage of contraceptives until they learned by chance that the district health center, just 10 km away, had oral contraceptives in stock. (See Guldner, 1995.) Administrative costs may actually increase because of the loss of economies of scale, because of the creation of additional layers of bureaucracy, or because of the inability of the central administration to reduce personnel after transferring functions to local governments. Decentralization in Papua New Guinea has resulted in provincial health administrations that are quite top-heavy.

Requirements for Successful Devolution. Case studies on devolution provide some possible ways to deal with the problems identified above and to make devolution efficient. Such solutions can be grouped into four areas: (1) the management capacity of the receiving government(s); (2) regional planning; (3) fiscal sustainability, and (4) the management responsibilities of the MOH.

Capacity of Receiving Organization or Government. A prerequisite for successful devolution is that the receiving organization have the managerial and technical capacity to manage the devolved responsibilities. In the absence of this capacity, there is no way to attain the hoped-for increases in efficiencies.

For example, in the Western Highlands Province of Papua New Guinea, there was an attempt in 1990 to further devolve health care from the province level down to the district level. Prior to 1990, there had been five districts. As part of the devolution, these were subdivided into a total of 14. District administrators were given responsibility for all budgetary and personnel decisions for all programs within their districts. However, only 4 of the 14 appointees to this position had been health care workers prior to this appointment and none of the appointees received any training. The districts did not have separate elected government structures to provide political oversight of the district administrators' operations. There was no clear delegation of responsibilities for system operation and a lack of system support. As a result, health workers at all levels (including the new district administrators) had negative opinions about the results of this devolution, and objective data suggest that fewer services were provided. (See Campos-Outcalt et al., 1995.)

Personnel administration is one aspect of management capacity that is particularly important to efficiency. In the Philippines, local governments have been more susceptible to political interference in personnel matters, which can increase the costs of producing health services. (See World Bank, 1994h.)

It is particularly worth noting that when governments retain central control over personnel placement, devolution is unlikely to work. It introduces confusion about lines of control, leading to inconsistency and/or organizational paralysis. Local government units need, at least eventually, to have the hiring and firing authority consistent with their responsibilities.

Regional Planning. Two regional planning issues are important to devolution plans and operations. First, authority over public health-care provisions must rest in a large enough region to cover the first referral hospital. Only then can the trade-offs be made between putting resources into primary-care clinics and putting them into hospitals. One study reports the case of Nigeria, where state governments are responsible for the first referral hospital, and local governments are responsible for primary care. (See Kutzin, 1994.) Because the budgets of state and local governments are distinct, there is no way to reallocate resources across levels of care.

Second, when there are separate national and/or international vertical programs that are not under the control of local governments in a devolved system, a regional planning system must be created to allow coordination across programs. The lack of such a regional planning system is clear in much of China. China has three separate vertical systems involved in planning, financing, and organizing urban hospital facilities: the public health system, the state-owned enterprise system, and the traditional Chinese medicine system. Each system protects its own institutional interests and has little incentive to coordinate with others.

Further, public hospitals in China are managed by different levels of government—national, provincial, and county—which results in duplication of facilities and equipment and enormous waste. Recent initiatives in regional health planning have begun to remedy this problem in three regions, each of which agreed on a five-year development plan. As one example of efficiency gains, managers accepted centralization of high-technology diagnostics in one hospital to serve the other area facilities. They also created better networks for assessment and maintenance of equipment. (See World Bank, 1997c.)

Fiscal Sustainability. Fiscal sustainability must be a paramount consideration in the planning of devolution. Will the devolution include enough funds to cover devolved services? Will the poorest governments be the worst hit? Will they need external budgets and support, or will they need to mobilize additional health resources? What about the impact of resource mobilization? In planning the local government's strategy for fiscal sustainability, it is important to pay attention to the incentives for equity and public health in the devolved system. For example, as we discussed more fully in Chapter 4, user fees can affect the availability of curative or public health services.

The solution, of course, is for the central government to maintain a role in financing the health care sector so that it can subsidize poorer regions. To provide a minimum standard of health care in rural areas, the Vietnamese MOH is seeking funds to support at least two workers in each commune. (See World Bank, 1995c.) In the Philippines, the central government historically accounted for about 90 percent of total government spending, with local governments covering only about 10 percent. In the early 1990s, 50 percent of the central Department of Health (DOH) responsibilities were transferred to local governments. The central government maintains its taxing policies and allocates revenues to local government units on a revenue-sharing, non-earmarked basis, thus allowing it to subsidize poorer regions. The World Bank estimated that the actual revenue-sharing formula has not disadvantaged governments in poorer regions, thus showing that devolution of operations need not cause equity problems when the central government maintains fiscal responsibility. (See World Bank, 1994h.) Adequate funding is possible if the central government (1) retains control of substantial resources and (2) is willing to defer obtaining savings from the devolution until operating efficiencies have actually generated the savings.

The Role of the MOH. The essential process of devolution requires that the MOH develop guidelines for policy and simultaneously relinquish control over operations. To obtain the hoped-for benefits of devolution, the MOH must be able to influence local health policy and implementation without compromising the autonomy of local decisionmaking from which many of the benefits of a devolved system would be expected to flow. An evaluation of one aspect of the Philippines' devolution found that local government units were unable to develop or implement their own plans either because they lacked national policies or because the policies were out of date since they applied only to the pre-devolution situation. (See Family Planning Management Development (FPMD), 1995.) As one researcher said in discussing the Vietnamese experience, "decentralization without direction appears to undermine health system effectiveness." (Guldner, 1995, p. 60.) One way to provide direction is through planning guidelines. When formulated by the MOH, they should place limits on acceptable behavior by local actors and must be accompanied by some means of enforcement.

If it is to retain influence over policies implemented by local governments, the central MOH must retain a substantial role in heath policy beyond the planning role. This can involve allocating a substantial proportion of health care resources, coordinating resources with local government licensing and accrediting functions, evaluating and monitoring programs, or providing technical support to local governments.

Resource allocation can be done either by a revenue-sharing formula or by project support. The choice here is a trade-off. The first maximizes the flexibility of the local governments, while the second maximizes the influence of the central government on expenditures. A mixed strategy, where project support is given for essential public health projects and additional revenue-sharing is provided to support curative services, may be appropriate when the central government has previously subsidized curative services heavily. In the example of the Philippines discussed above, the DOH of the Philippines retained partial control of such essential public health projects as malaria, tuberculosis, and schistosomiasis control programs. (See World Bank, 1994h.)

The World Bank argued strongly that the Philippines' DOH should establish itself as a full partner with local governments to deliver and coordinate affordable, equitable health services. (See World Bank, 1994h.) It argued that each level of government should trade the services it produces most efficiently for other services required to produce a nationally complete health care system. The ultimate success of this approach is not yet clear because of the time scale required to accomplish so much devolution.

The MOH can provide technical support through information systems or logistic systems where economies of scale favor central system development. It can also procure specialized items that are not available through local distribution systems, for which substantial volume discounts can be obtained, or for which technical knowledge is required.

Finally, the MOH can provide technical assistance on management issues. A variety of strategies have been proposed (and also studied), but only some of the approaches seem to mitigate the lack of management capacity at the level to which devolution is aimed. These include training, using temporary regional or central personnel to help with the transition, and technical management strategies. For example, longitudinal evaluation of a government-run community health worker project in South Africa helped managers understand client perception of services. The study results were used to modify the operational strategy and integrate the project into the health district. (See van der Walt and Matthews, 1995.)

Another project in The Gambia sought to improve district-level management by teaching management skills. Problem-solving and a participating study for planning and implementing were introduced. The evaluation phase showed some improvement in management, but the training was limited by government and donor policy that interfered with motivation and adhered to a preconceived management model. In any case, it is important that the pace and sequencing of devolving functions accommodate the need to build management capacity. (See Conn et al., 1996.)

One high-quality study showed that better management can lead to better quality of care. Loevinsohn conducted a controlled field trial to study the effect on quality of care of a supervision checklist for midwives in rural Philippine health posts. The checklist measured 20 process-of-care indicators for maternal and child health, such as percentage of pregnant women with more than three prenatal visits and tetanus immunization. The study design incorporated experimental and control sites that had equivalent performance at baseline. (Randomization of sites was not possible because of logistical and management considerations.) The experimental sites showed a significantly greater improvement on the measured indicators after six months (42 percent versus 18 percent). Although the study did not examine whether performance improvements were sustained beyond the initial follow-up period, its results indicate that structured supervision using a concise checklist of key process indicators can improve the quality of primary care. (See Loevinsohn et al., 1995.)

PRIVATE PROVISION OF SERVICES

One of the biggest management and organizational challenges an MOH faces is deciding which services it should provide directly and which services it should delegate to the private sector. Decisions about public finance are distinct from decisions about how to organize the actual provision of care. In particular, public goods need to be financed by the government, but they need *not* be directly provided by the government. Issues related to how health services should be financed were discussed in Chapter 4. Here, we begin by discussing criteria for public- and private-sector *provision* of health care. Then, we discuss the challenges of implementing private-sector provision, focusing on the regulatory and contracting functions the government must undertake to ensure acceptable performance by the private sector.

Criteria for Public or Private Provision of Health Care

Much has been written on the issue of which kinds of tasks are better suited for the private sector and which are better suited for the public sector. Experience shows that the decision between public and private cannot be made simply by dividing tasks into those better suited for one type of financing or the other. Rather, it requires considering the entire environment in which the tasks are undertaken. As Musgrove observed, decisions about whether the public sector should provide a service are largely analogous to the "make or buy" decisions of a private firm. (See Musgrove, 1996.) Thus, they should turn on costs or efficiency: Is it less expensive to buy from the outside or to produce the service internally?

Although efficiency is usually the relevant criteria for deciding between public and private provision, sometimes the decision may require a trade-off between efficiency and other public goals such as equity. In such circumstances, the correct answer depends both on policy and on implementation constraints. For example, the AIDS project in Burkina Faso was a joint public-private venture. The government mounted an education campaign to increase use of contraceptives and to change behaviors that spread STDs, educated traditional providers about STDs, and decided to supply private distributors and NGOs with condoms at a subsidized rate. Indeed, the program will supply 75 percent of all demand for condoms and therefore is expected to suppress the private market. It was judged that the short-run goals of improving access outweighed the long-run efficiency that would be provided by the private market. (See van der Gaag, 1995.)

Competition, When It Exists, Can Make the Private Sector More Efficient. When the private sector is driven by competition, it tends to be more efficient. When competition among private providers occurs in a market, providers strive to reduce their costs, hospitals pay attention to the demands of consumers, and consumers choose the provider that provides the best quality for the price. The separation of provision from finance through a purchase arrangement increases the transparency of resource allocation decisions, avoiding the kinds of hidden subsidies and irrational allocations that occur in many government-run operations.

It seems well established that the private sector will be more efficient when real competition is possible. Although perfect competition is not possible for most activities within the health care sector, there are "efficiency" circumstances where the private sector is likely to actually deliver more-efficient services.

Effective competition requires multiple private contractors, who compete to efficiently deliver services and, therefore, lower the costs of production. Private providers in the health sector do not necessarily face direct competition from other practitioners. Many authors speak of "contestability" as a suitable substitute for actual competitors. (See Broomberg, 1994.) In a contestable market, although there is no actual competition, there are providers or organizations that *could* enter the market and compete. An example is a private organization with a contract to run the only tertiary-care hospital in town. Although there is no competition after the contract has been awarded, the theory is that the threat of competition for the next contract will cause the existing contractor to behave as if it had competitors and, therefore, will create and maintain efficiency. Although the theory is clear, actual experience with contestable markets provides little evidence for or against the theory.

Even when there are competitors, the conditions for a competitive market are rarely fulfilled. Providers possess an information advantage—an information asymmetry—that lets them respond to competitive pressure in inefficient ways that are to their advantage. For example, private hospitals have been shown to engage in competition in which they increase costs without a commensurate improvement in quality. Thus, a second general requirement for private provision to be more efficient is that the government must have the skills and information required to adequately regulate the market or to negotiate contracts with providers. Whether purchasing is done by the government or by individuals, the government must obtain adequate information to monitor the costs and performance of the private sector.

Because competitive or even contestable markets are so rare in the health sector, there is only a small range of services where one can expect, a priori, that the private sector will usually perform more efficiently. These include ancillary services in larger urban areas—such as supplies for health clinics or non-health-care hospital activities like laundry, catering, or maintenance. (See Bennett, 1992.) The latter have been successfully contracted out in a variety of Asian countries, including laundry services in Bangladesh, India, Indonesia, Malaysia, Pakistan, Sri Lanka, and Thailand. In other parts of the world, cleaning services and canteens have been contracted out in Mexico, and maintenance of high-tech equipment, staff catering services, and maintenance of steam boilers have been contracted out in Uganda. (See Kutzin, 1994.)

In Most Cases, the Choice Depends on Local Culture and Circumstances. Beyond obvious choices for private provision, the best public-private balance for a particular country or region still depends on local culture and local circumstances. Even with this caveat, the appropriate division of the health care system between the public and private sectors can be determined only after also evaluating how the economic incentives will operate. For example, the extent of private-sector participation will be affected by the extent of constraints on private behavior and on the community rewards for community-spirited activity. One element of local circumstances—corruption—should also be considered. If there is widespread tolerance of endemic public corruption, it would be highly undesirable for there to be many government officials with access to large amounts of government funds.

There are examples that counteract almost all rules that have been proposed for determining the correct balance of activities. Some have argued that private-sector provision leads to inequities. But with the proper incentives, private doctors have been shown to provide very acceptable access to preventive and curative care. For example, in Namibia, private surgeons receive contracts to provide services in remote areas. The amount of their contractual payments is based on their workload. This is less expensive than hiring full-time government doctors for these sparsely settled areas. It provides improved continuity of care because turnover rates are low in private practice; in addition, the doctors are highly experienced. There may be a problem in that the doctors might give preference to their private patients; nevertheless, the government can provide more services to the poor in this way than it could otherwise. (See Kutzin, 1994.)

Another example showing that private-sector provision need not lead to inequities concerns private hospitals in the Philippines. (See World Bank, 1994h.) Although in the early 1970s private hospitals were concentrated in the richest cities and provinces, this is no longer the case. By 1990, the distribution of private and public hospitals across provinces was very similar.

The government can also offer incentives to private providers to locate where the government has no providers of its own. Alternatively, it can subsidize private providers or NGOs who care for the disadvantaged, perhaps providing staff to private facilities. To increase equity, the government must obtain agreement that the poor will have access to the subsidized services. However, these arrangements do not involve competition and, thus, may not increase efficiency. For example, NGOs often are efficient when small, but they can develop the same bureaucratic inefficiencies as governments as they become larger. In the end, the performance of the subsidized agency with respect to either efficiency or equity depends more on goodwill and monitoring by the government than on market forces. (See Kutzin, 1994.)

Hospitals have been repeatedly singled out by donors as candidates for privatization. Developing-country governments frequently spend too much on hospitals. Because hospitals are often more used by urban than rural residents and sometimes more by the middle class than the poor, the government money spent on operating hospitals hinders attainment of equity. In addition, public hospitals are sometimes used by consultants for their own private gain. Consequently, selling public hospitals might be a better choice than encouraging the development of new private hospitals. (See Griffin, 1989.)

The government may be better off directly providing services in cases where transaction costs involved in private provision are high. These transaction costs include the costs of obtaining information necessary to regulate or monitor the private providers. A different kind of cost that should be considered is when private control of an expensive asset puts the government in poor negotiating condition as a purchaser. For example, the government might wish to retain control over the sole tertiary-care hospital in a region and only encourage private providers to operate primary-care facilities, where competition for consumers is possible. The latter would be particularly true if there were multiple private-sector purchasers of care to create a real market.

Challenges of Private Provision

If a government decides that it wishes to encourage greater activity by private providers, it will need to consider whether there are substantial barriers to expanding private health care. For example, as discussed in Chapter 4, there must be some financing mechanism to pay for the services of private providers. Capital markets may also make it impossible to obtain the equipment required to open hospitals or clinics. Provider associations may need to be encouraged to take on professional education roles. Ground rules for the use of public hospitals by private doctors may need to be developed. For example, in Papua New Guinea, the desire to expand the private sector is hampered by barriers to private insurance, the absence of licensing and regulation, and a legal inability to admit a private patient to a hospital. (See Thomason, 1994.)

A variety of considerations must be addressed during the transfer of any function to the private sector. For example, the arrangements should result in an adequate return to the public treasury for the value of the assets involved. This will allow the capital that is thus freed up to be used for higher-priority purposes.

If the operation is to continue to serve the public good, it is important to ensure that the purchaser has adequate funds to both operate and maintain the privatized operation. Thus, the contractor must have available either third-party payments or some other accepted, sustainable method of obtaining funds. It must have sufficient reserves if cash flow is a problem. Similarly, the purchaser must also have the administrative capacity to operate and finance the facility.

When candidate organizations for privatization perform some functions that are basically public goods, extra care will have to go into the negotiations to ensure that these programs are continued or that adequate substitutes are found. Examples include such hospital programs as doctor training and blood bank facilities.

Unintended consequences frequently follow many public policy changes, but they are particularly likely in privatization projects unless a systematic approach is taken to considering all possible results of the transfer. It is especially important to consider the effect of the transfer on distributional goals. For example, will some portion of the population receive less care? Are there income groups or geographic groups or ethnic groups that are likely to be disadvantaged? And as we discussed above, it is also important to consider and plan for resistance to change from existing stakeholders.

In addition, while managing the provision of health services is difficult in both the public and private sector, it is even more challenging in the private sector, requiring many skills not present in a traditional developing-country MOH. (See Kutzin, 1994; Musgrove, 1996; Broomberg, 1994.) Such skills are needed specifically in the areas of economic analysis, regulation/standard setting, and contracting. (See the subsequent discussion on managing human resources.)

Regulation and Standard Setting. Regulation of the training, licensing, and operation of private providers, such as hospitals, physicians, and pharmacies, is essential to ensure quality and deter fraud. As a national agency, the MOH can set standards and enforcement mechanisms more uniformly than provinces or regions. In cases where authority over some services has been delegated to provinces or regions, the MOH can still retain the ability to set and enforce minimum standards for quality and access.

The need for regulation of private providers can be derived from theories of behavior, such as those discussed in Chapters 4 and 6. But it also is clear from observing behavior in either the developed or developing world. Newspapers regularly report serious quality problems at hospitals throughout the United States—even at prestigious institutions. (See Wolfe et al., 1994.) There is a widespread perception of serious problems, including the lack of basic hygiene and inadequate staffing, record keeping, and facilities at many of Bombay's private nursing homes, which include small surgical facilities and medical facilities and maternity homes. (See Yesudian, 1994.)

In addition to problems with quality, the for-profit motivation of some private providers, combined with a lack of information on the part of consumers, leads many individuals to believe there is a need for regulation to control excess profits. Although nonprofit providers do not have the same profit-maximizing goal, the goals of increasing their size and influence may lead to inappropriate expansion of activities, and thus may also require cost-containment regulation. A particular problem is the accumulation of high-cost technologies that raise health care costs and encourage unnecessary care. In Thailand, for example, a facility survey revealed 10 CT scanners per million population (1988) in Bangkok, a level only exceeded by the United States (14.7) and Japan (29.2). (See Nittayaramphong and Tangcharoensathien, 1994.)

In dealing with the subject of controlling the private sector, we should make an important distinction between regulation by incentive and regulation by directive. (See Rutten, 1996a.) In regulation by incentive, the health care system is set up so that key actors (e.g., doctors, rural health workers, hospital managers) face incentives that stimulate them to act efficiently. Regulation by directive involves setting up procedures that must be followed (e.g., licensing requirements, staffing requirements for a hospital) and that are enforced by threat of fines or removal from the market.

Both kinds of regulation are necessary to ensure a well-run private health care sector. Because people and organizations are complex and information is not always available, no set of incentive structures will always produce correct behavior. Thus, incentive structures need to be supplemented by directives and regulatory behavior. Some people will ignore rules that are not to their advantage in many situations; others will ignore rules only when they gain a large advantage. Thus, enforcing regulations will be much easier and much more successful if the incentive structure does not provide many opportunities for gains from contrary behavior.

Regulations themselves must meet certain conditions if they are to be successful. First, what the regulation demands must be clear and unambiguous. Vagueness in a regulation, such as mandating "adequate facilities," led to ambiguities that defied enforcement and were not successful in Bombay. (See Yesudian, 1994.) Licensing requirements for institutional providers should include minimum standards for a hygienic environment and minimum standards for qualified personnel. Second, regulations must be feasible, and complying with the regulations must not be too costly for the regulated. This is necessary to lower incentives for persons to ignore the regulations. Finally, the government must have both the will and a credible mechanism to enforce regulations and to detect and punish infringements.

Although governments frequently rely on professional associations to regulate their members, the inherent conflict of interest between serving their members and serving the public good has often led to complete lack of enforcement, as in the case of Bombay. (See Yesudian, 1994.) Foster et al. argue that "[e]ffective regulation of the private sector is possible but requires funds, qualified people, and a legal framework and political culture that makes enforcement possible." (Foster et al., 1994, p. 176.)

Contracting. The government can transfer some of its work to the private sector by contracting with private firms for specific services. Insofar as the resultant services, including the government's costs to administer and monitor the contract, are cheaper than services the government could produce, funds can be freed up for other uses. Contracting can also free up scarce skilled government personnel, who can then devote their time to management tasks that only the government can do.

In setting up contracts, it is important to ensure that the government is really purchasing services at costs that are lower than when it provided the service itself. The comparison should include, as part of the costs of the contract, the effort that the government must incur in negotiating, monitoring, and enforcing the contract. Determining the level of savings is difficult if the government has poor accounting systems. Nevertheless, it is crucial to any decisions about whether to contract.

Contracting may produce additional benefits beyond cost savings in an environment in which there is a separate private market for health care (funded, for example, by employers or through a social security fund, as in Latin America). Contracting can strengthen (or even produce) infrastructure, such as distributors or manufacturers, that the private sector can then use. And by having contract clauses that ensure efficient provision (e.g., the use of generic drugs), contracting can influence private-market practices or prices.

Contracting has also been used for clinical services, some examples of which were discussed above. The managed care program for government workers in the Philippines shows the elements of a comprehensive approach to contracting. The government allows its employees to enroll in private HMOs. Enrollment is voluntary, thus forcing the HMOs to compete on quality to attract members. The HMOs must also meet a series of government requirements. They must provide a better benefit package than the government's Medicare program with no increased price to the government or to the beneficiary. The government enforces a minimum standard for the number of hospital beds required. It also requires a performance bond. Finally, the government monitors both contractual and service performance.

Direct contracting for service provision by the MOH calls for such skills as writing requests for proposals and contracts, soliciting and evaluating proposals, and monitoring the performance of the winning vendors.

MANAGING TECHNOLOGY AND DEVELOPING HUMAN CAPITAL

Another key implementation issue has to do with deciding which pieces of the health infrastructure the MOH needs to manage. One relatively simple way to do this is to look at two inputs into health care that, when combined, are transformed into better health—the health care system's technologic capital and its human resources.

Managing Medical Technologies

As we showed in Chapter 1, medical technologies are an important tool for improving health outcomes and hold much promise for improving health in the future. However, such technologies are not without their problems. As a result, when it comes to actually choosing medical technologies and applying them within a country, the MOH needs to ensure that the process of selection in the public sector is managed efficiently and that the overall use of technologies is carefully regulated. Below, we examine some of the problems of medical technology and discuss approaches for managing them.

The Problems of Medical Technology. Despite the promise of medical technologies, their benefits have failed to reach the overwhelming majority of the Asian population. While doctors in the major hospitals in large urban areas enjoy the use of CT scanners and other expensive diagnostic equipment, basic medical devices such as intravenous catheters are frequently in short supply in the rural hospital and clinics to which most people have ready access. Underlying this tragic failure in health care delivery are three related problems. They arise at various points in the overall process that begins with the design of a medical product and ends with its replacement or disposal.

Lack of Availability of Appropriate Medical Devices. Because of their high cost and complexity, many commercially available medical devices are poorly suited to the needs of developing countries. (See Free, 1992; Heuck and Deom, 1991; Schmitt and Al-Fadel, 1989.) As a result, purchasing and maintaining a few pieces of equipment for a specialized application consume a large proportion of the allocated funds. And even this equipment may lie unused, because personnel are not trained to operate and maintain it properly.

Although there is a vast array of new technologies and medicines, the technologies are the result of research in wealthier countries; as a result, they need to be evaluated locally for use in developing countries. Because there is no single "answer" that determines what technology is most cost-effective for everyone, this is the natural domain of national cost-effectiveness and cost-benefit studies. Any valuation of benefits and effectiveness, however, includes a subjective measure that varies across cultures and societies.

Another appropriateness issue has to do with whether medical technologies are useful outside the environment they were designed to operate in. Developing countries rely on industrialized nations—particularly the United States and Japan—to supply the bulk of their medical equipment needs. For example, the results of a survey of major teaching hospitals in China indicate that more than 50 percent of the medical equipment with a value greater than U.S. $3,000 was purchased from U.S. and Japanese manufacturers alone. (See Peabody and Schmitt, 1992.) Such industrialized countries, with sufficient indigenous design and manufacturing capability, often lack incentives to manufacture products tailored for developing countries.

As a result, most medical equipment sold on the international market was designed originally for application in highly organized tertiary-care institutions by trained physicians and nurses, not for low-volume application in primary health care by medical workers who have had little exposure to modern medical technology. Unfortunately, the high price of a piece of medical equipment offers no guarantee that it can operate under the adverse environmental conditions encountered in hospitals and clinics in undeveloped tropical areas. For example, few instruments on the market today have been designed to withstand the electrical power fluctuations and high temperatures and humidity that are common in these areas.

Irrational Procurement and Application. To derive the maximum benefit from medical devices, careful assessment and selection are essential. Short-sighted procurement decisions lead to underutilization and waste valuable resources. The root of this problem can often be traced to the selfishness of a few who regard medical equipment as a status symbol rather than as a means of satisfying an established need. (See Bloom, 1989.) Encouraged by aggressive suppliers, a medical doctor may demand the purchase of an expensive instrument without considering more cost-effective alternatives. The confidence of one or two key proponents in the value of a new piece of equipment does not guarantee its utility. The appropriateness of medical equipment with respect to health needs of the patient population is often disregarded. An equally serious problem results from overestimating the ability of nurses and other support personnel to operate sophisticated instruments without having first received specialized training.

Inadequate Infrastructure for Long-Term Maintenance. As the purchasing power of the newly industrialized regions of Asia grows, a trend toward the purchase of increasingly sophisticated medical equipment has become evident. The alarming fact is that the infrastructure for maintenance and repair of these instruments already lags far behind present needs. (See Bloom, 1989; Murthy and Laxminarayan, 1986.) This situation has left a shameful proportion of medical equipment in a state of disrepair. According to one survey, even in some of the best teaching hospitals in China, one-third of the most expensive equipment purchased between 1979 and 1987 was judged to be in "poor" operating condition. (See Peabody and Schmitt, 1992.) More-recent evidence suggests that this maintenance problem persists in China and may, in fact, have worsened in some areas. (See Schmitt, 1993.)

The state of disrepair of existing medical equipment in other areas of Asia, notably the islands of Micronesia, has seriously affected patient care. (See Schmitt, 1990.) Although part of this problem can be attributed to inherent design insufficiencies that make instruments ill-suited for use outside of climate-controlled environments, improper use and lack of maintenance are the major culprits. Networks for obtaining spare parts promptly have not yet been established and technical support personnel are scarce.

How the MOH Can Manage Medical Technologies Appropriately. The preceding discussion shows that the failure of available technology to fulfill its promise in Asia is not primarily a failure of the hardware that we associate with high-technology medicine; rather, it is a failure to match this hardware with the needs and capabilities in the region. The obvious interdependency of the key problems identified above implies that transforming the present failure into success requires changes in the attitudes and policies on which the structure of the present MOH health care system is based.

The appropriateness of a specific type of medical technology should be judged from the perspective of both the user and the patient. Above all, it must meet a demonstrated need, as determined by its potential health benefits. The impact of a technology on the disease burden of the target population can be measured, for example, in terms of the expected number of DALYs gained as a result of its use. (See Chapter 3 for a discussion of DALYs.) Such measures are useful for evaluating the relative merits of health technologies having similar applications. (See WHO Ad Hoc Committee, 1996.)

Another important consideration is whether an institution can afford to purchase and maintain a particular medical device. The potential health benefit of the device is also a factor in this decision. Simply stated, the goal is to choose technologies with the potential to yield the greatest health benefit per unit cost. In some cases, the best decision may be to select a less-advanced medical device simply because the more-advanced device is not affordable. For example, one may discover that the latest model of an automated ventilator has added features that improve oxygen delivery in certain patients compared to the older generation, but it consumes more oxygen, which is an expensive imported commodity. Similarly, one may be faced with the choice of purchasing several cheaper devices that would serve the needs of several small hospitals or a single expensive device for use in an urban teaching hospital. Making the right decision in these cases requires an accurate assessment of the costs and benefits.

Unfortunately, as discussed above, health technologies appropriate for many applications in developing countries do not exist. Therefore, doing without certain medical devices may be the only viable option. Of course, any technology is worthless if the medical staff does not have adequate technical skills to apply it, so the training required to ensure effective use must be part of the cost-effectiveness decision.

> **Box 7.3: The Medical Equipment Maintenance Problem:**
> **Some Disturbing Findings in Truk, Micronesia**
>
> Even when medical technology is sound in itself, maintaining it can cause serious problems that diminish its effectiveness. As part of a 1990 effort sponsored by the WHO to conduct medical-equipment repair courses in Truk, Micronesia, researchers discovered firsthand just how much of a problem maintenance can be.
>
> The 140-bed Truk State Hospital, the principal medical-care facility serving Truk island in Micronesia, was equipped with a few hundred pieces of medical equipment purchased or received as donations when Truk was a UN Trust Territory. Until 1987, a Hawaiian contracting firm maintained the equipment, but when the contract ended, the responsibility fell on the hospital's technical staff—a head technician and his assistant, neither of whom had any formal training in engineering technology or medicine. By 1990, there was no regular maintenance system, and nearly every piece of the equipment in the hospital was inoperable.
>
> **The Overheating Incubator.** As in most tropical hospitals, the clinical laboratory was indispensable in diagnosing infectious diseases—relying on manual microbiological and biochemical analysis techniques that require only simple reagents and basic equipment, such as microscopes and centrifuges. The laboratory director asked the researchers about an incubator that would heat to the desired temperature, but would continue to rise beyond the set point, despite the front panel's indication that the heater had turned off. For several months, the staff had coped with the problem by pulling out the plug when the temperature climbed too high and plugging it in again when it fell too low. After confirming that the heater was indeed turning off properly at the right temperature, the researchers pulled the unit apart and discovered the hidden source of heat—a fan at the base of the unit whose blades were caked with layers of dust and dirt.
>
> **The "Broken" Fluoroscopy Unit.** The hospital's radiology department relied on a South Korean–made X-ray unit, the sole piece of radiological equipment that still functioned. The unit had its share of problems—including an X-ray table that could not move and a burned-out exposure meter—both of which could have been prevented if the unit had received regular maintenance. More interesting, however, was the report that the one fluoroscopy attachment had suddenly failed and the other showed poor image quality. When the radiologist pointed out the failed screen, the researchers reached down to a joystick-like control at the base of the unit to open the motorized collimator, and the screen instantly lit up. Turning to the other fluoroscopy unit with the poor image, the researchers opened a small door on the side of the monitor, tweaked the contrast and focus knobs, and the image sharpened and brightened.
>
> These two examples show that regular maintenance is critical when equipment designed in industrialized nations to operate in clean, climate-controlled hospital environments is brought into tropical locations. In addition, they also show the importance of matching equipment purchases with local needs and capabilities. The South Korean–made fluoroscopy unit had no English-language operating and service manuals, and no source for spare parts had been identified.

The Role of Clinical Engineering in Selecting, Applying, and Maintaining Medical Technologies. With such a large number of competing financial and technical issues involved in selecting, applying, and maintaining new medical technologies, it is not surprising that hospital administrators often avoid planning responsibilities related to acquiring medical technology. Choosing appropriate technologies is indeed a difficult task. One approach that has alleviated this difficulty in large U.S. hospitals is to delegate the decisionmaking authority for purchasing expensive medical equipment to a committee of experts. Serving on this committee are senior administrators, medical doctors and nurses from various departments, and a clinical engineer. Trained to understand all technical aspects of medical equipment, the clinical engineer typically assumes a leading role. As the head of the biomedical engineering department, he or she is responsible for collecting technical specifications and records that may influence a purchasing decision, as well as for maintaining and repairing equipment after it is purchased.

Although there is no simple formula for choosing and applying health technologies, costly mistakes can be avoided by following established guidelines. Drawing on its 20 years of experience in the United States, the discipline of clinical engineering has formulated a program for optimal utilization of medical equipment over its entire life cycle. (See Bronzino, 1992.) Figure 7.2 shows such a program, which has as its cornerstones prepurchase evaluation and regular maintenance.

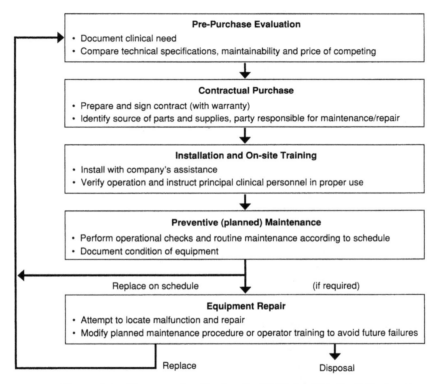

Figure 7.2—Program for Optimally Utilizing Medical Technology Over Its Entire Life Cycle

Despite the modest resources required to establish a department for medical-equipment maintenance, most hospitals in developing areas of Asia still do not have one. (See Schmitt and Qing, 1987.) The problem is compounded in primary-care clinics that have less equipment—though the equipment represents a large fraction of the budget—and cannot sustain a clinical engineering department. In China, some clinical engineering departments have been organized and are in operation in Chinese teaching hospitals in Beijing, Hangzhou, Xian, and Shanghai. (See Peabody and Schmitt, 1992.) Evidence suggests that clinical-engineering departments, when given adequate support from the hospital administration, reduce maintenance costs and promote better equipment utilization. (See Schmitt, 1993.) As technology advances and the purchase of imported medical instrumentation accelerates, the demand for clinical-engineering services in Asia is growing stronger.

Developing Human Resources

If health care activities are to be implemented and sustained over the long term, it is critical that human resources be developed. Developing human resources is a classic public good and, hence, the responsibility of the MOH. In this section, we examine human resources in terms of health professionals and health administrators.

Developing Health Professionals. Large strides have been made throughout Asia in developing well-trained health professionals, even in some of the poorer countries. For example, in 1975 at the conclusion of the war in Southeast Asia, Laos had only 90 doctors for its population of 3 million people, or 0.03 doctors per 1,000 persons. (See Holland and Phimphachanh 1995.) Since then, the number of doctors has increased about 14-fold, so that, despite the population growth, there are now 0.23 doctors per 1,000 persons.

Still, while there is a reasonable total supply of health professionals in developing countries in Asia (see the data in Chapter 2), many developing countries have problems *retaining* the doctors and nurses they train. Many developing countries subsidize the education of all physicians—even those who will spend their careers in private practice dealing with a profitable specialty. The costs of this training are even higher because of the migration of physicians and nurses from developing to developed countries. Both the Philippines and India have large outward doctor migrations. The Philippines also exports 2,000 to 3,000 nurses a year, mostly to North America. (See World Bank, 1993a.) Policies that would avoid this subsidy include eliminating the subsidy or replacing it with student loans. For example, a country might require that individuals repay the cost of state-financed education either directly or through a bond that they could work off in underserved areas.

Even if the overall supply of health professionals is reasonable, shortages remain in rural areas. Professional isolation, lack of additional work opportunities, substandard housing, and other disamenities make staffing rural health facilities difficult. However, primary health care workers with limited training can succeed in delivering needed care, as was shown in a study of using aid workers to deliver primary health care in Vanuatu. (See Harris, 1991.) China also uses many nonphysicians in rural areas. One study argues that the Chinese experience with village health workers shows that health care personnel with six months to two years of training after junior middle school could competently provide preventive and basic services. (See Hsiao, 1995a.) However, one must be careful not to expect those with limited training to be able to master all technical requirements of all public health programs. The Philippines' experience in the early 1980s was that the technical integrity of preventive programs deteriorated without specialized expertise. (See World Bank, 1995d.)

Developing Health Administrators. There is substantial agreement on the skill mix required to run a health care system in a developing country. One study, looking at implementing the activities described in the *World Development Report*

Table 7.1

Management Skill Areas for Health Care Systems

Categories	Management Skill Areas
Traditional management	Health care financing and budgeting Economic principles applied to health Planning methods Restructuring organizations
Interpersonal and communication skills	Listening skills Motivating people to work toward shared goals Identifying/working with resistance to change Fostering communication among people/organizations
Analytic thinking	Scientific and statistical thinking Defining processes and problems Using data to set priorities and monitor/evaluate performance
Data collection and manipulation	Developing and testing hypotheses Collecting and displaying data Interpreting data
Clinical skills	Clinical medicine

1993, organized this skill mix into five broad categories, shown above in Table 7.1. (See Cretin et al., 1995, for a more complete discussion of the study summarized here.)

This agreement is clearly shown in a survey of 107 health leaders from developing countries in Asia, Latin America, Africa, and the Middle East. They were asked about the importance of the skills shown in Table 7.1 and about the competence in those skills of those who were actively involved in health reform efforts in the developing world at each of three governmental levels in the health system: national, district (or provincial), and local.

Traditional management skills (such as finance and budgeting or applying economic principles to health care), interpersonal and communication skills, and analytic thinking skills were all rated as very to extremely important, whereas data collection and manipulation skills were rated as slightly less important (useful for district or local leaders who might need to be involved in "hands on" work with data or the design of experiments to test hypotheses, but not for national leaders). In terms of competence, however, leaders at all levels consistently rated skills in all four categories as fair to poor; national leaders received slightly better ratings than district leaders, and local leaders rated lowest. Clinical skills received the highest competence ratings at all levels, but were seen as only somewhat important.

Training for managers is thus a requirement for successful health care reform. Respondents' most frequently cited ideas for meeting the management development needs of health leaders included some traditional and some new approaches:

- Training designed to increase communication effectiveness for leaders at every level, to help them use local and national media to communicate high-level policy decisions and affect public and professional opinion.

- Expert consultation in the form of one-on-one long-term relationships between national leaders and experts. Tying the consultation to direct assistance in specific projects was seen as an effective way to structure consultation and training designed to assist leaders in planning, setting goals, and implementing change.

- Health policy or analytic support units designed to provide technical support for leaders in planning methods. National leaders might best be served not by developing technical skills themselves but by access to better technical advice. District and local leaders were also identified as needing this type of support.

- Training political and health leaders in the principles of analytic thinking or economic theory (as opposed to technical, analytic skills). This helps them use data to set priorities and to plan, pilot-test, and evaluate new policies.

- Executive seminars for national leaders in areas such as finance and organizational restructuring. Exposure to other systems through both classroom work and site visits was also suggested to improve leaders' motivational skills and their understanding of how to restructure organizations.

- Classroom and on-the-job training for district-level leaders, especially in financing, using and interpreting data, planning methods, and restructuring organizations. National or district-level trainers could work with local leaders to help them identify and overcome barriers to change. Longer-term programs with repeated contact and follow-up were seen as very useful for helping local leaders develop their analytic thinking, planning, and data skills.

- Interlevel training bringing together leaders from national, district, and local levels to improve communication and collaboration.

Improving the management and leadership skills of health leaders in the developing world should be a key component of any health care plan. As the survey revealed, leaders themselves are keenly aware of their management development needs and have many ideas about how to improve their skills. Unfortunately, funding for management training and education falls far behind that for technical equipment, construction, or even clinical training.

Box 7.4: Meeting Rural Needs for Health Care Providers: Two Different Approaches

Despite urbanization in Asia, the United Nations Development Program predicts the population growth in cities will slow, implying that in the next 20 years the majority of the population in the countries that the ADB supports will still live in rural areas. (See Loevinsohn, 1996.) More problematic, this rural majority continues to bear a disproportionate burden of the region's health problems. While there are a number of reasons for this urban-rural health status gap, one reason is not having enough providers to serve rural populations. Here, we look at two approaches Asian governments have used to remedy the problem.

One fairly straightforward approach is to encourage the growth in the overall number of physicians and then induce those physicians to locate in rural areas. This is the approach that India, Pakistan, and the Philippines have pursued. Unfortunately, these efforts have not met with much success. For example, Pakistani medical schools greatly increased their production of physicians in the 1980s in the hope that more physicians would choose to locate in rural areas. However, low salaries in rural areas, poor rural medical infrastructure, and lack of management training did not induce many newly trained doctors to relocate; this led to massive physician unemployment and, as a result, to the substantial emigration of doctors out of the country. (See World Bank, 1988b, 1993 l, 1994c, 1994h.)

Health officials in Papua New Guinea took a fundamentally different approach to the problem. Instead of relying on producing more doctors who would be willing to relocate to rural areas, the country created a new class of health professionals who came primarily from rural areas in the first place. In the 1970s, the College of Allied Health Sciences began training health extension officers (HEOs), who require less training and have lower salaries than physicians. Once in place at rural health centers, the HEOs are responsible for managing both primary care nurses and community health workers providing environmental and preventive health services.

HEOs receive clinical and public health training, supplemented by specific field experiences in health center management at health centers and provincial headquarters. In addition, the provincial government has installed radio links between remote health posts, district health centers, and provincial hospitals that afford the HEOs and other managers more regular contact. Provincial authorities have begun to use the radios to institute basic management procedures, such as requiring remote personnel to report in daily so that workers do not abandon their posts. Hospital-based physicians use the radios to conduct in-service educational seminars designed to improve primary-care quality. And the HEOs use the radios to make complex case presentations to physicians and receive advice about treatment or referral.

The program has not been without difficulties. Recent economic difficulties have delayed payment of rural health personnel, and the security situation in the provinces has deteriorated. In addition, in-service management training programs have faltered because of funding shortages. (See Asch and Peabody, 1996.) Still, despite these difficulties, the program has successfully placed HEOs in over 75 percent of the rural health centers.

Evidence from these two sets of experiences suggests that initiatives to get more providers in rural areas work best if they do not depend on physicians alone, if they include specific management training, and if they build communication links to ensure both oversight and ongoing support.

PAYMENT MECHANISMS

There is no universally "right" way to pay providers. Rather, each option has advantages and disadvantages, some of which vary based on the ways in which the payment system will be used. The value placed on each of these advantages and disadvantages depends on the goals of reform. Therefore, changes in the existing payment system must be tailored to the particular environment and policy goals. In this section, we discuss how payment systems can be used, the options available, and the pros and cons of these options.

The MOH needs payment systems to manage its own health delivery operations; to pay for care delivered by private providers to government beneficiaries (e.g., government workers, or the poor, or the beneficiaries of a government-run social insurance plan); and to regulate private providers, no matter who is financing the care (e.g., to prevent private providers from receiving excess profits by overcharging or to limit the total amount of resources spent on health care). Note that the issue of what the provider receives in payment is different from the finance issue, which we discussed in Chapter 4. The provider payment can be a mixture of a government-provided amount and either a user charge or copayment.

The design of price controls or of a system of administered prices should be directed at achieving an incentive system that results in greater efficiency. When prices are used to allocate funds within a system run entirely by the government, they should provide the managers of government health care facilities with the same signals that firm managers in a market economy receive when they observe market prices.

Determining the unit of service to be priced is important. Many developing countries price very small units of services (e.g., a single drug prescription, a laboratory test, a visit to the doctor). This can defeat the goal of cost containment if providers increase volume to increase profits. As a result, an FFS payment system may encourage technical efficiency but is also likely to encourage allocative inefficiency. Payments for larger bundles of services, such as a case or an episode of care, are intended to discourage unnecessary services. Global budget systems are frequently used by developing countries to allocate resources to hospitals or clinics. In a global budget, a total amount of money is allocated to a facility to cover all expenses; the unit being priced is all services provided by the facility. If global budgets are allocated without careful accounting for the level of output of different providers, they provide no incentives for technical efficiency. Per-capita payment systems, which are a fixed amount for all the care delivered to a person in a fixed time interval, are usually viewed as a way of encouraging both allocative and technical efficiency.

There is substantial interest in many developing countries in more sophisticated payment systems than FFS and global budgets and even some attempts at implementation. Because this interest is so recent, little is known about actual as opposed to theoretical effects. Nevertheless, we believe that a review of what is known, mostly from theory and from developed-country experience, is an important foundation for ongoing attempts at implementation. We begin below with a discussion of per-capita payment systems. Then, we consider a variety of ways of paying for hospital services, looking at their advantages and disadvantages.

Per-Capita Payment

Some developed countries want providers who will care for all the health care needs of a person for a fixed per-capita payment (capitation). When the providers are allowed to keep the difference between the payment amount and expenses as profit (or salary or bonuses), economic theory predicts that such per-capita payments provide strong incentives for both technical and allocative efficiency. There is some evidence from developed countries that health maintenance organizations (HMOs) that use this system do control the volume of services better than an FFS system. (See Luft and Morrison, 1991, and Manning et al., 1984.)

The theoretical attractiveness of per-capita payments has led many developing countries to consider such payment systems. The Philippines is one of the few developing countries that has operating HMOs. They are also being considered in Ecuador and in Columbia. (See Peabody et al., 1995a.)

Although HMO per-capita payments usually cover all medical services including both inpatient and outpatient care, per-capita payments also can be used for particular kinds of care. For example, the ZdravReform Project is conducting a demonstration project in the Issyk-Kul Oblast of the Kyrgyz Republic in which family practice groups will be paid on a per-capita basis for each person that they enroll. Because the primary-care doctor will get a single payment to cover all the primary care required by a patient, the doctor will try to provide these services as efficiently as possible. The doctor will be able to be efficient, because he will have authority to use the payment to purchase supplies and equipment and referral services that are frequently needed or delivered in the particular practice. A primary care per-capita system might encourage doctors to enter primary care rather than specialty medicine. It also might increase utilization of primary care compared to a system in which primary-care providers lack supplies and refer almost all care to polyclinics, such as the one the demonstration project will replace.

To date, there is little experience with capitation for primary care in developing countries, so it is not yet clear whether the theoretical advantages will be realized in practice. Most of the efficiency advantages HMOs have demonstrated in developing countries come from eliminating unnecessary hospitalizations, and a primary-care capitation payment system has no strong incentives with respect to hospitalizations. Furthermore, capitation payments might encourage primary-care physicians to refer as many patients as possible to specialists so as to reduce their own workload. Systems where physicians are at some financial risk for the cost of specialist care for their patients are used in developed countries to counter this threat.

A major issue in a per-capita payment system is determining the payment amounts. Although the idea of setting rates through a competitive bidding process has been discussed in the literature, there are few real examples in either developing or developed countries. Instead, prices are determined through an administrative process that allows the government to set prices compatible with its budget. The process begins with estimates of actual per-capita health care costs in each population segment.

In systems that provide universal coverage of a diverse population, the setting of per-capita rates faces a special obstacle. As we discussed in Chapter 5, utilization varies substantially in almost all developed and developing countries, with poor and rural persons receiving fewer services. In many cases, the poor and rural populations have a higher burden of illness despite the lower utilization. Nevertheless, one cannot deal with this underutilization merely by paying the same per-capita amount in all regions. Although providers might enter these areas in the long run, the costs to be borne in the interim will likely be catastrophic. There would be windfall gains to the HMOs serving rural areas. If the payment rate is set at the urban average, then costs will rise substantially—perhaps to unsustainable levels. However, if the payment is set at the national average, urban providers and patients will be seriously harmed and the system is unlikely to be politically sustainable. (See Peabody, 1996a.)

A more practical approach to setting rates is to use a relatively small deviation from regional averages, with the deviation being positive in poor or rural areas to encourage additional providers to settle there and negative in urban areas to encourage economy in the production of health care.

Unfortunately, other incentives can arise from per-capita payment systems. The same ability to retain earnings that provides the efficiency incentive can also produce an economic incentive to provide less care. If there is only one HMO for a well-defined population, monopolistic capitated providers have incentives to give low-quality care. Using the payment system in a market that contains several competitive HMOs will help with this problem, but it will not solve it, because information problems may prevent patients or their purchasing agents from realizing they are being undertreated.[9]

Per-capita payments in a competitive market provide incentives for plans to select only patients whose costs are likely to be less than the payment amount ("cream skimming"). Plans in which costly people are concentrated will be at a disadvantage regardless of how efficiently they provide care. So plans will have incentives to select people whose expected cost is less than the payment and make themselves unattractive to people whose expected cost is greater than the payment. However, if each person's payment reflects what an average provider would spend on the individual (so is higher for people who need more care), these incentives to select disappear, and plans can even afford to specialize in particular kinds of expensive patients.

Such risk-adjusted payment systems have been the subject of much recent work in the United States. (See Weiner et al., 1996; Ellis et al., 1996.) However, they have very high data requirements and are unlikely to be practical in developing countries. Note that competition will not help money-losing patients; unless firms are properly compensated, they may not want their business. Thus, systems of regulation to ensure that patients are not discriminated against must be part of any competitive HMO market.

---

[9] In the United States, much research effort is going into the development of indicators of outcomes for HMO firms. At this time, these indicators are not comprehensive enough to form the basis for purchasing decisions related to quality of care.

Hospital Payments

Because hospitals consume such a large share of health care dollars, hospital payment is frequently a major focus of reform efforts. In this section, we discuss the pros and cons of alternative ways of paying for hospital services.

Global budget is the generic name for any hospital payment system in which the hospital is allocated a fixed amount of funds to operate over a fixed period of time, usually a year. Global budgets are used in the hospital sector in many Asian countries. In some countries, parts of the global budget are restricted to particular kinds of use, such as salaries. For example, in the Kyrgyz Republic, the global budget is partitioned according to budget categories called Chapters—Chapter 1 is wages, Chapter 2 is payroll-related taxes, Chapter 9 is pharmaceuticals, and so forth. At the time of independence, spending in any category was not allowed to exceed the budgeted amount. This form of payment, with its focus on inputs rather than outputs, provides no incentives for efficiency. Insofar as the Chapters prevent the flexible use of funds, the payment system actually inhibits the efficient use of resources. However, it provides the government with complete budget control, because it determines exactly what will be spent. (See Carter, 1995.)

An FFS that pays for individual services delivered in the hospital also provides no incentive for efficiency and lacks even the value of cost containment. In South Korea, hospitals and physicians are reimbursed on an FFS basis according to a relative-value scale. Hospitals are paid a per diem plus additional reimbursement for services such as drugs. The per diem is reduced to 80 percent for days beyond 16. A plus factor is used as a case-mix adjuster for payments. General community hospitals receive fee plus 13 percent, multispecialty hospitals receive fee plus 20 percent, and university hospitals receive fee plus 30 percent. (See De Geyndt, 1991.) This FFS system provides little incentive for efficiency; as a result, it is one of the reasons costs have been rising over time. In 1990, health care spending reached 5.4 percent of the GDP. (See De Geyndt, 1992.) As shown in the data section in Chapter 2, this is at the higher end of the range for larger Asian countries.

Table 7.2 compares a traditional global budget system with alternative hospital payment systems, which do provide some incentives for efficiency. When hospitals are paid on a per-case basis or on an all-inclusive per-day basis and managers are allowed to retain the difference between payment and costs, they have substantial incentives to control costs. Per-diem payments encourage longer hospital stays than per-case payment methods. The incentives to increase length of stay (LOS) found in a per-diem payment system are quite strong and have been found to have measurable effects on LOS throughout the world, including recent experience in the Ukraine. (See Wouters, 1992.) This effect can overpower the efficiency incentives in the system.

To account for differences in case mix across hospitals, a per-case discharge system usually groups patients with relatively similar costs. The system can be as simple as separating medical and surgical patients or as complicated as DRGs, which classify patients into hundreds of categories based on the disease that caused the hospitalization and the procedures received in the hospital. Per-diem payment systems should also be adjusted for case mix (e.g., providing a higher payment for days in an intensive care unit and/or extra payment for surgery).

Table 7.2

Comparison of Inpatient Payment Systems

Area of Comparison	Global Budget	Per Diem	Per Case	Case-Based Global Budget
Incentives for length of stay	Incentive to increase	Strong incentive to increase	Strong incentive to decrease	Incentive to decrease, which is weaker than for per-case payment because impact delayed
Incentives for efficient management	None	Strong	Strong	Delayed
Incentives to hospitalize	None	Depends on level of occupancy achieved by LOS	Positive incentive to hospitalize and to discharge and readmit. Strong incentive when case classification system is weak	Delayed positive incentive to hospitalize and to discharge and readmit. Strong incentive when case classification system is weak
Access for the very ill	None	Some incentive to avoid patients who require more than average services per day. Strongest when per-diem classification system is weakest Incentive is weaker than in per case because profit can often be made up by longer LOS	Incentive to avoid patients who require more than average services per case and the larger group that require long LOS Strongest when case classification system is weakest Can be mitigated by outlier payments	As in per-case system, except effect is weakened by delayed impact
Upcoding incentives	Least	Generally weak because classification system usually has only a few, well-defined categories	Strong incentives exist, but could be mitigated by regulatory oversight	As in per-case system, except effect is weakened by delayed impact
Data requirements	Least	Patient discharge abstracts for payment, hospital cost report for rate setting	More clinical detail on discharge abstract for case classification, more resource utilization on discharge abstract besides hospital cost report for rate setting	Same as per-case payment
Uncertainty for hospital managers	Least	Some	More	Less
Uncertainty for payer	Least	Some	Some	Less

Whether payment is per day or per case, efficient behavior is encouraged when prices are set at a level to efficiently produce a bundle of services. Then, when a provider's cost structure differs from his payments, he has an incentive either to become more efficient or to reduce his frequency of delivery of the services for which his costs exceed the payment. The resultant specialization should improve the efficiency of the health delivery system as a whole. Considerations of beneficiary access and provider equity also imply that prices should be proportional to costs so that beneficiaries with all conditions will be able to find treatment and so that hospitals with all possible case mixes will receive adequate payment. (See Carter and Rogowski, 1992.) Finally, prices that are not proportional to cost encourage inefficient behavior on the part of providers (as the Chinese experience discussed at the beginning of this chapter illustrates).

Per-case payments are usually calculated as rate times weight, where the weight for a DRG (or other group) reflects the cost of caring for the typical case in the DRG relative to the cost of caring for the overall typical case. Thus, a case in a DRG with a weight of 2 typically costs twice as much as a case in a DRG with a weight of 1. Note that it is not expected that the payment for a particular case will exactly equal the costs of the case. It is intended only that average payments will equal average costs for the patients in a DRG. The rate can be set to control the total growth in hospital costs, since the weights are set to average 1.

However, pricing at cost is difficult. Different providers use different production functions and face slightly different input prices. Accounting methods are needed to estimate costs at the level of detailed clinical groups such as DRGs, and these estimate only average cost, not marginal cost.[10] To avoid encouraging the overproduction of services, one would theoretically prefer to price at marginal cost rather than average cost and use a different method of reimbursing fixed costs. Price regulation can also result in shifting costs among payers in a multipayer environment.

Per-case payment systems have bad incentives to provide unnecessary hospitalizations, to avoid caring for a patient whose cost is more than the payment, and to "upcode" (i.e., to claim to have sicker patients than one actually has in order to obtain extra reimbursement). The difficulties of price regulation have been the subject of much research on the DRG payment system used by the U.S. government to pay private hospitals. On average, there is evidence that the use of DRGs encourages hospital efficiency and has small or no effects on quality, although problems with the system remain. (See Coulam and Gaumer, 1991.)

Global budgets are usually adjusted incrementally every year. When some hospitals experience changes in workload because of a change in the volume of cases or in their case mix, incremental changes are not adequate to provide a payment system that is fair to the personnel of all hospitals and their patients. The last column in Table 7.2 concerns an alternative form of global budget in which the budget amount is based on hospital output in the previous year—a case-based global budget that would provide payments to a set of similar hospitals that are proportional to hospital output as measured by the sum of the weights for the cases discharged in the previous year. This form of global budget is market-oriented, since hospitals compete to attract patients to increase their budget for the next year.

[10]Barnum and Kutzin provide a good discussion of how different hospital costing methods are used. (See Barnum and Kutzin, 1993.) Algorithms for calculating DRG weights are discussed in the literature. (See Carter and Rogowski, 1992.)

Choosing a Policy

As we said at the beginning of this section, a payment system must be tailored to the particular policy goals and environment of the reform being carried out. The first step in choosing a payment system must be to determine the problems in the current environment and assess what objectives are to be attained through changing the payment system. As we have just seen, payment options differ with respect to the incentives they provide for cost control and for efficient production of health care, as well as in terms of how much they ensure equity across providers. Only when the priorities assigned to these competing goals are known, can a policymaker begin to evaluate the different payment options. Other policies and political, social, and institutional factors will affect how providers, patients, and government employees respond to the incentives within the payment system options. Another important consideration is the administrative cost entailed in using the system. Are data available that distinguish the resources needed by different patients? If not, what would it cost to collect such data? Are trained personnel available who could collect them? Would the data be valuable for other purposes?

In many ways, the choice of a particular payment system resembles most of the health policy problems discussed throughout this book. For each problem, there is some information from theory, experiment, or other countries' experience that sheds light on the value of alternatives. In every case, however, there is a need to particularize this information to fit a particular decision. Each situation must be examined to determine the problems to be ameliorated, choose goals for reform, determine the factors that will affect outcomes, and estimate the results of alternative policy options. After implementation, outcomes must be monitored for unexpected occurrences and evaluated for possible improvements. Thus, the information we have provided in this book is merely the tiniest of first steps in the process of improving health in developing countries. The rest is in the hands of those men and women charged with managing their health sectors.

POLICY IMPLICATIONS

When we look across the findings in this chapter, what can we say policymakers should focus on? First, whatever planning process is used, it should transform the government's political goals into operational programs that can be conducted within budget constraints and assessed by objective, measurable criteria. While the PPBS system discussed above is not the ideal planning process, it does have the advantage of formalized planning and evaluation, programming, and budgeting phases. Given the complexity of the health care planning process—and what is at stake in terms of people's lives—it makes no sense to operate with an informal system that does not deliberately connect values, priorities, goals, and programs. Discontinuities or misalignments within such a system can lead not only to wasted resources but to lost lives.

Second, when information is collected and analyzed, it should be tailored to the needs of managers at all levels of the MOH, rather than merely providing statistical summaries. Computerized information collection and analytical activities can save immense amounts of time and money, but they have not clearly been shown to improve health status and they are not a substitute for taking the time to make the information useful to policymakers.   Information systems should be purchased, designed, and used so that they help with program decisions and evaluate the effectiveness of those programs. Indeed, the very fact that computers enable MOH staff to collect and analyze vast amounts of information may lead them to believe that their task is done when the data have been entered and processed. To the contrary, it is essential to think through the role of information and data and then formulate them in a way that is useful to policymakers.

Third, if the MOH devolves responsibility for providing health care services, it should only do so after ensuring that local capabilities are in place—specifically, that local services are fiscally sustainable and that local personnel have the skills required to deliver and manage the services—and that the central government's goals for equity and efficiency is likely to be met. This is another way of saying that the decision to devolve must be based on more than the allure of efficiency that such activities promise—it must also be consistent with the values and priorities and goals that drive a country's health-sector policy. Implementation and follow-through are the key to successful devolution.

Fourth, if the MOH decides to delegate the provision of hospital services or other services (clinics, nursing homes, or physician care) to the private sector, it should not do so unless an effective system for regulating institutional providers is in place. While there are examples where private providers have provided services without creating feared inequities—indeed, we discuss some examples in this chapter—it is nonetheless true that private providers and public providers have very different motivations. Therefore, before implementing any form of private provision, policymakers must ensure that a consistent set of regulations is in place—both regulations that are driven by incentives and those that are guided by directives. Ultimately, values like equity are public goods, and it is the government's responsibility—even if it delegates the provision of services to the private sector—to ensure that the public good is met.

Fifth, the MOH needs to integrate the private practice of medicine into its planning and regulatory activities. Too often this is ignored—data are harder to collect and often not available. This is ironic because private providers represent an important political force. With the right combination of incentives and regulations, they will readily support some of the government's policy objectives. Where possible, data are needed to monitor policy response. Decisions between enforcement and reward strategies, while naturally based on evidence of their relative efficacy, should also consider administrative costs. Value mandates or imprecise prescriptions that are difficult to enforce are common regulatory problems that need to be identified and eliminated.

Finally, all regulatory systems should contain enforcement mechanisms that reward conforming behavior and credibly punish violations.

ADB	Asian Development Bank
ADL	activity of daily living
AIDS	auto immune deficiency syndrome
ARIs	acute respiratory tract infections
BCG	bacillus of Calmette-Guérin
BOPH	Bureau of Public Health
BPS	*Biro Pusat Statistik*
CT	computered tomography or (CAT) computerized axial tomography
CD-ROM	compact disk—read only memory
CME	continuing medical education
CPG	clinical practice guidelines
CQI	continuous quality improvement
DALYs	Disability Adjusted Life Years
DCS	Department of Census and Statistics
DHS	Demographic Health Survey
DTP	diphtheria-tetanus-pertussis
E&C	education and communication
ECG	electrocardiogram
EHI	Employees Health Insurance
EMPs	*Empresas de Medicina Prepagada*
EPI	Expanded Program on Immunization
FBS	(Pakistan) Federal Bureau of Statistics
FFS	fee for service
FPMD	Family Planning Management Development
GDP	gross domestic product
GNP pc	gross national product per capita
HeaLYs	Health Adjusted Years
HFS	Health, Financing and Sustainability (household survey)

HIS	health information system
HIV	human immunodeficiency virus
HMO	health maintenance organization
IABD	Inter-American Development Bank
IDT	*Inpres Desa Tertinggal*
IDU	intravenous drug users
IEEE	Institute of Electrical and Electronic Engineers
IIPS	International Institute for Population Sciences
IMF	International Monetary Fund
IMR	infant mortality rate
IPA	Independent Practice Association
IRD	Institute for Resources Development/Westinghouse
ISAPRE	*Institutos de Salud Previsional*
km	kilometer
Korea DPR	Korea Democratic People's Republic of Korea (North Korea)
Lao PDR	People's Democratic Republic of Lao
LOS	length of service
LSMS	Living Standards Measurement Surveys
MCH	maternal and child health
MCH-FP	Maternal and Child Health—Family Planning
MCO	managed care organization
MOH	Ministry of Health
MOPH	Ministry of Public Health
MRI	magnetic resonance imaging
MSA	medical savings account
NGO	nongovernmental organizations
NHA	National Health Account
NHI	National Health Insurance
NHS	National Health Service
NHS	National Health Service (Centre for Reviews and Dissemination)
NIH	(National Institutes of Health) Technology Assessment
NIPS	National Institute of Population Studies

NSO	National Statistics Office
NTB	*Nusa Tenggara Barat*
OECD	Organization for Economic Cooperation and Development
ORS	oral rehydration solution
ORT	oral rehydration therapy
PAP	Papanicolaou (smear)
PATH	Program for Appropriate Technology in Health
PCS	prospective cohort study
PEM	protein-energy malnutrition
PNG	Papua New Guinea
PODES	*Potensi Desa* (Census of Village Potential)
PPBS	Policy, Programming and Budgeting System
PPO	preferred provider organization
PPP	purchasing power parity
PPRC	Physician Payment Review Commission
QOL	quality of life
RCT	randomized control trials
RHF	recommended home fluid
Rp.	rupiah (Indonesia)
SI	social insurance
SSC	social security contributions
STDs	sexually transmitted diseases
SUSENAS	*Survey Sosiala Ekonomi Nasional* (Indonesia National Socio-Economic Survey)
TM	transtheoretical model
TPA	tissue plasminogen activator
TQM	total quality management
UNAIDS	(Joint) United Nations Programme on HIV/AIDS
UNDP	United Nations Development Program
UNESCO	United Nations Educational, Scientific and Cultural Organization
UNFPA	United Nations Fund for Population Affairs
UNICEF	United Nations International Children's Emergency Fund

USAID	United States Agency for International Development
USDHHS	U.S. Department of Health and Human Services
WHO	World Health Organization
WHO/SEARO	World Health Organization/Southeast Asia Regional Office
WHO/TDR	World Health Organization/Special Programme for Research and Training in Tropical Disease
WHO/WPRO	World Health Organization/Western Pacific Regional Office
WID	women in development

In Chapter 2, we discussed seven categories of data policymakers need to make informed health care interventions and presented the status of the data in a series of tables within each of the seven data categories. Here, we examine the sources for the quantitative data in the tables, along with the definitions for the measures/indicators used in the tables.

One of the lessons we learned in constructing the tables in this chapter is that the data are difficult to come by. No single source or clearinghouse existed for data used to make the cross-country comparisons. Rather, we had to consolidate data from over 70 sources—both from routinely collected information systems and from specially designed studies. Most of the aggregated routine data used comes from the World Bank, WHO, and UNICEF annual reports. These were supplemented by data from regional sources, such as the ADB, and from policy research groups, such as RAND, USAID (e.g., the HFS project), and the United Nations Economic and Social Council.

Sources of the special studies are generally found in research reports, such as the medical and social science (e.g., economics and management sciences) literature. They are also found in consultant (as opposed to research) reports from the World Bank Staff Appraisal Reports, WHO Program Reports, WHO Regional reports, UN Reports, private consultant reports (such as ABT Associates-HFS reports) and peer-reviewed journal articles.

DEMOGRAPHIC AND SOCIOECONOMIC FACTORS

Within this data category, we present three tables, which are discussed below.

Table 2.2: Population Structure and Dynamics in 44 Asian Countries

Population and Projected Populations (millions): Considers all residents regardless of legal status or citizenship, with refugees normally considered part of the population of their home country. For this indicator, we used estimates and 2025 population projections from the World Bank's 1996 World Development Report and reports from WHO's Regional Offices in the Western Pacific and Southeast Asia.

Annual Average Population Growth (percent). We define this indicator as the new population in a given year divided by the population of the previous year. The indicator itself provides a ten-year average of this growth rate.

Crude Birth Rate. Number of births per 1,000 population.

Crude Death Rate. Number of deaths per 1,000 population.

Fertility Rate. Number of newborn babies per number of women of childbearing age (15–49).

Table 2.3: Population Distribution by Region in 44 Asian Countries

Urban Population as a Percentage of Total Population. Represents the share of the country's population that lives in urban areas. In general, urban areas are defined as metropolitan areas with one million or more population. The indicator is given for three time periods—1980, 1990–1992, and 1995. The main sources of information were from data in the World Bank's 1993 and 1996 World Development Reports and the 1995 WHO/WPRO Regional Office.

Urban Population Average Annual Growth Rate (percent). Given for two time periods—1980–1990 and 1990–1994.

Concentration in Capital (percent). Examines the population living in the capital city. It gives the capital population as a percentage of the urban total and of the entire population. The time period reported is 1990.

Table 2.4: Distribution of Income in 44 Asian Countries

Gross National Product Per Capita (GNP pc). This indicator measures the total domestic and foreign value added generated by residents of a country. It is equal to the GDP plus the net factor income (wages and investment income received from abroad by residents of a country minus those earned by nonresidents in a country). The GNP per capita is simply GNP divided by the total population. The GNP per capita should not be considered a good measure of welfare. The time period reported is 1994.

Gini Index. The Gini index is a measure of inequality in income distribution. It has a maximum value of 100 (the case when one household receives all the national income), and a minimum value of 0 (the case when there is perfect equality).

Percentage Share of Income or Consumption by Percentile and Income Quintile. This is the share of total income that is held by a given subgroup of the population. These subgroups or percentiles are ranked by level of per capita income, or household income.

We relied on four main sources of information: (1) the World Development Reports, 1993, 1996 and 1997; (2) the World Bank's 1997 Sector Strategy paper; (3) recent mission reports from the World Bank; and (4) consulting reports from RAND. The World Bank based its calculations on representative national surveys for various years between 1981 and 1991. The results of these surveys were compiled by government statistical agencies or by the World Bank in the case of the LSMS. The RAND data come from national surveys done in Bangladesh, India, Indonesia, and Malaysia.

MEASURES OF ACCESS TO HEALTH CARE AND OTHER BASIC NEEDS

Within this data category, we present two tables, which are discussed below.

Table 2.5: Access to Basic Necessities in 44 Asian Countries

Child Malnutrition. Two different criteria are used to measure this indicator: less than 80 percent of standard weight for age, or more than minus two standard deviations from the 50th percentile of the weight for age of population. The indicator is reported over the time period 1989–1995. The sources of information for this indicator were the 1996 World Development Report, WHO's 1994 *Progress*

Towards Health for All and WHO/SEARO's 1995 *Health Situations in the Southeast Asia Region.*

Adult Literacy Rate for Both Sexes and for Females. This indicator, used as a proxy measure of access to education, is defined as the proportion of the population 15 years and older who can read and write a short simple statement with understanding. The main sources of information were the projections prepared in 1995 by UNESCO.

Access to Safe Water. Represents the percentage of the population with "reasonable" access to a safe water supply (from treated surface waters to untreated but uncontaminated sources such as sanitary wells and protected boreholes). In rural areas, reasonable access implies that household members do not have to spend a disproportionate part of the day fetching water. The time period reported is 1994–1995. The main source of information was the World Bank development reports. Data were available in WHO's 1994 *Progress Towards Health for All,* and the 1995 World Health Report for the countries not considered by the World Bank.

Access to Sanitation. Refers to the percentage of the population with at least adequate excreta-disposal facilities that can prevent human, animal, and insect contact with excreta. The sources of information for this indicator and the time period reported were the same as those for access to safe water.

Table 2.6: Access to Health Care in 44 Asian Countries

General Access to Health Care. Measured as the percentage of the population with access to health services in no more than one hour. The time period reported for the indicator is 1989–1995. Data came from a variety of sources: the 1993 and 1997 World Development Reports, WHO's 1994 *Progress Towards Health for All,* and the 1995 WHO/SEARO and WHO/WPRO regional reports.

Contraceptive Prevalence. This indicator, used as a proxy of access to family planning services, defines the percentage of women age 15 to 49 who are practicing, or whose husbands are practicing, any form of contraception. The time period reported is 1986–1994. Our data came from the United Nations Department for Economic and Social Information and Policy Analysis (United Nations, 1994).

Prenatal Care. Measures the percentage of women who visited a health professional during pregnancy. The time period reported is 1980–1990. The indicator is based on estimates from WHO's regional office and World Bank figures. As primary data, these institutions used health and demographic household surveys, as well as routinely collected information systems, such as hospital records.

Immunization. This indicator represents the percentage of children that have received the following vaccines: BCG, three doses of DTP, three doses of polio, and the vaccine for measles. The time period reported is 1994–1995. Information on coverage was generally available through the EPI Information System and the 1996 World Health Report.

AN INVENTORY OF PUBLIC AND PRIVATE RESOURCES

Within this data type, we present two tables, which are discussed below.

Table 2.7: Health Expenditures in 44 Asian Countries

Per Capita Expenditures in Health (dollars). In this indicator, total expenditures are divided into expenditures from the public sector (i.e., from the government budget), the private sector (i.e., household consumption), and from social security. We divide each of these categories of expenditures by the total population to obtain per capita values. The time period reported is 1990–1991.

Health Expenditures As a Percentage of GDP. In this indicator, we divide total health expenditures, public health expenditures (including social security), and private health expenditures by total GDP. The time period reported is 1990.

The sources used to compute these indicators were the tables in the 1993 and 1996 World Development Report and the Western Pacific Regional Office; the 1994 *Progress Towards Health for All* Program Report; and the International Monetary Fund 1995 Annual Report. Data about the distribution of these resources by type of use are available in Table 1.2.

Table 2.8: Health Infrastructure and Manpower in 44 Asian Countries

Hospital Beds, Physicians, and Nurses Per 1,000 Population. These three indicators are obtained by dividing the total number of hospitals, physicians, and nurses by the total population, and then multiplying by 1,000. The indicators came from the World Bank Development Report, WHO reports and DHS surveys between 1987 and 1994.

MEASURES OF HEALTH OUTCOMES

Within this category, we present one table, which is discussed below.

Table 2.10: Aggregate Version of the Most Commonly Used Health Outcome Measures in 44 Asian Countries

Life Expectancy at Birth. Defined as the number of years a newborn would live if the mortality rates observed at the time of its birth were to remain constant during his/her life. The time period reported is 1995. The main sources were the 1996 and 1997 World Development Reports, and WHO's 1994 and 1995 global and regional *Progress Towards Health for All* reports, which used data collected from the United Nations Population Division.

Under-Five Mortality Rate and Infant Mortality Rate. The first indicator measures the probability of a newborn dying before reaching age five. These probabilities are derived from life tables of estimated life expectancy at birth and from infant mortality rates. The second indicator is the probability of dying between birth and exactly one year of age. Both indicators are expressed per 1,000 live births. The time period reported is 1995. Both indicators were compiled on the basis of the World Bank's 1996 World Development Report, WHO reports on *Progress Towards Health for All;* DHS reports for Asia from 1987–1994; and UNICEF's 1992 Report on the *State of the World's Children.*

Maternal Mortality Rate. This indicator refers to the number of female deaths that occur during childbirth per 100,000 live births. The time period reported is 1989–1995. The data came from the 1996 World Development Report and WHO's *Progress Towards Health for All* and from the Regional Office situation reports. The World Bank based its numbers on the estimates of fertility and mortality provided by the U.N. Population Division and on country statistical offices. In general, the estimates are generated from the last population census. When the World Bank does not provide this information, we used estimates from the Western Pacific Region Databank on Socioeconomic and Health indicators published by WHO. In general, WHO and World Bank numbers closely corroborate each other.

Abdussalam M and F Kaferstein. 1994. Food Safety in Primary Health Care. *World Health Forum*. 15(4): 393-399.

Abel-Smith B. 1994. *An Introduction to Health: Policy, Planning and Financing*. New York: Longman Group.

Abel-Smith B and E Mossialos. 1994. Cost Containment and Health Care Reform: A Study of the European Union. *Health Policy*. 28: 89-132.

Acton J. 1975. Nonmonetary Factors in the Demand for Medical Services: Some Empirical Evidence. *Journal of Political Economy*. 83(3): 595-614.

Adair L and B Popkin. 1993. Growth Dynamics During the First Two Years of Life: A Prospective Study in the Philippines. *European Journal of Clinical Nutrition*. 47: 42-51.

Aday LA and RM Andersen. 1974. A Framework for the Study of Access to Medical Care. *Health Services Research*. 9: 208-220.

Ainsworth M. 1983. The Demand for Health and Schooling in Mali: Results of Community and Service Provider Survey. In *Financing Health Services in Developing Countries, an Agenda for Reform*. World Bank. Washington, DC.

Aiyer S, D Jamison and J Londono. 1995. Health Policy in Latin America: Progress, Problems and Policy Options. *Cuadernos de Economia*. 32(95): 11-28.

Ajzen I and M Fishbein. 1980. *Understanding Attitudes and Predicting Social Behavior*. Englewood Cliffs, NJ: Prentice-Hall.

Akanov A. 1996. *Kazakhstan: Health Care System in Transition*. Final Meeting on Social Sector Issues in Asian Transition Economies. Asian Development Bank. Manila, Philippines.

Akin J, N Birdsall and D De Ferranti. 1987. *Financing Health Services in Developing Countries: an Agenda for Reform*. A World Bank Policy Study. World Bank.

Akin J, C Griffin, DK Guilkey, et al. 1985. *The Demand for Primary Health Services in the Third World*. Totowa, New Jersey: Rowman and Allenheld.

Akin J, DK Guilkey and EH Denton. 1993a. *Multinomial Probit Estimation of Health Care Demand: Ogun State, Nigeria*. Working Draft. University of North Carolina.

_____. 1993b. Quality of Services and Demand for Health Care in Nigeria: A Multinomial Probit Estimation. *Social Science and Medicine*. 40(11): 1527-1537.

Akram D and M Agboatwalla. 1992. A Model for Health Intervention. *Journal of Tropical Pediatrics*. 38: 85-87.

Al-Krenawi A, J Graham and B Maoz. 1996. The Healing Significance of the Negev's Bedouin Dervish. *Social Science and Medicine*. 43(1): 13-21.

Alderman H. 1991. Food Subsidies and the Poor. In G Psacharopoulos, ed. *Essays on Poverty, Equity, and Growth*. Oxford University Press.

_____. 1992. *Pakistan Integrated Household Survey, Final Results, 1991*. UNDP, World Bank. Washington, DC.

Alderman H and P Gertler. 1989. *The Substitutability of Public and Private Medical Care Providers in the Treatment of Children's Illnesses in Urban Pakistan*. LSMS Working Paper. 57. World Bank. Washington, DC.

Alderman H and J Lavy. 1996. Household Responses to Public Health Services: Cost and Quality Tradeoffs. *The World Bank Research Observer*. 11(1): 3-22.

Alexander JA, HS Zuckerman and DD Pointer. 1995. The Challenges of Governing Integrated Health Care Systems. *Health Care Management Review*. 20(4): 69-81.

Ali SW. 1996. Health Sector Reform and the Reasons for Public Investment in Health Care. *Health Sector Priorities Strategic Planning Workshop*. Manila: Asian Development Bank.

Aljunid S. 1995. The Role of Private Medical Practitioners and Their Interactions with Public Health Services in Asian Countries. *Health Policy and Planning*. 10(4): 333-349.

_____. 1996. Computer Analysis of Qualitative Data: The Use of Ethnograph. *Health Policy and Planning*. 11(1): 107-111.

Aljunid S and I Norhassim. 1992. Utilization of Health Facilities by the Malays of Kuala Selangor. *Journal of UKM Medical Faculty*. 14(1): 43-52.

Allen H. 1984. Consumers and Choice: Cost Containment Strategies for Health Care Provision. *Health Psychology*. 3(5): 411-430.

Allison T. 1996. Identification and Treatment of Psychosocial Risk Factors for Coronary Artery Disease. *Mayo Clinic Proceedings*. 71: 817-819.

Alonso P, S Lindsay, J Armstrong, et al. 1991. The Effect of Insecticide Treated Bed-Nets on Mortality of Gambian Children. *Lancet*. 337: 1499-1515.

Amlet R and HB Dull, eds. 1987. *Closing the Gap: The Burden of Unnecessary Illness*. New York: Oxford University Press.

Anand S and K Hanson. 1995. *Disability Adjusted Life Years: A Critical Review*. Working Paper Series. 95.06. Harvard Center for Population and Development Studies. Cambridge, MA.

Andersen R and J Newman. 1973. Societal and Individual Determinants of Medical Care Utilization. *Milbank Memorial Fund Quarterly.* 51: 95-124.

Andersen RM. 1968. *Behavioral Model of Families' Use of Health Services.* Research Series. 25. Center for Health Administration Studies.

_____. 1995. Revisiting the Behavioral Model and Access to Medical Care: Does It Matter? *Journal of Health and Social Behavior.* 36(March): 1-10.

Anderson IB, WH Mullen, JE Meeker, et al. 1996. Pennyroyal Toxicity: Measurement of Toxic Metabolite Levels in Two Cases and Review of the Literature. *Annals of Internal Medicine.* 124: 726-734.

Anderson PP, S Burger, JP Habicht, et al. 1993. Protein-energy Malnutrition. In DT Jamison, WH Mosley, et al., eds. *Disease Control Priorities in Developing Countries.* New York: Oxford University Press.

Appleton S and P Collier. 1996. On Gender Targeting of Public Transfers. In van de Walle D and Nead K (eds.). *Public Spending and the Poor.* Baltimore: Johns Hopkins University Press.

Arrow J. 1996. Estimating the Influence of Health as a Risk Factor on Unemployment: a Survival Analysis of Employment Durations for Workers Surveyed in the German Socio-economic Panel (1984-1990). *Social Science and Medicine.* 42(12): 1651-1659.

Arrow K. 1963. Uncertainty and the Welfare Economics of Medical Care. *American Economic Review.* 53: 941-973.

Asch S and JW Peabody. 1996. *Papua New Guinea. Institutional Plan for the College of Allied Health Services: The National Context and Training Responsibilities.* DRU-1376-ADB. RAND, Santa Monica, CA.

Asch S, E Sloss, R Kravitz, et al. 1995. Unpublished research on access to care for the elderly. RAND. Santa Monica, CA.

Ashworth A and R Feachem. 1985. Interventions for the Control of Diarrhoeal Diseases in Young Children: Weaning Education. *Bulletin of the World Health Organization.* 63: 1115-1127.

Asian Development Bank (ADB). 1991. *Health, Population and Development in Asia and the Pacific.* Manila, Philippines: Asian Development Bank.

_____. 1992. Regional Technical Assistance Project on Rural and Urban Poverty. Country Studies. *Asian Development Review.* 10(1): 1-164.

_____. 1994a. *Regional Cooperation for Development, Opportunities and Challenges.* ADB Theme Paper. 2. Asian Development Bank, Manila, Philippines.

_____. 1994b. *Population Policy: Framework for Assistance in the Population Sector.* Asian Development Bank, Manila, Philippines.

_____. 1994c. Regional Technical Assistance Project on Rural and Urban Poverty. Country Studies. *Asian Development Review*. 12(1): 1-204.

_____. 1995a. *Annual Report*. Asian Development Bank. Manila, Philippines.

_____. 1995b. *Asia: Development Experience and Agenda*. ADB Theme Paper. 3. Asian Development Bank. Manila.

_____. 1996a. *Basic Facts of Developing Member Countries of ADB*. Asian Development Bank. Manila, Philippines.

_____. 1996b. Kazakhstan: Health Care System in Transition. *Final Meeting on Social Sector Issues in Asian Transition Economies*. Manila, Philippines: Asian Development Bank.

Asthana S. 1995. Variations in Poverty and Health Between Slum Settlements: Contradictory Findings from Visakhapatnam, India. *Social Science and Medicine*. 40(2): 177-188.

_____. 1996. AIDS-Related Policies, Legislation and Programme Implementation in India. *Health Policy and Planning*. 11(2): 184-197.

Atkinson AB. 1996. On Targeting Social Security: Theory and Western Experience with Family Benefits. In van de Walle D and Nead K (eds.). *Public Spending and the Poor*. Baltimore: Johns Hopkins University Press.

Attah E and N Plange. 1993. *Quality of Health Care in Relation to Cost Recovery in Fiji: Focus Group Study Report*. Small Applied Research Paper. 6. Abt Associates, Inc. Bethesda, MD.

Avriel D, B Aronson and I Bertrand. 1993. Appropriate Information: New Products and Services. *World Health Forum*. 14(4): 410-417.

Awynski E and M Gallivan. 1992. *The Global Medical Device Market Report*. Washington, DC: Health Industry Manufacturers Association.

Azudova L. 1992. Health Service in the Network of Public Sector in the Period of Transition to Market Economy in the Slovak Republic. *Ekonomicky Casopis*. 40(6): 478-484.

Babunakis M. 1976. *Budgets: An Analytical and Procedural Handbook for Government and Nonprofit Organizations*. Westport, CT: Greenwood Press.

Bachmann M. 1994. Would National Health Insurance Improve Equity and Efficiency of Health Care in South Africa? Lessons from Asia and Latin America. *South African Medical Journal*. 84(3): 153-157.

Bailar JC and F Mosteller. eds. 1992. *Medical Uses of Statistics*. Boston, MA: NEJM Books.

Baker J and J van der Gaag. 1993. Equity in Health Care and Health care Financing: Evidence from Five Developing Countries. in E Van Doorslaer, Wagstaff, et al., eds. *Equity in the Finance and Delivery of Health Care.* New York: Oxford University Press.

Baldessarini R, B Cohen and M Teicher. 1990. Pharmacological Treatment. In S Levy and P Ninan, eds. *Schizophrenia Treatment.* New York: American Psychiatric Press.

Banerji D. 1992. Health Policies and Programmes in India in the Eighties. *Economic and Political Weekly.* 27(12): 599.

Bangladesh Health and Demographic Survey. 1995. *Morbidity, Health, Social and Household Environment Statistics.* Dhaka, Bangladesh: Bangladesh Bureau of Statistics and UNICEF.

Barbieri M. 1993. Seminar on Causes and Prevention of Adult Mortality in Developing Countries, Santiago, Chile, October 7-11, 1991. *Population.* 48(2): 512-515.

Barlow R and F Diop. 1995. Increasing the Utilization of Cost-Effective Health Services Through Changes in Demand. *Health Policy and Planning.* 10(3): 284-295.

Barlow R and L Grobar. 1985. *Costs and Benefits of Controlling Parasitic Diseases.* Washington, DC: World Bank Population, Health, and Nutrition Department.

Barns T. 1991. Obstetric Mortality and its Causes in Developing Countries. *British Journal of Obstetrics and Gynaecology.* 98(4): 345-348.

Barnum H. 1987. Evaluating Healthy Days of Life Gained from Health Projects. *Social Science Medicine.* 24(10): 833-841.

Barnum H and ER Greenberg. 1993. Cancers. In D Jamison, W Mosley, et al., eds. *Disease Control Priorities in Developing Countries.* New York: Oxford University Press.

Barnum H and J Kutzin. 1993. *Public Hospitals in Developing Countries: Resource Use, Cost, Financing.* Baltimore: Johns Hopkins University Press.

Barnum H, J Kutzin and H Saxenian. 1995. Incentives and Provider Payment Methods. *International Journal of Health Planning and Management.* 10: 23-45.

Barr D. 1996. The Current State of Health Care in the Former Soviet Union: Implications for Health Care Policy and Reform. *American Journal of Public Health.* 86(3): 307-312.

Barr N. 1992. Economic Theory and the Welfare State: A Survey and Interpretation. *Journal of Economic Literature.* 30: 741-803.

Barro RJ. 1997. *Determinants of Economic Growth: A Cross-Country Empirical Study.* Cambridge, MA: MIT Press.

Barrett B. 1994. Medicinal Plants on Nicaragua's Atlantic Coast. *Journal of Economic and Taxonomic Botany*. 48: 8.

_____. 1996. Integrated Local Health Systems in Central America. *Social Science and Medicine*. 43(1): 71-82.

Bartlett A, M Debocaletti and M Bocaletti. 1993. Reducing Perinatal Mortality in Developing Countries: High Risk or Improved Labour Management. *Health Policy and Planning*. 8(4): 360-368.

Basta SS, D Soekirman and NS Scrimshaw. 1979. Iron Deficiency Anemia and the Productivity of Adult Males in Indonesia. *American Journal of Clinical Nutrition*. 32: 916-925.

Baumol W. 1985. Productivity Policy in the Service Sector. In RP Inman, *Managing the Service Economy: Prospects and Problems*. Cambridge University Press.

Beaton G, R Martorell, KA L'Abbe, et al. 1993. *Effectiveness of Vitamin A Supplementation in the Control of Young Child Morbidity and Mortality in Developing Countries: A Project of the International Nutrition Program*. University of Toronto Department of Nutritional Sciences.

Beaton GH and H Ghassemi. 1982. Supplementary Feeding Programs for Young Children in Developing Countries. *The American Journal of Clinical Nutrition*. 35: 864-916.

Beck T. 1994. Managing Rural Development: Health and Energy Programmes in India. *Pacific Affairs*. 67(2): 299-300.

Becker G. 1965. A Theory of the Allocation of Time. *Economic Journal*. 75(299): 493-517.

_____. 1993. *Policy Options for Financing Health Services in Pakistan, Volume II Hospital Quality Assurance Through Standards and Accreditation*. Abt Associates, Inc. Bethesda, MD.

Beebe J. 1995. Basic Concepts and Techniques of Rapid Appraisal. *Human Organization*. 54(1): 42-51.

Begum S and A. Salahuddin. 1991. Study on Quality Assessment of Neonatal Tetanus Cases Admitted in the Infectious Diseases Hospital, Dhaka. *Academy of Hospital Administration*. 3:25-8.

Behrman JR. 1990. *The Action of Human Resources and Poverty on One Another: What We Have Yet to Learn*. Living Standards Measurement Study Working Paper. 74.

Behrman JR, R Sickles, P Taubman, et al. 1991. Black White Mortality Inequalities. *Journal of Econometrics*. 50(1-2): 183-203.

Behrman JR and BL Wolfe. 1989. Does More Schooling Make Women Better Nourished and Healthier? *The Journal of Human Resources*. 24(4): 644-663.

Beilin L, I Rouse, B Armstrong, et al. 1988. Vegetarian Diet and Blood Pressure Levels. *American Journal Clinical Nutrition.* 48: 806-810.

Bell M and R Franceys. 1995. Improving Human Welfare Through Appropriate Technology: Government Responsibility, Citizen Duty or Customer Choice? *Social Science and Medicine.* 40(9): 1169-1179.

Belmarino S. 1994. The Role of the State in Health Systems. *Social Science and Medicine.* 39(9): 1315-1321.

Benefo K, A Tsui and J Johnson. 1994. Ethnic Differentials in Child-Spacing Ideals and Practices in Ghana. *Journal of Biosocial Science.* 26:311-26.

Bengoa JM. 1974. Problem of Malnutrition. *WHO Chronicle.* 28(1): 3-7.

Bennett FJ. 1995. Qualitative and Quantitative Methods: In-Depth or Rapid Assessment? *Social Science and Medicine.* 40(12): 1589-1590.

Bennett S. 1992. Promoting the Private Sector: A Review of Developing Country Trends. *Health Policy and Planning.* 7(2): 97-110.

Bennett S, A Radalowicz, V Vella, et al. 1994a. A Computer Simulation of Household Sampling Schemes for Health Surveys in Developing Countries. *International Journal of Epidemiology.* 23(6): 1282-1291.

Bennett S, G Dakpallah and P Garner. 1994b. Carrot and Stick: State Mechanisms to Influence Private Provider Behaviour. *Health Policy and Planning.* 9(1): 1-13.

Bennett S and V Tangcharoensathien. 1994. A Shrinking State? Politics, Economics and Private Health Care in Thailand. *Public Administration and Development.* 14: 1-17.

Beracochea E, R Dickson, P Freeman, et al. 1995. Case Management Quality Assessment in Rural Areas of Papua New Guinea. *Tropical Doctor.* 25(2): 69-74.

Berg C. 1995. Prenatal Care in Developing Countries: The World Health Organization Technical Working Group on Antenatal Care. *Journal of the American Medical Women's Association.* 50(5): 182-186.

Berkelman R and J Buehler. 1990. Public Health Surveillance of Non-Infectious Chronic Diseases: The Potential to Detect Rapid Changes in Disease Burden. *International Journal of Epidemiology.* 19(3): 628-635.

Berman P. 1997. National Health Accounts in Developing Countries: Appropriate Methods and Recent Applications. *Health Economics.* 6(1):11-30.

Berman P and A Bir. 1995. Health Sector Reform in Developing Countries: Making Health Development Sustainable, Introduction. *Health Policy.* 32(1-3): 3-11.

Berman P and RR Eliya. 1993. *Factors Affecting the Development of Private Health Care Provision in Developing Countries.* HFS USAID.

Berman P and L Rose. 1996. The Role of Private Providers in Maternal and Child Health and Family Planning Services in Developing Countries. *Health Policy and Planning*. 11(2): 142-155.

Berman P, Brotowasisto, M Nadjib, et al. 1989. The Costs of Public Primary Health Care Services in Rural Indonesia. *Bulletin of the World Health Organization*. 67(6): 685-694.

Berman P, C Kendall and K Bhattacharyya, eds. 1989. The Household Production of Health: Putting People at the Center of Health Improvement. In *Towards More Efficacy in Child Survival Strategies: Understanding the Social and Private Constraints and Responsibilities*. Baltimore: Johns Hopkins University School of Hygiene and Public Health.

Berman P, D Sisler and J Habicht. 1989. Equity in Public-Sector Primary Health Care: The Role of Service Organizations in Indonesia. *Economic Development and Cultural Change*. 37(4): 777-803.

Bernstein J and J Shuval. 1994. Emigrant Physicians Evaluate the Health Care System of the Former Soviet Union. *Medical Care*. 32(2): 141-149.

Bertrand W. 1988. Information as a Primary Health Care Intervention: The Impact of New Technology on Improving Health for All. In BE RG Wilson JH Bryant, A Abrantes, eds. *Management Information Systems and Microcomputers in Primary Health Care*. Geneva: Aga Khan Foundation.

Berwick DM. 1996. Payment by Capitation and the Quality of Care. *New England Journal of Medicine*. 335(16): 1227-1230.

Besley T. 1996. *Political Economy of Targeting: Theory and Experience*. Annual Bank Conference on Development Economics. World Bank. Washington, DC.

Besley T and S Coate. 1991. Public Provision of Private Goods and the Redistribution of Income. *American Economic Review*. 81(4): 979-984.

Besley T and M Gouveia. 1994. Alternative Systems of Health Care Provision. *Economic Policy*. 201-258.

Besley T and R Kanbur. 1990. *The Principals of Targeting*. Policy, Research and External Affairs Working Paper Series. 385. The World Bank Research Administrator's Office. Washington, DC.

_____. 1993. The Principles of Targeting. In M Lipton and J van der Gaag, eds. *Including the Poor*. Washington, DC: World Bank.

Bhan M, NK Arora, OP Ghai, et al. 1986. Major Factors in Diarrhoea Related Mortality Among Rural Children. *Indian Journal of Medical Research*. 83: 9-12.

Bhargava A and J Yu. 1992. *A Longitudinal Analysis of Infant and Child Mortality Rate in Africa and Non-African Developing Countries*. Background Paper. World Bank, Africa Technical Department. Washington, DC.

Bhat R. 1993. The Private Public Mix in Health Care in India. *Health Policy and Planning*. 8(2): 189-189.

Bhatia JC and J Cleland. 1995. Determinants of Maternal Care in a Region of South India. *Health Transition Review*. 5: 127-142.

Birdsall N. 1989. Thoughts on Good Health and Good Government. *Daedalus*. 188: 23.

_____. 1993. Pragmatism, Robin Hood, and Other Themes: Good Government and Social Well-Being in Developing Countries. In LC Chen, A Kleinman, et al., eds. *Health and Social Science in International Perspective*. Cambridge: Harvard University Press.

Birdsall N and R Hecht. 1995. *Swimming Against the Tide: Strategies for Improving Equity in Health*. Draft manuscript.

Birdsall N and E James. 1993. Efficiency and Equity in Social Spending: How and Why Governments Misbehave. In M Lipton and J van der Gaag, eds. *Including the Poor*. Washington, DC: The World Bank.

Birdsall N, D Ross and R Sabot. 1995. Inequality and Growth Reconsidered: Lessons from East Asia. *World Bank Economic Review*. 9(3): 477-508.

Biro Pusat Statistik-Republik Indonesia (BPS). 1992. *SUSENAS, PODES*. Central Bureau of Statistic, Republic of Indonesia. Jakarta, Indonesia.

_____. 1994. *SUSENAS, PODES*. Central Bureau of Statistic, Republic of Indonesia. Jakarta, Indonesia.

Bitran R. 1994. *A Supply-Demand Model of Health Care Financing with an Application to Zaire*. EDI Technical Materials. World Bank. Washington, DC.

Bitran R and DK McInnes. 1993. *The Demand for Health Care in Latin America: Lessons from the Dominican Republic and El Salvador*. Economic Development Institute Seminar Paper No. 46. Washington, DC: The World Bank.

Bjorkman J. 1991. The Politics of Health in India. *Journal of Health Politics Policy and the Law*. 16(3): 616-620.

Black R. 1991. Would Control of Childhood Infectious Diseases Reduce Malnutrition? *Acta Pediatrica Scandinavia*. 374(Supplement): 133-140.

Blendon R and R Leitman. 1992. Satisfaction with Health Systems in 10 Nations. *Health Affairs*. 9(2): 185-192.

Bloom G. 1989. The Right Equipment...In Working Order. *World Health Forum*. 10: 3-27.

Blum A and P Fargues. 1990. Rapid Estimations of Maternal Mortality in Countries with Defective Data: an Application to Bamako (1974-85) and Other Developing Countries. *Population Studies*. 44(1): 155-171.

Blum D and RG Feachem. 1983. Measuring the Impact of Water Supply and Sanitation Investments on Diarrhoeal Diseases: Problems of Methodology. *International Journal of Epidemiology*. 12(3): 357-365.

Blumenfeld SN. 1993. Quality Assurance in Transition. *Papua New Guinea Medical Journal*. 36(2): 81-89.

Bobadilla JL, P Cowley, P Musgrove, et al. 1994. Design, Content, and Financing of an Essential National Package of Health Services. *Bulletin of the World Health Organization*. 72(4): 653-662.

Boerma J, AE Sommerfelt, SO Rutstein, et al. 1990. *Immunization: Levels, Trends and Differentials*. Demographic and Health Surveys Comparative Studies No. 1. Columbia, MD: Institute for Resource Development/Macro Systems, Inc.

Bogg L, H Dong, K Wang, W Cai and D Vinod. 1996. The Cost of Coverage: Rural Health Insurance in China. *Health Policy and Planning*. 11:238-52.

Bongaarts J. 1987. Does Family Planning Reduce Infant Mortality? *Population and Development Review*. 13: 323-324.

_____. 1988. Does Family Planning Reduce Infant Mortality? Reply. *Population and Development Review*. 14: 188-190.

Booth P. 1992. Changing Provider Behavior—The New PRO Scope of Work. *Journal of Ahima*. 63(12): 11-12.

Bossert T. 1995. Decentralization. In K Janovsky, ed. *Health Policy and Systems Development*. Geneva: World Health Organization.

Bossert T, R Soebekti and N Rai. 1991. Bottom-Up Planning in Indonesia: Decentralization in the Ministry of Health. *Health Policy and Planning*. 6(1): 55-63.

Bovet P. 1995. The Epidemiologic Transition to Chronic Diseases in Developing Countries: Cardiovascular Mortality, Morbidity, and Risk Factors in Seychelles (Indian Ocean). *Sozial-und Praventivmedizin*. 40(1): 35-43.

Brauer AP, L Horlick, E Nelson, et al. 1979. Relaxation Therapy for Essential Hypertension. *Journal of Behavioral Medicine*. 2: 21-29.

Breyer F. 1995. The Political Economy of Rationing in Social Health Insurance. *Journal of Population Economics*. 8(2): 137-148.

Brieger WR, SA Adekunle and GA Oke. 1996. Culturally Perceived Illness and Guinea Worm Disease Surveillance. *Health Policy and Planning*. 11(1): 101-106.

Briend A, B Wojtyniak and M Rowland. 1988. Breastfeeding, Nutritional State and Child Survival in Rural Bangladesh. *British Medical Journal*. 296: 879-882.

Briscoe J. 1984. Water and Health: Selective Primary Health Care Revisited. *American Journal of Public Health*. 74: 1009-1013.

Briscoe J, JS Akin and DK Guilkey. 1990. People are Not Passive Acceptors of Threats to Health-Endogeneity and its Consequences. *International Journal of Epidemiology*. 19(1): 147-153.

Bronzino JD. 1992. *Management of Medical Technology: A Primer for Clinical Engineers*. Stoneham, MA: Butterworth.

Brook R and F Appel. 1973. Quality of Care Assessment: Choosing a Method for Peer Review. *New England Journal of Medicine*. 288: 1323-1329.

Brook R, C Kamberg and E McGlynn. 1996. Health System Reform and Quality. *Journal of the American Medical Association*. 276(6): 476-480.

Broomberg J. 1994. Managing the Health Market in Developing Countries: Prospects and Problems. *Health Policy and Planning*. 9(3): 237-251.

Broomberg J, C Debeer and M Price. 1990. The Private Health Sector in South Africa: Current Trends and Future Developments. *South African Medical Journal*. 78(3): 139-142.

Brotowasisto GO, R Malik and P Sudharto. 1988. Health Care Financing in Indonesia. *Health Policy and Planning*. 3(2): 131-140.

Brown RS, DG Clement, JW Hill, et al. 1993. Do Health Maintenance Organizations Work for Medicare? *Health Care Financing Review*. 15(1): 7-23.

Brown T, W Sittitrai, S Vanichseni and U Thisyakorn. 1994. The Recent Epidemiology of HIV and AIDS in Thailand. *AIDS*. 9(Supplement 2):S131-41.

Brundtland G, M Khalid, S Agnelli, et al. 1987. From One Earth to One World, An Overview by the World Commission on Environment and Development. In *Our Common Future*. Oxford University Press.

Bryant J, D Marsh, K Khan, et al. 1993. A Developing Country's University Oriented Toward Strengthening Health Systems: Challenges and Results. *American Journal of Public Health*. 83(11): 1537-1543.

Buekens P, M Boutsen, F Kittel, et al. 1993. Does Awareness of Rates of Obstetric Interventions Change Practice? *British Medical Journal*. 306(6 March 1993): 623.

Bulatao RA, E Bos, PW Stephens, et al. 1990. *World Population Projections, 1989-90 Edition: Short- and Long-Term Estimates*. Baltimore, MD: World Bank, Johns Hopkins University Press.

Bumgarner J and E Richard. 1992. *China: Long-Term Issues and Options in the Health Transition*. Washington, DC: World Bank.

Bundy DA, MS Wong, LL Lewis, et al. 1989. Control of Gastro-Intestinal Helminths by Age-Group Targeted Chemotherapy Delivered Through Schools. *Transactions of the Royal Society of Tropical Medicine and Hygiene*. 8: 115-120.

Burr M and BB BK. 1988. Heart Disease in British Vegetarians. *American Journal Clinical Nutrition*. 48: 830-833.

Buxton M and S Hanney. 1996. How Can Payback from Health Services Research Be Assessed? *Journal of Health Services and Resource Policy*. 1(1): 35-43.

Byass P. 1992. The Impact of Portable Technology on Health in Developing Countries: Recent Progress and Future Potential. In KC Lun, P Degoulet, et al., eds. *MEDINFO 92*. Amsterdam: North-Holland Elsevier.

Caiden N. 1980. Budgeting in Poor Countries: Ten Common Assumptions Re-examined. *Public Administration Review*. (January/February): 40-46.

Caldwell JC. 1986. Routes to Low Mortality in Poor Countries. *Population and Development Review*. 12(2): 171-220.

_____. 1990. Cultural and Social Factors Influencing Mortality Levels in Developing Countries. *Annals of the American Academy of Political and Social Science*. 510(July): 44-59.

_____. 1993. Health Transition: The Cultural, Social, and Behavioural Determinants of Health in the Third World. *Social Science and Medicine*. 36(2): 125-135.

Caldwell JC, S Findley, P Caldwell, et al. eds. 1989. *What We Know About Health Transition: The Cultural, Social and Behavioural Determinants of Health, Vol. 2*. Canberra, Australia: Health Transition Center, Australian National University.

Campion E. 1993. Why Unconventional Medicine? *New England Journal of Medicine*. 328(4): 282-283.

Campos-Outcalt D. 1991. Microcomputers and Health Information in Papua New Guinea: A Two Year Follow-Up Evaluation. *Health Policy and Planning*. 6(4): 348-353.

Campos-Outcalt D, K Kewa, and J Thomason. 1995. Decentralization of Health Services in Western Highlands Province, Papua New Guinea: An Attempt to Administer Health Service at the Subdistrict Level. *Social Science and Medicine*. 40(8): 1091-1098.

Carey J, M Oxtoby, L Nguyen, et al. 1997. Tuberculosis Beliefs Among Recent Vietnamese Refugees in New York State. *Public Health Rep*. 112(1): 66-72.

Carlos T, O Solon and PJ Gertler. May 1996. Estimating the Welfare Effects of Insurance Coverage. Paper presented at the Inaugural Conference of the International Health Economics Association. Vancouver, Canada.

Carnoy M, J Samoff, M Burris, et al. 1990. *Education and Social Transition in the Third World*. Princeton: Princeton University Press.

Carr-Hill RA. 1996. *From Health-for-Some to Health-for-All*. WHO Document. WHO/SHS/96.2. Geneva: World Health Organization.

Carter G. 1995. *Trip Report, Kyrgyz Republic*. Zdrav Reform Project. Abt Associates, Inc.

Carter G and J Rogowski. 1992. How Pricing Policies, Coding, and Recalibration Method Affect DRG Weights. *Health Care Financing Review*. 14(2): 83-96.

Carter WB, T Inui, W Kukull, et al. 1982. Outcome-based Doctor-Patient Interaction Analysis: II. Identifying Effective Provider and Patient Behavior. *Medical Care*. 20(6): 550-566.

Carter WB, TC Gayle and S Baker. 1990. Behavioral Intervention and the Individual. in K Holmes, P Mardh, et al., eds. *Sexually Transmitted Diseases, 2nd Edition*. New York: McGraw-Hill.

Cashier P and B Salary. 1995. Regional Economic Growth and Convergence in India. IMF Working Paper 95/58. Internal Migration Center—State Grants and Economic Growth in the States of India. Washington, D.C.

Cassels A. 1995. *Health Sector Reform Key Issues in Developed Countries*. WHO Document. WHO/SHS/NHP/95.4 Unpublished. World Health Organization. Geneva.

Cassels A and K Janovsky. 1991. Management Development for Primary Health Care: A Framework for Analysis. *International Journal of Health Planning and Management*. 6: 109-124.

Castro E and K Mokate. 1988. Malaria and Its Socioeconomic Meaning: The Study of Cunday in Colombia. In AN Herrin and PL Rosenfield, eds. *Economics, Health, and Tropical Diseases*. Manila: University of the Philippines School of Economics.

Cates W Jr and AR Hinman. 1992. AIDS and Absolutism—The Demand for Perfection in Prevention. *New England Journal of Medicine*. 327(7):492-4.

Central Bureau of Statistics (CBS) and State Ministry of Population/National Family Planning Coordinating Board and Ministry of Health and Macro International (MI). 1995. *Indonesia Demographic and Health Survey*. CBS and MI. Calverton, MD.

Chae YM, SI Kim, BH Lee, et al. 1994. Implementing Health Management Information Systems: Measuring Success in Korea's Health Centers. *International Journal of Health Planning and Management*. 9: 341-348.

Chalker J. 1995. Effect of a Drug Supply and Cost Sharing System on Prescribing and Utilization: A Controlled Trial from Nepal. *Health Policy and Planning*. 10(4): 423-430.

Chalmers I, K Dickersin and T Chalmers. 1992. Getting to Grips with Archie Cochrane's Agenda. *British Medical Journal*. 305(3): 786-788.

Chase E and R Carr-Hill. 1994. The Dangers of Managerial Perversion: Quality Assurance in Primary Health Care. *Health Policy and Planning*. 9(3): 267-278.

Chayovan N, P Kamnuansilpa and J Knodel. 1988. *Thailand Demographic and Health Survey 1987*. Institute of Population Studies, Chulalongkorn University and Institute for Resource Development/Westinghouse. Bangkok, Thailand.

Chen L, A Chowdhury and S Huffman. 1980. Anthropometric Assessment of Energy Protein Malnutrition and Subsequent Risk of Mortality Among Pre-school Aged Children. *American Journal of Clinical Nutrition*. 33: 1836-1845.

Chen L, A Hill, C Murray, et al. 1993. A Critical Analysis of the Design, Results and Implications of the Mortality and Use of Health Services Surveys. *International Journal of Epidemiology*. 22(5): s73-s80.

Chen L, A Kleinman and J Caldwell. eds. 1992. *Health and Social Change*. Westport, Conn.: Auburn House.

Cheng S and T Chiang. 1996. *The Impact of a Universal Health Insurance on Medical Care Utilization in Taiwan: Results from a Natural Experiment*. Draft. Graduate Institute of Public Health and Center for Health Policy Research National Taiwan University.

Chernichovsky D. 1991. Microcomputers and Health Information in Papua New Guinea: A Two Year Follow-up Evaluation. *Health Policy and Planning*. 6(4): 348-353.

_____. 1995a. Health Systems Reforms in Industrialized Democracies: An Emerging Paradigm. *The Milbank Quarterly*. 73(3): 339-371.

_____. 1995b. What Can Developing Countries Learn from Health System Reforms of Developed Countries? *Health Policy*. 32: 79-91.

Chetwynd J. 1993. Integration of Research and Decision Making: A Way to Enhance Communication [Abstract]. *Abstracts of the International Society of Technological Assessment in Health Care*. 9: 30.

Chi C. 1994. Integrating Traditional Medicine into Modern Health Care Systems: Examining the Role of Chinese Medicine in Taiwan. *Social Science and Medicine*. 39: 307.

Ching P. 1995. User Fees, Demand for Children's Health Care, and Access Across Income Groups: The Philippine Case. *Social Science and Medicine*. 41(1): 37-46.

Chinitz D. 1994. Reforming the Israeli Health Care Market. *Social Science and Medicine*. 39(10): 1447-1457.

Chu D. 1992. Global Budgeting of Hospitals in Hong Kong. *Social Science and Medicine*. 35(7): 857-868.

Chunming C. 1992. Disease Surveillance in China. *Morbidity and Mortality Weekly Report*. 41(Supplement): 111-122.

Cibulskis R and J Izard. 1996. Monitoring Systems. In K Janovsky, ed. *Health Policy and Systems Development: An Agenda for Research*. Geneva: World Health Organization.

Cichon M and C Gillion. 1993. The Financing of Health Care in Developing Countries. *International Labour Review.* 132(2): 173-186.

Cipolla CM. 1978. *The Economic History of World Population.* New York: Barnes and Noble.

Clancy C and D Kamerow. 1996. Evidence-Based Medicine Meets Cost-Effectiveness Analysis. *Journal of the American Medical Association.* 276(4): 329-330.

Clark R, R Dorwart and S Epstein. 1994. Managing Competition in Public and Private Mental Health Agencies: Implications for Services and Policy. *Milbank Quarterly.* 72(4): 653-678.

Cleland J and JV Ginneken. 1988. Maternal Education and Child Survival in Developing Countries: The Search for Pathways of Influence. *Social Science and Medicine.* 27(12): 1357-1368.

Cleland J, JF Phillips, S Amin, et al. 1994. *The Determinants of Reproductive Change in Bangladesh: A Success in a Challenging Environment.* Washington, DC: World Bank.

Clemens JD, B Stanton, B Stoll, et al. 1986. Breastfeeding as a Determinant of Severity of Shigellosis. *American Journal of Epidemiology.* 123: 710-720.

Clemens JD, BF Stanton, J Chakraborty, et al. 1988. Measles Vaccination and Childhood Mortality in Rural Bangladesh. *American Journal of Epidemiology.* 128: 1330-1339.

Cliff J. 1993. Donor Dependence or Donor Control? The Case of Mozambique. *Community Development Journal.* 28: 237-244.

Clough J. 1996. Can Medicine Serve Both Humanity and the Bottom Line? *Cleveland Journal of Medicine.* 63(5): 257-258.

Coates TJ and RJ Greenblatt. 1990. Behavioral Change Using Interventions at the Community Level. in K Holmes, P Mardh, et al., eds. *Sexually Transmitted Diseases, 2nd Edition.* New York: McGraw-Hill.

Cochrane Collaboration Informatics Methods Group and the Health Information Research Unit. 1996. *The Cochrane Collaboration Internet Homepage.* http://hiru.mcmaster.ca/cochrane/default.htm/. Hamilton, Ontario: McMaster University.

Cochrane S and DK Guilkey. 1995. The Effects of Fertility Intentions and Access to Services on Contraceptive Use in Tunisia. *Economic Development and Cultural Change.* 43(4): 779-804.

Cochrane S, J Hammer, B Janowitz, et al. 1990. *The Economics of Family Planning.* Population, Health, and Nutrition Division. Washington, DC: World Bank.

Cochrane S and F Sai. 1993. Excess Fertility. In D Jamison, W Mosley, et al., eds. *Disease Control Priorities in Developing Countries.* Oxford University Press.

Cockerham WC. 1990. A Test of the Relationship Between Race, Socioeconomic Status, and Psychological Distress. *Social Science and Medicine*. 31(12):1321-6.

Collins CD. 1994. *Management and Organization of Developing Health Systems*. Oxford: Oxford University Press.

_____. 1995. Decentralization. In K Janovsky, ed. *Health Policy and Systems Development: An Agenda for* Research. Geneva: World Health Organization.

Collins CD and C Barker. 1995. Health Management and Action Research: Bringing Them Together for the District Medical Officer. *Tropical Doctor*. 25(2): 75-79.

Collins CD, AT Green and DJ Hunter. 1994. International Transfers of National Health Service Reforms: Problems and Issues. *Lancet*. 344(8917): 248-250.

Comey XC, CG Barrios and XR Guerrero. 1996. Traditional Birth Attendants in Mexico: Advantages and Inadequacies of Care for Normal Deliveries. *Social Science and Medicine*. 43(2): 199-207.

Conly G. 1975. The Impact of Malaria on Economic Development: A Case Study. *Scientific Publication*. 297.

Conn CP, P Jenkins and SO Touray. 1996. Strengthening Health Management: Experience of Disctict Teams in the Gambia. *Health Policy and Planning*. 11(1): 64-71.

Cooper R and RS Kaplan. 1988. Measure Costs Right: Make the Right Decisions. *Harvard Business Review*. September-October: 96-103.

Cornia G, R Jolly and F Stewart. eds. 1987. *Adjustment with a Human Face*. Oxford: Oxford University Press.

Coulam RF and GL Gaumer. 1991. Medicare's Prospective Payment System: A Critical Appraisal. *Health Care Financing Review*. Annual Supplement: 45-77.

Cowley P and RJ Wyatt. 1993. Schizophrenia and Manic-depressive Illness. In DT Jamison, WH Mosley, et al., eds. *Disease Control Priorities in Developing Countries*. New York: Oxford University Press.

Cox C and K Roghmann. 1984. Empirical Test of the Interaction Model of Client Health Behavior. *Research in Nursing and Health*. 7(4): 275-285.

Cox C, J Sullivan and K Roghmann. 1983. A Conceptual Explanation of Risk-Reduction Behavior and Intervention Development. *Nursing Research*. 33(3): 168-173.

Creese A and J Kutzin. 1995. *Lessons from Cost-Recovery in Health*. Discussion Paper. WHO/SHS/NHP/95.5. World Health Organization. Geneva.

Cretin S, N Duan, A Williams, et al. 1990. Modeling the Effect of Insurance on Health Expenditures in the People's Republic of China. *Health Services Research*. 24(4): 667-685.

Cretin S, J Sine, M Klein, et al. 1995. *Transforming Health Systems in the Developing World: Barriers to Change*. The Rockefeller Foundation.

Cretin S, JJ Sine and AP Williams. 1997. Unpublished RAND research on the effects of coinsurance on health care expenditures in rural China: results of an experiment.

Culyer A. 1995. Need: The Idea Won't Do—But We Still Need It. *Social Science and Medicine*. 40(6): 727-730.

Curtale F, B Siwakoti and C Lagrosa. 1995. Improving Skills and Utilization of Community Health Volunteers in Nepal. *Social Science and Medicine*. 40(8): 1117-1125.

Cutler DM. 1996. *Public Policy for Health Care*. National Bureau of Economic Research Working Paper Series. 5591. Cambridge, MA: National Bureau of Economic Research.

Datt G and D Gunewardena. 1994. *Some Aspects of Poverty in Sri Lanka: 1985-90*. Washington, DC: World Bank;

Datt G and M Ravallion. 1993. Regional Disparities, Targeting, and Poverty in India. In M Lipton and J van der Gaag, eds. *Including the Poor*. Washington, DC: World Bank.

DaVanzo J and WP Butz. 1978. *Influences on Fertility and Infant Mortality in Developing Countries: The Case of Malaysia*. N-1166-AID. RAND. Santa Monica, CA.

Dave P. 1991. Community and Self-Financing in Voluntary Health Programmes in India. *Health Policy and Planning*. 6(1): 20-31.

Davidow S. 1996. Observations on Health Care Issues in the Former Soviet Union. *Journal of Community Health*. 21(1): 51-60.

Davies HM, A Hashim and E Talero. 1993. *Information Systems Strategies for Public Financial Management*. Discussion Paper. 193. World Bank. Washington, DC.

Davis D, M Thomson, A Oxman and R Haynes. 1995. Changing Physician Performance: A Systematic Review of the Effect of Continuing Medical Education Strategies. *Journal of the American Medical Association*. 274:700-705.

Davis DA, MA Thomson, AD Oxman, et al. 1992. Evidence for the Effectiveness of CME, A Review of 50 Randomized Controlled Trials. *Journal of the American Medical Association*. 268(9): 1111-1117.

Davis P and P Howden-Chapman. 1996. Translating Research Findings into Health Policy. *Social Science and Medicine*. 43(5): 865-872.

Dawson L, L Manderson and V Tallo. 1993. *A Manual for the Use of Focus Groups*. Boston: International Nutrition Foundation for Developing Countries.

de Ferranti D. 1985. *Paying for Health Services in Developing Countries: An Overview.* World Bank Staff Working Papers. 721. World Bank.

De Geyndt WD. 1991. *Managing Health Expenditures Under National Health Insurance: The Case of Korea.* Technical Paper. 156. World Bank. Washington, DC.

_____. 1992. *Staff Appraisal Report on the Republic of Korea Public Hospital Modernization Project.* World Bank. Washington, DC.

de Kadt E. 1989. Making Health Policy Management Intersectoral: Issues of Information Analysis and Use in Less Developed Countries. *Social Science and Medicine.* 29(4): 503-514.

Dean AG and JA Dean. 1991. Epi Info: A General-Purpose Microcomputer Program for Public Health Information Systems. *American Journal of Preventive Medicine.* 7(3): 178-182.

Dean PN. 1989. *Government Budgeting in Developing Countries.* New York: Rutledge.

Deaton A. 1994. Looking for Boy-Girl Discrimination in Household Expenditure Data. *World Bank Economic Review.* 3(1): 1-15.

Deaton A and C Paxson. 1994. Intertemporal Choice and Inequality. *Journal of Political Economy.* 102(2): 437-467.

DeGraff DS, JF Phillips, R Simmons, et al. 1986. Integrating Health Services into an MCH-FP Program in Matlab, Bangladesh: An Analytical Update. *Studies in Family Planning.* 17(5): 228-234.

DeJonghe E, C Murray, HG Chum, et al. 1994. Cost Effectiveness of Chemotherapy for Sputum Smear Positive Pulmonary Tuberculosis in Malawi, Mozambique, and Tanzania. *International Journal of Health Planning and Management.* 9(2):151-181.

Demographic and Health Surveys (DHS), http://www2.macroint.com/dhs.

Deolalikar AB. 1992. Does the Impact of Government Health Expenditures on the Utilization of Health Services and Health Outcomes of Individuals Differ Across Expenditure Classes? *World Bank Conference on Public Expenditures and the Poor: Incidence and Targeting.* World Bank.

Department of Census and Statistics (DCS) [Sri Lanka] and Institute for Resource Development/Westinghouse (IRD). 1988. *Sri Lanka Demographic and Health Survey 1987.* DCS. Colombo, Sri Lanka.

Department of Health. 1994. *Health and Vital Statistics I and II, 1993.* 62-84. Department of Health, Republic of China, The Executive Yuan. Taipei, Taiwan.

Dial T, S Palsbo, C Bergsten, et al. 1995. Clinical Staffing in Staff- and Group-Model HMOs. *Health Affairs.* Summer 1995. 168-180.

Diallo I, R Molouba and LC Sarr. 1993. Primary Health Care: From Aspiration to Achievement. *World Health Forum.* 14(4): 349-355.

Diop F and C Leighton. 1995. *Cost-effectiveness Analysis of Safe Motherhood Services in South Kalimantan, Indonesia.* Technical Note. 36. Abt Associates, Inc. Bethesda, MD.

Dixon J and C Sindall. 1994. Applying Logics of Change to the Evaluation of Community Development in Health Promotion. *Health Promotion International.* 9(4): 297-309.

Domar A, P Zuttermister and M Seibel. 1992. Psychological Improvement in Infertile Women after Behavioral Treatment. *Fertility and Sterility.* : 144-147.

Donabedian A. 1973. *Aspects of Medical Care Administration: Specifying Requirements for Health Care.* Cambridge, MA: Harvard University Press.

_____. 1980. *The Definition of Quality and Approaches to Its Assessment, Explorations in Quality Assessment and Monitoring.* Ann Arbor, MI: Health Administration Press

Donaldson C and K Gerard. 1989. Countering Moral Hazards in Public and Private Health Care Systems: A Review of Recent Evidence. *Journal of Social Policy.* 18(April): 234-251.

Dor A, P Gertler and J van der Gaag. 1987. Non-Price Rationing and the Choice of Medical Care Providers in Rural Cote d'Ivoire. *Journal of Health Economics.* 6: 291-304.

Douglas R. 1990. Acute Respiratory Infections: History, Medicine, and Behaviour. In J Caldwell, S Findley, et al., eds. *What We Know About Health Transition.* Australian National University Printing Service.

Dow WH, P Gertler, RF Schoeni, et al. 1997. *Health Care Prices, Health and Labor Outcomes: Experimental Evidence.* Labor and Population Working Paper Series. DRU 1588-NIA. RAND. Santa Monica, CA.

Dranove D and W White. 1987. Agency and the Organization of Health Care Delivery. *Inquiry.* 24(4): 405-415.

Dubois R. 1996. Reducing Costs: The Case for Disease Management. *Clinical Performance and Quality Health Care.* 4(4): 226-7.

Dundee J, W Chestnutt, R Ghaly, et al. 1986. Traditional Chinese Acupuncture: A Potentially Useful Antiemetic? *British Medical Journal.* 293: 583-584.

Duran-Arenas L, MB Asfura and JF Mora. 1992. The Role of Doctors as Health Care Managers: An International Perspective. *Social Science and Medicine.* 35(4): 549-555.

Durkin M, S Islam, Z Hasan, et al. 1994. Measures of Socioeconomic Status for Child Health Research: Comparative Results From Bangldesh and Pakistan. *Social Science and Medicine.* 38(9): 1289-1297.

Eastman SJ. 1987. *Vitamin A: Deficiency and Xeropthalmia: Recent Findings and Some Programme Implications.* New York: UNICEF.

Edwards SD. 1986. Traditional and Modern Medicine in South Africa: A Research Study. *Social Science and Medicine.* 22: 1273.

Eisenberg D, T Delbanco and C Berkey. 1993. Cognitive Behavioral Techniques for Hypertension: Are They Effective? *Annals of Internal Medicine.* 118: 964-972.

Eisenberg DM, RC Kessler and C Foster. 1993. Unconventional Medicine in the U.S. *New England Journal of Medicine.* 328: 246-252.

Eklund P and K Stavem. 1994. Community Health Insurance Through Prepayment Schemes in Guinea-Bissau. In P Shaw and M Ainsworth, eds. *Financing Health Services Through User Fees and Insurance: Lessons from Sub-Saharan Africa.* New York: World Bank.

El-Kholy A and S Mandil. 1984. The Relevance of Microcomputers to Health Improvement in Developing Countries. *Information & Management.* 8: 177-182.

el-Rafie M, W Hassouna, N Hirschhorn, et al. 1990. Effects of Diarrhoeal Disease Control on Infant and Childhood Mortality in Egypt. *Report from the National Control of Diarrhoeal Diseases Project.* 335(8690): 334-338.

Ellis R. 1987. The Revenue Generating Potential of User Fees in Kenyan Government Health Facilities. *Social Science and Medicine.* 25(9): 995-1002.

Ellis R and T McGuire. 1986. Provider Behavior Under Prospective Reimbursement. Cost Sharing and Supply. *Journal of Health Economics.* 5(2): 129-151.

Ellis R and T McGuire. 1993. Supply-Side and Demand-Side Cost Sharing in Health Care. *Journal of Economic Perspectives.* 7(4): 135-152.

Ellis R, G Pope, L Iezzoni, et al. 1996. Diagnosis-Based Risk Adjustment for Medicare Capitation Payments. *Health Care Financing Review.* 17(3): 101-128.

Ellwein LB, JM Lepkowski, RD Thulasiraj, et al. 1991. The Cost Effectiveness of Strategies to Reduce Barriers to Cataract Surgery. *International Ophthalmology.* 15(3): 175-183.

Elo IT. 1992. Utilization of Maternal Health-Care Services in Peru: The Role of Women's Education. *Health Transition Review.* 2(1): 49-69.

Elum D and R Feechum. 1983. Measuring the Impact of Water Supply and Sanitation on Diarrhoeal Diseases: Problems of Methodology. *International Journal of Epidemiology.* 12: 357-365.

Emerson JD and GA Colditz. 1992. Use of Statistical Analysis in the *New England Journal of Medicine.* In JC Bailar and F Mosteller, eds. *Medical Uses of Statistics.* Boston, MA: NEJM Books.

Engle P, P Menon and L Haddad. 1996. *Care and Nutrition: Concepts and Measurement.* FCND Discussion Paper. 18. International Food Policy Research Institute.

Ensor T. 1995. Introducing Health Insurance In Vietnam. *Health Policy and Planning*. 10(2): 154-163.

Enthoven AC. 1993. The History and Principles of Managed Competition. *Health Affairs*. Supplement 1993. 24-48.

Ernster V. 1994. The Impact of Social Factors on Disease. In *Harrison's Principles of Internal Medicine, Part One- Introduction to Clinical Medicine*. New York: McGraw-Hill, Inc.

Esman MJ. 1991. *Management Dimensions of Development: Perspectives and Strategies*. West Hartford, CT: Kumarian Press.

Esrey SA. 1996. Water, Waste, and Well-Being: A Multicountry Study. *American Journal of Epidemiology*. 143(6): 608-623.

Esrey SA and R Feachem. 1990. *Interventions for the Control of Diarrhoeal Diseases Among Young Children: Promotion of Food Hygiene*. CDD/89.30. World Health Organization.

Ewbank D and S Preston. 1990. Personal Health Behavior and the Decline in Infant and Child Mortality: The United States 1900-1930. In J Caldwell, S Findley, et al., eds. *What We Know About Health Transition: The Cultural, Social, and Behavioral Determinants of Health*. Canberra: Australian National University Printing Service.

Family Planning Management Development (FPMD). 1995. *Lessons Learned From the Family Planning Management Development Project, 1993-1995*. Management Sciences for Health. Manila, Philippines.

Fauveau C, M Siddiqui and A Briend. 1992. Limited Impact of a Targeted Food Supplementation Programme in Bangladeshi Urban Slum Children. *Annals of Tropical Paediatrics*. 12: 41-48.

Fauveau V, K Stewart, SA Khan, et al. 1991. Effects on Mortality of Community-Based Maternity Care Programme in Rural Bangladesh. *Lancet*. 338: 1183-1186.

Fawzy FI, NW Fawzy, CS Hyun, et al. 1993. Malignant Melanoma Effects of an Early Structured Psychiatric Intervention, Coping, and Affective State on Recurrence and Survival 6 Years Later. *Archives of General Psychiatry*. 50: 681-689.

Feachem R. 1997. Opening Remarks at World Bank International Conference, Innovations in Health Care Financing. Arlington, VA

Feachem R, W Graham and I Timaeus. 1989. Identifying Health Problems an Health Research Priorities in Developing Countries. *Journal of Tropical Medicine and Hygiene*. 92(3): 133-191.

Feachem R and MA Koblinksy. 1984. Interventions for the Control of Diarrhoeal Diseases Among Young Children: Promotion of Breast Feeding. *Bulletin of the World Health Organization*. 62: 271-291.

Feachem RG, T Kjellstrom, CJL Murray, et al. 1993. *The Health of Adults in the Developing World.* Oxford: Oxford University Press.

Feinstein A and C Wells. 1977. Randomized Trials vs. Historical Controls: The Scientific Plagues of Both Houses. *Transactions of the Association of American Physicians*. 90: 239-247.

Feldstein M and B Friedman. 1977. Tax Subsidies, The Rational Demand for Insurance, and the Health Care Crisis. *Journal of Public Economics*. 7: 155-178.

Feldstein P, T Wickizer and J Wheeler. 1988. Private Cost Containment, the Effects of Utilization Review Programs on Health Care Use and Expenditures. *New England Journal of Medicine*. 318(20): 1310-1314.

Feng X, GB S Tang, M Segall, et al. 1995. Cooperative Medical Schemes in Contemporary Rural China. *Social Science and Medicine*. 41(8): 1111-1118.

Ferreccio C, E Ortiz, L Astroza, et al. 1990. A Population-Based Retrospective Assessment of the Disease Burden Resulting From Invasive Haemophilus-Influenzae in Infants and Young Children in Santiago, Chile. *Pediatric Infectious Disease Journal*. 9(7): 488-494.

Ferrinho P, D Robb, H Cornielje, et al. 1993. Primary Health Care in Support of Community Development. *World Health Forum*. 14(2): 158-162.

Fiander A. 1991. Obstetric Mortality and its Causes in Developing Countries. *British Journal of Obstetrics and Gynaecology*. 98(8): 841-842.

Fiedler J. 1993. Increasing Reliance on User Fees as a Response to Public Health Financing Crises: A Case Study of El Salvador. *Social Science and Medicine*. 36(6): 735-747.

Field M. 1995. The Health Crisis in the Former Soviet Union: A Report from the Post-war Zone. *Social Science and Medicine*. 41(11): 1469-1478.

Fielding R, J Li and Y Tang. 1995. Health Care Utilization as a Function of Subjective Health Status, Job Satisfaction and Gender Among Health Care Workers in Guanghzou, Southern China. *Social Science and Medicine*. 41(8): 1103-1110.

Finau SA. 1994. National Health Information Systems in the Pacific Islands: In Search of a Future. *Health Policy and Planning*. 9(2): 161-170.

Fisher-Hoch S, O Tomori, A Nasidi, et al. 1995. Review of Cases of Nosocomial Lassa Fever in Nigeria: The High Price of Poor Medical Practice. *British Medical Journal*. 311(7009): 857-859.

Flood A. 1996. Scientific Bases Versus Scientism in Health Services. *Journal of Health Services and Resource Policy*. 1(2): 63-64.

Foege W and D Henderson. eds. 1986. *Management Priorities in Primary Health Care.* Chicago: University of Chicago Press.

Foltz A. 1994. Donor Funding for Health Reform: Is Non-Project Assistance the Right Prescription? *Health Policy and Planning.* 9(4): 353-370.

Ford K, P Fajans and DN Wirawan. 1994. AIDS Risk Behaviours and Sexual Networks of Male and Female Sex Workers and Clients in Bali, Indonesia. *Health Transiiton Review.* 4(Supplement): 125-152.

Foreman S. 1994. *Using Principal-Agent Theory to Establish Outcomes-Based Payment for Health Care.* [Abstract]. Presented at Association for Health Services Research/Foundation for Health Services Research Annual Meeting.

Forgia GL, C Griffin, N Homedes, et al. 1993. *Health Insurance in Practice: Fifteen Case Studies from Developing Countries.* HFS Small Applied Research Paper. 4. Abt Associates, Inc. Bethesda, MD.

Forgia GML. 1990. *Health Services for Low-Income Families: Extending Coverage Through Prepayment Plans in the Dominican Republic.* Health Financing and Sustainability Project Small HFS Technical Report. 2. Abt Associates, Inc. Bethesda, MD.

Forsberg B, JV Ginneken and N Nagalkerke. 1993. Cross-Sectional Household Surveys of Diarrhoeal Diseases—A Comparison of Data from the Control of Diarrhoeal Diseases and Demographic and Health Surveys Programmes. *International Journal of Epidemiology.* 22(6): 1137-1145.

Fortney JA. 1987. The Importance of Family Planning in Reducing Maternal Mortality. *Studies in Family Planning.* 18: 109-115.

Foster G. 1987. World Health Organization Behavioral Science Research: Problems and Prospects. *Social Science and Medicine.* 24: 709-715.

Foster S. 1990. *Improving the Supply and Use of Essential Drugs in Sub-Saharan Africa.* Policy Research and External Affairs Working Paper Series. Washington, DC: World Bank Population and Human Resources Department.

Foster S, C Normand and R Sheaff. 1994. Health Care Reform: The Issues and Role of Donors. *Lancet.* 344(8916): 175-177.

Foster SO, DA Mcfarland and AM Johh. 1993. Measles. In DT Jamison, WH Mosley, et al., eds. *Disease Control Priorities in Developing Countries.* New York: Oxford University Press.

Franke R and B Chasin. 1992. Kerala State, India, Radical Reform as Development. *International Journal of Health Services.* 22(1): 139-156.

Free MJ. 1992. Health Technologies for a Developing World: Addressing the Unmet Needs. *International Journal of Technology Assessment in Health Care.* 8: 623-634.

Free MJ, JA Green and MM Morrow. 1993. Health Technologies for a Developing World: Promoting Self-Reliance Through Improving Local Procurement and Manufacturing Capabilities. *International Journal of Technology Assessment in Health Care.* 9: 623-634.

Freeman HE and MF Shapiro. 1993. *A Contemporary Perspective on Access to Health Care*. Los Angeles: UCLA School of Medicine.

Freemantle N, R Grilli, J Grimshaw, et al. 1995. Implementing Findings of Medical Research: The Cochrane Collaboration on Effective Professional Practice. *Quality in Health Care*. 4: 45-47.

Frenk J. 1993. The Public/Private Mix and Human Resources for Health. *Health Policy and Planning*. 8(4): 315-326.

Frenk J. 1995. Comprehensive Policy Analysis for Health System Reform. In P Berman, ed. *Health* Sector *Reform in Developing Countries*. Cambridge: Harvard University Press.

Frenk J, JL Bobadilla, J Sepulveda, et al. 1989. Health Transition in Middle-income Countries: New Challenges for Health Care. *Health Care Policy and Planning*. 4(1): 29-39.

Frerichs R and TT Khin. 1989. Computer-Assisted Rapid Surveys in Developing Countries. *Public Health Report*. 104:14-23.

Friedman G. 1974. *Primer of Epidemiology*. New York: McGraw-Hill.

Fuchs V. 1978. The Supply of Surgeons and the Demand for Operations. *Journal of Human Resources*. 13: 35-56.

Fuchs V. 1990. The Health Sectors Share of the Gross National Product. *Science*. 247(4942): 534-538.

Fuchs V. 1991. National Health Insurance Revisited. *Health Affairs*. 10(4): 7-17.

Fuchs V. 1992. The Best Health Care System in the World. *Journal of the American Medical Association*. 268(7): 916-917.

Fuchs V. 1994a. Health System Reform: A Different Approach. *Journal of the American Medical Association*. 272(7): 560-563.

Fuchs V. 1994b. A Conversation About Health Care Reform. *Western Journal of Medicine*. 161(1): 83-86.

Fuchs V. 1996. Economics, Values, and Health Care Reform. *American Economic Review*. 86(1): 1-24.

Fuchs V and R Zeckhauser. 1987. Valuing Health—A 'Priceless' Community. *AEA Papers and Proceedings*. 77(2): 268.

Fukukawa S. 1995. The Need for Analysis on Values and Characteristics Shared by Asians. *Human Studies*. 15(September 1995): 2-3.

Fuller T, J Edwards, S Sermsri, et al. 1993. Gender and Health: Some Asian Evidence. *The Journal Of Health and Social Behavior*. 34(3): 252-271.

Gaiha R and A Deolalikar. 1993. Persistent, Expected, and Innate Poverty: Estimates for Semi-Arid Rural South India, 1975-1984. *Cambridge Journal of Economics.* 17(4): 101-104.

Galloway R and J McGuire. 1994. Determinants of Compliance with Iron Supplementation: Supplies, Side Effects, or Psychology? *Social Science and Medicine.* 39(3): 381-390.

Ganatra B and S Hirve. 1994. Male Bias in Health Care Utilization for Under Fives in a Rural Community in Western India. *Bulletin of the World Health Organization.* 72(1): 101-104.

Garber A. 1994. Can Technology Assessment Control Health Spending? *Health Affairs.* Summer 1994: 115-126.

Garber A and V Fuchs. 1991. The Expanding Role of Technology Assessment in Health Policy. *Stanford Law and Policy Review.* 3(Fall): 203-209.

Garfinkel M, H Schummacker, A Husain, et al. 1994. Evaluation of a Yoga Based Regimen for Treatment of Osteoarthritis of the Hands. *Journal of Rheumatology.* 21: 1341-1343.

Garner P and I Thaver. 1993. Urban Slums and Primary Health Care: The Private Doctor's Role. *British Medical Journal.* 306: 667.

Gauss C and L Simpson. 1995. Reinventing Health Services Research. *Inquiry.* 32: 130-134.

Gelbach JB and LH Pritchett. 1995. *Does More for the Poor Mean Less for the Poor? The Politics of Tagging.* Policy Research Working Paper. 1523. World Bank. Washington, DC.

Gerhard I and F Postneek. 1992. Auricular Acupuncture in the Treatment of Female Infertility. *Gynecological Endocrinology.* 6(3): 171-181.

Gertham U, J Sogaard, F Andersson, et al. 1992. An Econometric Analysis of Health Care Expenditure: A Cross-Section Study of the OECD Countries. *Journal of Health Economics.* 11: 63-84.

Gertler PJ, ed. 1994a. *Poverty Alleviation Strategies.* Indonesian Economic Memorandum. Washington, DC: World Bank.

_____. 1994b. *Changing Pricing Policy in the Social Sectors.* Indonesia Public Expenditures and the Poor. Washington, DC: World Bank.

Gertler PJ. 1995a. Financing Health Care in Asia: Policy Issues and Responses. *Workshop on Financing Human Resource Development in Asia, July 11-14.* Manila, Philippines: Asian Development Bank.

_____. 1995b. On the Road to Social Insurance: Lessons from and for Asian Economies. *Conference on Human Resources Development.* Manila, Philippines: Asian Development Bank.

_____. 1996. *On the Road to Social Health Insurance: Lessons from and for Asian Economics*. Asian Development Bank.

Gertler P and J Gruber. 1997. *Insuring Consumption Against Illness*. National Bureau of Economic Research, Cambridge, MA.

Gertler P and J Hammer. 1997. Strategies for Pricing Publicly Provided Health Services. In Schieber G, ed. *Innovations in Health Care Financing*. Washington, DC: World Bank.

Gertler PJ, J Litvack and N Prescott. 1997. Access to Health Care During Transition: The Role of the Private Sector in Viet Nam. In D Dollar, L Litavak, et al., eds. *Poverty and the Transition to the Market in Viet Nam*. New York: Oxford University Press.

Gertler PJ, L Locay and W Sanderson. 1987. Are User Fees Regressive? The Welfare Implications of Health Care Financing Proposals in Peru. *Journal of Econometrics*. 36: 67-88.

_____. 1988. *Health Care Financing and the Demand for Medical Care*. LSMS Working Paper. 37. World Bank. Washington, DC.

Gertler PJ and JW Molyneaux. 1994. How Economic Development and Family Planning Programs Combined to Reduce Indonesian Fertility. *Demography*. 31(1): 33-63.

_____. 1996a. Unpublished research on Financing Public Health Sector Expenditures Through User Fees: Theory and Evidence from an Explicit Social Experiment in Indonesia. RAND. Santa Monica, CA.

_____. 1996b. Pricing Public-Provided Private Health Care Services: Theory and Evidence from an Actual Experiment. *American Economic Association Meeting*. San Francisco.

Gertler PJ and O Rahman. 1994. Social Infrastructure and Urban Poverty, Chapter 4. In EM Pernia, ed. *Urban Poverty in Asia: A Survey of Critical Issues*. Hong Kong: Oxford University Press.

Gertler PJ and O Solon. 1996. *Who Benefits from Social Health Insurance in Low Income Countries?* Unpublished paper. RAND. Santa Monica, CA.

Gertler PJ and R Sturm. 1997. Private Health Insurance and Public Expenditures in Jamaica. *Journal of Econometrics*. 77:237-257.

Gertler PJ and J van der Gaag. 1990. *The Willingness to Pay for Medical Care: Evidence from Two Developing Countries*. Baltimore: Johns Hopkins University Press.

Gertler PJ, BM Yang, D Lee, et al. 1996. Unpublished research on financing health care in an aging society: a crisis on Korea's horizon. RAND. Santa Monica, CA.

Ghana Health Assessment Project Team. 1981. A Quantitative Method of Assessing the Health Impact of Different Diseases in Less Developed Countries. *International Journal of Epidemiology*. 10: 73-80.

Gillett JD. 1987. The Harnessing of Artificial Satellites for Prevention of Disease in the Tropics: Flights of Fancy or Fact? *Transactions of the Royal Society of Tropical Medicine and Hygiene*. 81: 350-351.

Gillis M, DH Perkins, M Roemer, et al. 1983. *Economics of Development*. New York: W. W. Norton & Company.

Gillman MW, LA Cupples, D Gagnon, et al. 1995. Protective Effect of Fruits and Vegetables on Development of Stroke in Men. *Journal of the American Medical Association*. 273: 1113-1117.

Gilson L. 1993. Health-Care Reform in Developing Countries. *Lancet*. 342(8874): 800.

Gilson L, M Alilio and K Heggenhougen. 1994. Community Satisfaction with Primary Health Care Services: An Evaluation Undertaken in the Morogoro Region of Tanzania. *Social Science and Medicine*. 39(6): 767-780.

Gilson L, S Jaffar, S Mwankusye, et al. 1993. Assessing Prescribing Practice: A Tanzanian Example. *International Journal of Health Planning and Management*. 8: 37-58.

Gilson L, PD Sen, S Mohammed, et al. 1994. The Potential of Health Sector Non-Governmental Organizations: Policy Options. *Health Policy and Planning*. 9(1): 14-24.

Ginsburg J. 1996. Medical Savings Accounts. *Annals of Internal Medicine*. 125(4): 333-340.

Gish O, R Malek and P Sudharto. 1988. Who Gets What? Utilization of Health Services in Indonesia. *International Journal of Health Planning and Management*. 3: 185-196.

Gittelsohn J and ME Bentley. 1996. Development and Use of the Women's Health Protocol in India. *Practicing Anthropology*. 18(3): 7-9.

Glassman P, K Model, JW Peabody, et al. 1996. The Role of Medical Necessity and Cost-Effectiveness in Making Medical Decisions. *Annals of Internal Medicine*. 126(2): 152-156.

Glewwe P. 1990. The Measurement of Income Inequality Under Inflation: Correction Formulae for 3 Inequality Measures. *Journal of Development Economics*. 32(1): 43-67.

Glewwe P. 1991. Household Equivalence Scales and the Measurement of Inequality Transfers from the Poor to the Rich Could Decrease Inequality. *Journal of Public Economics*. 44(2): 211-216.

Glewwe P and HG Jacoby. 1995. An Economic Analysis of Delayed Primary School Enrollment in a Low Income Country: The Role of Early Childhood Nutrition. *The Review of Economics and Statistics*. 77(1): 156.

Glewwe P and J van der Gaag. 1990. Identifying the Poor in Developing Countries: Do Different Definitions Matter? *World Development*. 18(6): 803-814.

Goldman DP, SD Hosek, LS Dixon, et al. 1995. The Effects of Benefit Design and Managed Care on Health Care Costs. *Journal of Health Economics*. 14(4): 401-418.

Golembiewski RT and J Rabin. eds. 1983. *Public Budgeting and Finance: Behavioral, Theoretical, and Technical Perspectives*. New York: M Dekker.

Goodwin K and K Jamison. 1990. *Manic-Depressive Illness*. New York: Oxford University Press.

Gotzsche PC. 1989. Methodology and Overt and Hidden Bias in Reports of 196 Double-Blind Trials of Nonsteroidal Antiinflammatory Drugs in Rheumatoid Arthritis. *Controlled Clinical Trials*. 10: 31-56.

Government of Pakistan Ministry of Health. 1995. *Situation Analysis of Health Sector in Pakistan*. Government of Pakistan Ministry of Health. Islamabad, Pakistan.

Govindaraj R, C Murray and G Chellaraj. 1995. *Health Expenditures in Latin America*. World Bank Technical Paper. 274. World Bank. Washington, DC.

Gray BH and MJ Field. eds. 1989. *Controlling Costs and Changing Patient Care? The Role of Utilization Management*. Washington, DC: National Academy Press.

Green A. 1995. The State of Health Planning in the '90s. *Health Policy and Planning*. 10(1): 22-28.

Greenhalgh T. 1987. Drug Prescription and Self-Medication in India: An Exploratory Survey. *Social Science and Medicine*. 3: 307-318.

Grell G. 1993. The University, the Private Sector, and the Health of the Caribbean People. *West Indian Medical Journal*. 42(1): 3-9.

Gribble JN and SH Preston. 1993. The Epidemiological Transition: Policy and Planning Implications for Developing Countries. *National Research Council Workshop Proceedings, Workshop on the Policy and Planning Implications of the Epidemiological Transition in Developing Countries, November 20-22*. Washington, DC: National Academy Press.

Griffin C. 1989. *Strengthening Health Services in Developing Countries Through the Private Sector*. Washington, DC: International Finance Corporation.

Griffin C. 1992a. *Health Care in Asia: A Comparative Study of Cost and Financing*. World Bank Regional and Sectoral Studies. Washington, DC: World Bank.

Griffin C. 1992b. Welfare Gains from User Charges for Government Health Services. *Health Policy and Planning*. 7(2): 177-180.

Griffin C. 1994. Health Care in Asia: A Comparative Study of Cost and Financing. *Social Indicators Research*. 321(1): 94-96.

Griffin CC and VB Paqueo. 1993. The Development, Growth and Distribution of Public and Private Medical Resources in the Philippines. In A Mills and K Lee, eds. *Health Economics Research in Developing Countries*. Oxford University Press.

Grimshaw JM and IT Russell. 1993. Effect of Clinical Guidelines on Medical Practice: A Systematic Review of Rigorous Evaluations. *Lancet*. 342: 1317-1322.

Grogan C. 1995. Urban Economic Reform and Access to Health Care Coverage in the People's Republic of China. *Social Science and Medicine*. 41(8): 1073-1084.

Grol R. 1993. Development of Guidelines for General Practice Care. *British Journal of General Practice*. 43(369): 146-151.

Grosh ME. 1996. *Administering Targeted Social Programs in Latin America: From Platitudes to Practice*. Aldershot, England: Ashgate Publishing Ltd, Published in Association with the World Bank.

Gu X, S Tang and S Cao. 1995. The Financing and Organization of Health Services in Poor Rural China: A Case Study in Donglan County. *International Journal of Health Planning and Management*. 10(4): 265-282.

Gu X, S Tang, S Cao, et al. 1993. Financing Health Care in Rural China: Preliminary Report of a Nationwide Study. *Social Science and Medicine*. 36(4): 385-391.

Guldner M. 1995. Health Care in Transition in Vietnam: Equity and Sustainability. *Health Policy and Planning*. 10(Supplement): 49-62.

Gupta PC. 1988. Health Consequences of Tobacco SSE in India. *World Smoking and Health*. 13: 5-10.

Gupta R, B Jain and P Keswani. 1993. Awareness of Cholesterol as Coronary Risk Factor Among General Practicioners at Jaipur. *Journal of the Association of Physicians of India*. 41(11): 717-719.

Guy C, ed. 1992. *Strategies for Health Care Finance in Developing Countries: With a Focus on Community Financing in Sub-Saharan Africa*. New York: St. Martin's Press.

Gwatkin DR, ed. 1993. *Distributional Implications of Alternative Strategic Responses to the Demographic-Epidemiological Transition: An Initial Inquiry*. Washington, DC: National Academy Press.

Haaga JG. 1989. Mechanisms for the Association of Maternal Age, Parity, and Birth Spacing with Infant Health. In *Contraceptive Use and Controlled Fertility*. Washington, DC: National Academy Press.

Haak H and HV Hogerzeil. 1995. Essential Drugs for Ration Kits in Developing Countries. *Health Policy and Planning*. 10(1): 40-49.

Hall J, D Roter and N Katz. 1988. Meta-Analysis of Correlates of Provider Behavior in Medical Encounters. *Medical Care*. 26(7): 657-675.

Hall P, H Land, R Parker, et al. 1975. *Change, Choice and Conflict in Social Policy*. London: Heinemann.

Hammer JS. 1997a. Economic Analysis for Health Projects. *World Bank Research Observer*. 12(1): 47-72.

_____. 1997b. Prices and Protocols in Public Health Care. *World Bank Economic Review*. 11(3):409-432.

Hammer JS and P Berman. 1995. Ends and Means in Public Health Policy in Developing Countries. *Health Policy*. 32(1-3): 29-45.

Hanson K. 1992. AIDS: What Does Economics Have to Offer? *Health Policy and Planning*. 7(4): 315-328.

Harris M. 1991. The Politics of Aid in the Third World. *Health Policy and Planning*. 6(1): 86-89.

Harvard School of Public Health and UNAIDS. 1996. *The Status and Trends of the Global HIV/AIDS Pandemic Symposium Final Report*. AIDSCAP/Family Health International. Vancouver, B.C.

Hawe P. 1994. Capturing the Meaning of "Community" in Community Intervention Evaluation: Some Contributions from Community Psychology. *Health Promotion International*. 9(3): 199-210.

Haynes R, D Davis, A McKibbon and P Tugwell. 1984. A Critical Appraisal of the Efficacy of Continuing Medical Education. *Journal of the American Medical Association*. 251:61-64.

Haynes RB, DW Taylor and DL Sackett. 1979. *Compliance in Health Care*. Baltimore: Johns Hopkins University Press.

Hayward R, B Haynes and A Jadad. eds. 1996. *Cochrane Overview: Preparing, Maintaining, and Disseminating Systematic Reviews of the Effects of Health Care*. Ontario, Canada: McMaster University.

Heisler M and J Richmond. 1994. Lessons from Finland's Successful Immunization Program. *New England Journal of Medicine*. 331(21): 1446-1447.

Hellandendu J. 1993. Damaging Effects of Micro-Politics on the Management of Health Posts. *World Health Forum*. 14(4): 398-399.

Henderson G, J Akin, L Ahiming, et al. 1994. Long-Term Issues and Options in the Health Transition World Bank. *China Quarterly*. (138): 532-532.

Henderson G, SG Jin, J Akin, et al. 1994. Distribution of Medical Insurance in China. *Social Science and Medicine*. 41(8): 1119-1130.

Henderson PL. 1995. Donor and Government Constraints to Sustainability in Nepal. *Health Policy and Planning*. 10(Supplement): 17-27.

Henderson R and T Sunderesan. 1982. Cluster Sampling to Assess Immunisation Coverage: A Review of Experience with a Simplified Method. *Bulletin of the World Health Organization*. 60: 253-260.

Herbert V. 1986. Unproven (Questionable) Dietary and Nutritional Methods in Cancer Prevention and Treatment. *Cancer*. 58: 1930-1941.

Herrin AN, O Solon and R Racelis. May 1996. National Health Accounts in the Philippines. Paper presented at the Inaugural Conference of the International Health Economics Association. Vancouver, Canada.

Herz B and AR Measham. 1987. *The Safe Motherhood Initiative: Proposals for Action*. World Bank Discussion Paper. 9. World Bank. Washington, DC.

Hesketh TM, WX Zhu and KH Zheng. 1994. Improvement of Neonatal Care in Zhejiang Province, China Through a Self-Instructional Continuing Education Programme. *Medical Education*. 28: 252-259.

Heuck CC and A Deom. 1991. Health Care in the Developing World: Need for Appropriate Laboratory Technology. *Clinical Chemistry*. 37(4): 490-496.

Higgins W. 1994-95 Winter. Supplementing Managed Competition. *Inquiry*. 31(4):385-93.

Hill AG and DF Roberts. eds. 1989. *Health Interventions and Mortality Change in Developing Countries*. Cambridge, England: Parkes Foundation.

Hill K and A Pebley. 1989. Child Mortality in the Developing World. *Population and Development Review*. 15(4): 657-687.

Hira SK and RS Hira. 1987. Congenital Syphillis. In AO Osoba, ed. *Sexually Transmitted Diseases in the Tropics*. London: Bailliere's Tindall.

Hiscock J. 1995. Looking a Gift Horse in the Mouth: The Shifting Power Balance Between the Ministry of Health and Donors in Ghana. *Health Policy and Planning*. 10(Supplement): 28-39.

Ho LS. 1995. Market Reforms and China's Health Care System. *Social Science and Medicine*. 41(8): 1065-1072.

Hobcraft J. 1987. Does Family Planning Save Children's Lives? Paper prepared for the International Conference on Better Health for Women and Children Through Family Planning. Nairobi.

Hobcraft J. 1993. Women's Education, Child Welfare and Child Survival: A Review of the Evidence. *Health Transition Review*. 3(2): 159-175.

Hobcraft JN, JW McDonald and SO Rutstein. 1985. Demographic Determinants of Infant and Early Child Mortality: A Comparative Analysis. *Population Studies*. 39(3): 363-386.

Hojman D. 1996. Economic and Other Determinants of Infant and Child Mortality in Small Developing Countries: The Case of Central America and the Caribbean. *Applied Economics*. 28(3): 281-290.

Holland S and C Phimphachanh. 1995. *Impact of Economic and Institutional Reforms on the Health Sector in Laos*. Institute of Development Studies.

Hollman CDJ, RJ Donovan, B Corti, et al. 1996. Evaluating Projects Funded by the Western Australian Health Promotion Foundation: First Results. *Health Promotion International*. 11(2): 75-88.

Holmes K, P Mardh, P Sparling, et al. 1990. *Sexually Transmitted Diseases*, 2nd Edition. Tropical and Geographical Medicine. New York: McGraw-Hill.

Hoque BA and MM Hoque. 1994. Partnersip in Rural Water Supply and Sanitation: a Case Study from Bangladesh. *Health Policy and Planning*. 9(3): 288-293.

Hornbrook M. 1995. *Promise and Performance in Managed Care*. Portland.

Horngren CT. 1982. *Cost Accounting: A Managerial Emphasis, Fifth Edition*. Englewood Cliffs, NJ: Prentice-Hall, Inc.

Hornic RC. 1988. *Development Communication; Information, Agriculture, and Nutrition in the Third World*. Lanham, MD: University Press of America.

Hotchkiss D. 1993. *The Role of Quality in the Demand for Health Care in Cebu, Philippines*. Small Applied Research Paper. 12. Abt Associates, Inc. Bethesda, MD.

Hsiao W and Y Liu. 1996. Economic Reform and Health- Lessons from China. *New England Journal of Medicine*. 335(6): 430-432.

Hsiao WC. 1995a. The Chinese Health Care System: Lessons for Other Nations. *Social Science and Medicine*. 41(8): 1047-1055.

Hsiao WC. 1995b. Medical Savings Accounts—Lessons from Singapore. *Health Affairs*. 14(2): 260-266.

Hsiao WC, M Herrera, T Bossert, et al. 1995. Managed Competition with Universal Insurance: The Colombian Health Sector Reform. Presented at the Association of Health Services Research Conference.

Hsiao WC-L, C-L Yuang and J-FR Lu. 1989. *Current System of Health Care Financing and Delivery in R.O.C. and Its Challenge for Future Development*. Draft. Harvard University School of Public Health, National Taiwan University, Insitute of Public Health.

Htoon MT, J Bertolli and LD Kosasih. 1993. Leprosy. In DT Jamison, WH Mosley, et al., eds. *Disease Control Priorities in Developing Countries.* New York: Oxford University Press.

Huber JH. 1993. Ensuring Access to Health Care with the Introduction of User Fees—A Kenyan Example. *Social Science and Medicine.* 36(4): 485-494.

Hudelson P, T Huanca, D Charaly, et al. 1995. Ethnographic Studies of ARI in Bolivia and Their Use by the National ARI Programme. *Social Science and Medicine.* 41(2): 1677-1683.

Huffman SL and C Combest. 1988. *Promotion of Breastfeeding: Yes, It Works.* Bethesda: Center to Prevent Childhood Malnutrition.

Hully SB and SR Cummings (eds.) 1988. Designing a New Study: II. Cross-Sectional and Case-control Studies. *Designing Clinical Research: An Epidemiologic Approach.* Baltimore: Williams and Wilkins.

Humphrey J. 1992. Vitamin A Deficiency and Attributable Mortality Under-5-Year-Olds. *Bulletin of the World Health Organization.* 70(2): 225-232.

Huntington D and S Schuler. 1993. The Simulated Client Method: Evaluating Client-Provider Interactions in Family Planning Clinics. *Studies in Family Planning.* 24(3): 187-193.

Husein K, O Adeyi, J Bryant, et al. 1993. Developing a Primary Health Care Information System that Supports the Pursuit of Equity, Effectiveness, and Affordability. *Social Science and Medicine.* 36(5): 585-596.

Hussey GD and M Klein. 1990. A Randomized, Controlled Trial of Vitamin A in Children with Severe Measles. *New England Journal of Medicine.* 323(3): 160-164.

Huttin C. 1994. The Chinese Medicines Market: Moving Towards a Market System? *Health Policy.* 29: 247-259.

Huttly S. 1990. The Impact of Inadequate Sanitary Conditions on Health in Developing Countries. *World Health Statistics Quarterly.* 43: 118-126.

Hyder A, G Rotllant and R Morrow. 1998. Measuring the Burden of Disease: Healthy-Life Years. *American Journal of Public Health.* 88:196.

Iglehart JK. 1992. The American Health Care System: Managed Care. *New England Journal of Medicine.* 327(10): 742-7.

Iglehart JK. 1995. Medicaid and Managed Care. *New England Journal of Medicine.* 332(25): 1727-1731.

Ikegami N. 1991. Japanese Health Care: Low Cost Through Regulated Fees. *Health Affairs.* 10(3): 87-109.

Ikegami N and J Campbell. 1995. Medical Care in Japan. *New England Journal of Medicine.* 333(19): 1295-1299.

Imai M. 1986. *Kaizen: The Key to Japan's Competitive Success*. New York: Random House.

Indonesia Central Bureau of Statistics NFPCB Ministry of Health, and Macro International Inc.,. 1992. *Demographic and Health Survey 1991*. Calverton, MD: Macro International, Inc.

Indrayan A. 1995. Informatics: The Key to Efficiency. *World Health Forum*. 16: 305-311.

Ingram G. 1992. *Social Indicators and Productivity Convergence in Developing Countries*. Policy Research Working Papers Development Economics. WPS 894. World Bank. Washington, DC.

Institute of Medicine (U.S.). 1990. Committee to Design a Strategy for Quality Review and Assurance in Medicare. Division of Health Care Services. In KN Lohr, ed. *Medicare: A Strategy for Quality Assurance*. Washington, DC: National Academy Press.

Inter-American Development Bank (IABD). 1988. *Summary of the Ex-post Evaluations of Public Health Programs*. IADB, Operations Evaluations Office.

International Insititute for Population Sciences (IIPS). 1995. *National Family Health Survey (MCH and Family Planning), India, 1992-1993*. IIPS. Bombay.

International Monetary Fund (IMF). 1995. Annual Report, 1995, of the Executive Board for the Financial Year Ended April 30, 1995. Washington, DC.

Jablensky A, N Sartorius, G Ernberg, et al. 1992. Schizophrenia: Manifestations, Incidence, and Course in Different Cultures: A World Health Organization Ten Country Study. *Psychological Medicine*. 20(Supplement): 1-97.

Jamison DT. 1985. China's Health Care System: Policies, Organization, Inputs, and Finance. In JAW Scott B. Halstead and Kenneth S. Warren, eds. *Good Health at Low Cost*. New York: Rockefeller Foundation.

_____. 1993. An Overview. In DT Jamison, WH Mosley, et al., eds. *Disease Control Priorities in Developing Countries*. New York: Oxford University Press.

_____. 1996. *Health Finance Issues in Asia*. Manila. Asian Development Bank.

Jamison DT and J-P Jardel. 1994. Comparative Health Data and Analyses. In C Murray and A Lopez, eds. *Global Comparative Assessments in the Health Sector: Disease Burden, Expenditures and Intervention Packages*. Geneva: World Health Organization.

Jamison DT and J Leslie. 1990. Health and Nutrition Considerations in Educational Planning: The Cost and Effectiveness of School-Based Intervention. *Food and Nutrition Bulletin*. 12: 204-214.

Jamison DT and W Mosley. 1991. Selecting Disease Control Priorities in Developing Countries. Health Policy Responses to Epidemiological Change. *American Journal of Public Health*. 81(1): 15-22.

Jamison DT, WH Mosley, AR Measham, et al. 1993. *Disease Control Priorities in Developing Countries*. Oxford University Press. New York.

Jamison DT, J Wang, K Hill, and JL Londono. 1996. Income, Mortality and Fertility in Latin America: Country-Level Performance, 1960-90. *Analisis Economico*. 11:219-261.

Janovsky K, ed. 1996. *Health Policy and Systems Development, an Agenda for Research*. Geneva: World Health Organization.

Janseen R and J Vandermade. 1990. Privatisation in Health Care—Concepts, Motives and Policies. *Health Policy*. 14(3): 191-202.

Japanese Ministry of Health and Welfare. 1986. *1985 National Health Survey*. Kousei, Tokiei, Kyokai. Tokyo.

Jara JDL and T Bossert. 1995. Chile's Health Sector Reform: Lessons from 4 Reform Periods. In P Berman, ed. *Health Sector Reform in Developing Countries*. Cambridge: Harvard University Press.

Jarlais DD, N Padian and W Winkelstein. 1994. Targeted HIV-prevention Programs. *New England Journal of Medicine*. 331(21): 1451-1453.

Javitt JC. 1993. Cataracts. In DT Jamison, WH Mosley, et al., eds. *Disease Control Priorities in Developing Countries*. New York: Oxford University Press.

Javitt JC, G Venkataswamy and A Sommer. 1983. The Economic and Social Aspect of Restoring Sight. In P Henkind, ed. *ACTA: 24th International Congress of Opthalmology*. New York: J. B. Lippincott.

Jilek WG and TN Jilek. 1974. Witch Doctors Succeed Where Doctors Fail; Psychotherapy Among the West Coast Salish Indians. *Canadian Psychology Association Journal*. 19: 351.

Jimenez E. 1986. The Public Subsidization of Education and Health in Developing Countries: A Review of Equity and Efficiency. *World Bank Research Observer*. 1: 111-129.

Jimenez E. 1987. *Pricing Policy in the Social Sectors: Cost Recovery for Education and Health in Developing Countries*. Baltimore: Johns Hopkins University Press.

Jimenez E. 1994. The Role of Physical and Human Infrastructure in Development. In J Behrman and T Srinivasan, eds. *Handbook of Development Economics*. Amsterdam: North Holland Press.

Jingheng H, X Yindi, J Yongxin, et al. 1994. Evaluation of a Health Education Programme in China to Increase Breast-Feeding Rates. *Health Promotion International*. 9(2): 95-98.

Johanssen SR. 1990. Cultural Software, Institutional Hardware, and Health Information Processing in Social System. In J Caldwell et al., eds. *What We Know About Health Transition*. Canberra, Australia: Australian National University Printing Service.

Joseph RM. 1982. *Budgeting in Third World Countries: An Annotated Bibliography*. P-893. Vance Bibliographies.

Kabat-Zinn J, L Lipworth and R Burney. 1985. The Clinical Use of Mindfulness Meditation for the Self-Regulation of Chronic Pain. *Journal of Behavioral Medicine*. 8: 163-190.

Kaewsonthi S and AG Harding. 1986. Cost and Performance of Malaria Surveillance: The Patients' Perspectives. *Southeast Asian Journal of Tropical Medicine and Public Health*. 17: 406-412.

Kafle KK, RP Gartoulla and Y Pradhan. 1992. Drug Retailer Training: Experiences from Nepal. *Social Science and Medicine*. 35(2): 1015-1025.

Kamat VR. 1995. Reconsidering the Popularity of Primary Health Centers in India: A Case Study from Rural Maharashtra. *Social Science and Medicine*. 41(1): 87-98.

Kanaaneh H. 1977. Health Education in Developing Countries. *Public Health Reviews*. 6(3): 239-275.

Kark S, E Kark and J Abramson. 1993. Commentary: In Search of Innovative Approaches to International Health. *American Journal of Public Health*. 83(11): 1533-1536.

Kartman B, N Stalhammar and M Johannesson. 1996. Valuation of Health Changes with the Contingent Valuation Method: A Test of Scope and Question Order Effects. *Health Economics*. 5(6):531-41.

Katz A and J Thomson. 1996. The Role of Public Policy in Health Market Change. *Health Affairs*. 15(2): 77-91.

Kaufman A, J Hamilton and JW Peabody. 1988. Medical Education in China for the 21st Century: The Context for Change. *Journal of Medical Education*. 22: 253-260.

Kaufman J, Z Zhang, X Quiao, et al. 1992. The Quality of Family Planning Services in Rural China. *Studies in Family Planning*. 23(2): 73-84.

Keller A. 1991. Management Information Systems in Maternal and Child Health/Family Planning Programs: A Multi-Country Analysis. *Studies in Family Planning*. 22(1): 19-30.

Kerr E, B Mittman, R Hays, et al. 1995. Managed Care and Capitation in California: How Do Physicians at Financial Risk Control Their Own Utilization? *Annals of Internal Medicine*. 123: 500-504.

Keusch G. 1986. Control of Infections to Reduce Malnutrition. *Reviews of Infectious Diseases*. 8(2): 298-312.

Keyou G, J Akin and G Henderson. 1994. Equity and the Utilization of Health Services: Report of an 8-province Survey in China. *Social Science and Medicine*. 39(5): 687-699.

Khan A. 1996. Policy-making in Pakistan's Population Programme. *Health Policy and Planning*. 11(1): 30-51.

Khan ME and L Manderson. 1992. Focus Groups in Tropical Diseases Research. *Health Policy and Planning*. 7(1): 56-66.

Khare RS, Dava, Daktar, et al. 1996. Anthropology of Practiced Medicine in India. *Social Science and Medicine*. 43(5): 837-848.

Kielman AA and C McCord. 1977. Home Treatment of Childhood Diarrhoea in Punjab Villages. *Journal of Tropical Paediatrics and Environmental Child Health*. 23: 197-201.

Kinghorn AWA. 1996. Implications of the Development of Managed Care in the South African Private Health Care Sector. *South African Medical Journal*. 86(4): 335-338.

Kipp W, A Kielman, E Kwered, et al. 1994. Monitoring of Primary Health Care Services: An Example from Western Uganda. *Health Policy and Planning*. 9(2): 155-160.

Kleijnen J, P Knipschild and G Riet. 1991. Clinical Trials of Homeopathy. *British Medical Journal*. 302: 316-323.

Kleinman A. 1978. Concepts and a Model for the Comparison of Medical systems as Cultural Systems. *Social Science and Medicine*. 12(2B): 85-93.

Kleinman A. 1980. *Patients and Healers in the Context of Culture: an Exploration of the Borderland Between Anthropology, Medicine, and Psychiatry*. Berkeley: University of California Press.

Knowles J. 1996. *Partnerships for Health Reform*. Trip Report. Abt Associates, Inc. Bethesda, MD.

Kochweser D and A Yankauer. 1991. What Makes Infant Mortality Rates Fall in Developing Countries? *American Journal of Public Health*. 81(1): 12-13.

Koenig MA, MA Khan, B Wojtyniak, et al. 1990. Impact of Measles Vaccination on Childhood Mortality in Rural Bangladesh. *Bulletin of the World Health Organization*. 59: 901-908.

Koenig MA, JF Phillips, RS Simmons, et al. 1987. Trends in Family Size Preferences and Contraceptive Use in Matlab, Bangladesh. *Studies in Family Planning*. 18(3): 117-127.

Komori T, R Fujiwara, M Tanida, et al. 1995. Effects of Citrus Fragrance on Immune Function and Depressive States. *Neuroimmunomodulation*. 2: 174-180.

Kongstvedt PR. 1993. *The Managed Health Care Handbook*. Gaithersburg, MD: Aspen.

Kosecoff J, DE Kanouse, WH Rogers, et al. 1987. Effects of the National Institutes of Health Consensus Development Program on Physician Practice. *Journal of the American Medical Association*. 258(19): 2708-2713.

Kristein MM, CB Arnold and EL Wynder. 1977. Health Economics and Preventive Care. *Science*. 195(4277): 457-462.

Kroeger A. 1983. Health Interview Surveys in Developing Countries: A Review of the Methods and Results. *International Journal of Epidemiology*. 12(4): 465-481.

Kuo WH. 1989. Book Review, M M Rosenthal: Health Care in the People's Republic of China—Moving Toward Modernization. *Contemporary Sociology*. 18(1): 128-129.

Kutty VR. 1991. The Role of Planning in Health Care—What It Should Be in India. *Current Science*. 60(4): 277-281.

Kutzin J. 1994. *Experience with Organizational and Financing Reform of the Health Sector*. Current Concerns, SHS Paper No. 8. WHO/SHS/CC/94.3. Geneva: World Health Organization.

Kutzin J and H Barnum. 1992. Institutional Features of Health Insurance and Their Effects on Developing Country Health Systems. *International Journal of Health Planning and Management*. 7(1): 51-72.

Kwast BE, W Kidane-Mariam, EM Saed, et al. 1984. *Report on Maternal Health in Addis Ababa, Sept. 1981-Sept. 1983: A Community Based Survey on the Incidence and Etiology of Maternal Mortality and the Use of Maternal Services, and Confidential Inquiries into Maternal Deaths in Addis Ababa, Ethiopia*. Save the Children Federation.

Kwon S. 1994. *The Role of Public and Private Transfers to Vulnerable Groups with Special Reference to Experiences of the Eastern Asian Countries*. Mimeo. World Bank. Washington, DC.

Lafond A. 1995a. Improving the Quality of Investment in Health: Lessons on Sustainability. *Health Policy and Planning*. 10(Supplement): 63-72.

Lafond A. 1995b. No Incentive for Change: The Influence of Local Interests in Northwest Frontier Province, Pakistan. *Health Policy and Planning*. 10(Supplement): 40-48.

Lafond A. 1995c. Sustainability in the Health Sector: The Research Study. *Health Policy and Planning*. 10(Supplement): 1-5.

Laga M, AZ Meheus and P Piot. 1989. Epidemiology and Control of Gonococcal Opthalmia Neonatorum. *Bulletin of the World Health Organization*. 67: 471-477.

Lam C, M Catarivas, C Munro, et al. 1994. Self-Medication Among Hong Kong Chinese. *Social Science and Medicine*. 39(12): 1641-1647.

Lanata C, G Stroh, R Black, et al. 1990. Lot Quality Assurance Sampling in Health Monitoring. *Lancet*. 1: 122-123.

Langenbrunner J, M Borowitz, J Haycock, et al. 1994b. *Technical Assistance in Developing a Health Insurance Reform Demonstration in Issyk-kul Oblast, Kyrgyzstan: Progress, Problems, and Prospects.* Technical Report. 15. Abt Associates, Inc. Bethesda, MD.

Langenbrunner J, I Sheiman, S Zaman, et al. 1994a. *Evaluation of Health Insurance Demonstration in Kazakhstan: Dzeskasgan and South Kazakhstan Oblasts.* Technical Report. 14. Abt Associates, Inc. Bethesda, MD.

Larsen JV. 1992. Reducing the Perinatal Mortality Rate in Developing Countries. *Tropical Doctor*. 22(2): 49-51.

Lavy V and J Germain. 1994. *Quality and Cost in Health Care Choice in Developing Countries.* LSMS Working Paper No.105. Washington, DC: The World Bank.

Lavy V and JM Quigley. 1993. *Willingness to Pay for the Quality and Intensity of Medical Care: Low-income Households in Ghana.* LSMS Working Paper. 94. World Bank. Washington, DC.

Lawson JS and V Lin. 1994. Health Status Differential in the People's Republic of China. *American Journal of Public Health*. 84(5): 737-741.

Lee M. 1994. The Politics of Pharmaceutical Reform: The Case of the Philippine National Drug Policy. *International Journal of Health Services*. 24(3): 477-494.

Lerman SJ, DS Shepard and RA Cash. 1985. Treatment of Diarrhoea in Indonesian Children: What it Costs and Who Pays for It. *Lancet*. 2: 651-654.

Leslie C. 1976. Pluralism and Integration in the Indian and Chinese Medical Systems. In AK R Alexander and P Kunstadter, eds. *Medine in Chinese Cultures*. Washington, DC: The John E. Fogarty International Center, National Institutes of Health.

Lettenmeier C, L Liskin, CA Church, et al. 1988. *Mother's Lives Matter: Maternal Health in the Community.* Population Information Program. 7. Johns Hopkins University.

Levin HM. 1987. Economic Dimensions of Iodine Deficiency Disorders. In BS Hetzel, JT Dunn, and JB Stanbury, eds. *The Prevention and Control of Iodine Deficiency Disorders.* New York: Elsevier.

Levin HM, E Pollitt, R Galloway, et al. 1993. Micronutrient Deficiency Disorders. In DT Jamison, WH Mosley, et al., eds. *Disease Control Priorities in Developing Countries.* New York: Oxford University Press.

Levin J. 1996. How Religion Influences Morbidity and Health: Reflections on Natural History, Salutogenesis and Host Resistance. *Social Science and Medicine*. 43(5): 849-864.

Levin LS and E Ziglio. 1996. Helath Promotion as an Investment Strategy: Considerations on Theory and Practice. *Health Promotion International*. 11(1): 163-169.

Levine A and J Luck. 1994. *The New Management Paradigm: A Review of Principles and Practices*. MR-458-AF. RAND. Santa Monica, CA.

Levine M, G Losonsky, D Herrington, et al. 1986. Paediatric Diarrhoea: The Challenge of Prevention. *Paediatric Infectious Disease Journal*. 5: S29-S43.

Levit KR, HC Lazenby, BR Braden, CA Cowan, PA McDonnell, L. Sivarajan, JM Stiller, DK Won, CD Donham, AM Long and MW Stewart. 1996. National Health Expenditures, 1995. *Health Care Financing Review*. 18(1):175-214.

Lewis M. 1995. Private Payers of Care in Brazil: Characteristics, Costs and Coverage. *Health Policy and Planning*. 10(4): 362-375.

Lieberman S, B Stout and A Nyamete. 1994. *Indonesia's Health Work Force*. World Bank Report. 12835-IND. World Bank. Washington, DC.

Lindblom CE. 1977. *Politics and Markets*. New York: Basic Books.

Linn B. 1980. Continuing Medical Education: Impact on Emergency Room Burn Care. *Journal of the American Medical Association*. 244: 565-570.

Linsenmeyer W. 1989. Foreign Nations, International Organizations, and Their Impact on Health Conditions in Nicaragua Since 1979. *International Journal of Health Services*. 19: 509-529.

Litvack JI and C Bodart. 1993. User Fees Plus Quality Equals Improved Access to Health Care—Results of a Field Experiment in Cameroon. *Social Science and Medicine*. 37(3): 369-383.

Liu XZ and W Hsiao. 1995. The Cost Escalation of Social Health Insurance Plans in China—Its Implication for Public Policy. *Social Science and Medicine*. 41(8): 1095-1101.

Loevinsohn BP. 1990. Health Education Interventions in Developing Countries: A Methodological Review of Published Articles. *International Journal of Epidemiology*. 19(4): 788-794.

Loevinsohn BP. 1996. *Specific Challenges Facing the Health Sector in Asia*. Strategic Planning Workshop on Health Sector Policy Priorities. Asian Development Bank. Manila, Philippines.

Loevinsohn BP, ET Guerrero and SP Gregorio. 1995. Improving Primary Health Care Through Systematic Supervision: A Controlled Field Trial. *Health Policy and Planning*. 10(2): 144-153.

Lok SH. 1995. Market Reforms and China's Health Care System. *Social Science and Medicine*. 41(8): 1065.

Lomas J. 1991. Words Without Action? The Production, Dissemination, and Impact of Consensus Recommendations. *Annual Review of Public Health.* 12: 41-65.

Lomas J, GM Anderson, K Domnick-Pierre, et al. 1989. Do Practice Guidelines Guide Practice? *The New England Journal of Medicine.* 321: 1306-1311.

Long M. 1982. An Integrated Theory of Provider Behavior in Health Maintenance Organizations. *Journal of Community Health.* 8(2): 119-129.

Love RR. 1994. Clinical Trials and Practice Guidelines as Educational Methods in Developing Countries. *Journal of Cancer Education.* 9(4): 200-201.

Lowell J, C Richard Neu, and D Tong. 1998. Financial Crisis and Contagion in Emerging Market Countries. MR-962. RAND. Santa Monica, CA.

Luft H. 1978a. *Poverty and Health. Economic Causes and Consequences of Health Problems.* Cambridge, MA: Ballinger Press.

_____. 1978b. How Do Health Maintenance Organizations Achieve Their "Savings"? Rhetoric and Evidence. *New England Journal of Medicine.* 298(24): 1336-1343.

Luft H and E Morrison. 1991. Alternative Delivery Systems. In E Ginzberg, ed. *Health Services Research.* Cambridge, MA: Harvard University Press.

Lutter C. 1992. The Relationship Between Energy Intake and Diarrhea Disease in Their Effects on Child Growth: Biological Modelling, Evidence, and Implications for Public Health Policy. *Food and Nutrition Bulletin.* 14(1): 36-42.

Lwanga S and C Tye. eds. 1986. *Teaching Health Statistics, Twenty Lesson and Seminar Outlines.* Geneva: World Health Organization.

Lyttleton C. 1996. Health and Development: Knowledge Systems and Local Practice in Rural Thailand. *Health Transition Review.* 6(1): 25-48.

Maclure R. 1995. Primary Health Care and Donor Dependency: A Case Study of Nongovernment Assistance in Burkina Faso. *International Journal of Health Services.* 25(3): 539-558.

MacQueen KM, T Nopkesorn, MD Sweat, et al. 1996. Alcohol Consumption, Brothel Attendance, and Condom Use: Normative Expectations Among Thai Military Conscripts. *Medical Anthology Quarterly.* 10(3): 402-423.

Maine D. 1981. *Family Planning: Its Impact on the Health of Women and Children.* New York: Columbia University, Center for Population and Family Health.

Maine D, A Rosefield, M Wallace, et al. 1987. Prevention of Maternal Death in Developing Countries: Program Options and Practical Considerations. Paper presented at the International Safe Motherhood Conference, Feb. 10-13. Nairobi.

Makinen M. 1993. *Policy Options for Financing Health Services in Pakistan.* Summary Report. Volume 1. Abt Associates, Inc. Bethesda, MD.

Malaysia Ministry of Health. 1988. *National Health and Morbidity Survey 1986-87. Overview of Findings and Recommendations*. Malaysian Family Life Survey (MFLS-2). Ministry of Health. Kuala Lumpur.

Manderson L and PA Aby. 1992. Can Rapid Antropological Procedures Be Applied to Tropical Diseases? *Health Policy and Planning*. 7(1): 46-55.

Manderson L, T Mark and N Woelz. 1995. *Women's Participation In Health and Development Project*. Resource Paper. World Health Organization.

Manderson L, LB Valencia and B Thomas. 1992. *Bringing the People in: Community Participation and the Control of Tropical Disease*. Resource Papers for Social and Economic Research in Tropical Diseases. 1. World Health Organization.

Manning W, A Leibowitz, G Goldberg, et al. 1995. *A Controlled Trial of the Effect of a Prepaid Group Practice on the Utilization of Medical Services*. R-3029-HHS. RAND. Santa Monica, CA.

Manning WG. 1987. Health Insurance and the Demand for Medical Care: Evidence from a Randomized Experiment. *American Economic Review*. 77(3): 251-277.

Manning WG, A Leibowitz, GA Goldberg, et al. 1984. A Controlled Trial of the Effect of a Prepaid Group on the Use of Services. *New England Journal of Medicine*. 310(23): 1505-10.

Manning WG, JP Newhouse, N Duan, et al. 1988. *Health Insurance and the Demand for Medical Care: Evidence from a Randomized Experiment*. R-3476-HHS. RAND. Santa Monica, CA.

Mansergh G, A Haddix, R Steketee, et al. 1996. Cost-effectiveness of Short-Course Zidovudine to Prevent Perinatal HIV Type 1 Infection in a Sub-Saharan African Developing Country Setting. *Journal of the American Medical Association*. 276(2): 139-145.

Martines J, M Phillips and R Feachem. 1993. Diarrheal Diseases. In DT Jamison, WH Mosley, et al., eds. *Disease Control Priorities in Developing Countries*. New York: Oxford University Press.

Massaro TA and YN Wong. 1995. Positive Experience with Medical Savings Accounts in Singapore. *Health Affairs*. 14(2): 267-272.

Matejski M. 1982. Ethical Issues in the Health Care System. *Journal of Allied Health*. 11(2): 131-139.

Mathews P. 1993. Socio-Economic Determinants of Health Systems in India Under the Aspect of Colonial Structures—Kaifi, Ak. *Journal Of Contemporary Asia*. 23(2): 278-280.

Maticka-Tyndale E, M Haswell-Elkins and T Kuyyakonon. 1994. A Research-Based HIV Intervention in Northeast Thailand. *Health Transition Review*. 4(Supplement): 349-367.

Maung KU, M Khin and NN Wai. 1993. Risk Factors for Persistent Diarrhoea and Malnutrition in Burmese Children. *International Journal of Epidemiology*. 21(5): 1021-1029.

Maurice J. 1995. Malaria Vaccine Raises Dilemma. *Science*. 267(January 20): 320-323.

Max E and DS Shepard. 1989. Productivity Loss Due to Deformity from Leprosy in India. *International Journal of Leprosy*. 57(2): 476-482.

Maynard A. 1994. Can Competition Enhance Efficiency in Health Care? Lessons from the Reform of the U.K. National Health Service. *Social Science and Medicine*. 39(10): 1433-1445.

McDivitt JA, RC Hornik and CD Carr. 1994. Quality of Home Use of Oral Rehydration Solutions: Results from Seven Healthcom Sites. *Social Science and Medicine*. 38(9): 1221-1234.

McFarland D. 1993. *Health Insurance in Fiji*. Technical Note. 20. Abt Associates, Inc. Bethesda, MD.

McGeary M and PM Smith. 1996. The R&D Portfolio: A Concept for Allocating Science and Technology Funds. *Science*. 274: 1484-1485.

McHorney C and A Tarlov. 1995. Individual-Patient Monitoring in Clinical Practice: Are Available Health Status Surveys Adequate? *Quality of Life Research*. 4: 293-307.

Mckinlay J and S Mckinlay. 1977. The Questionable Contribution of Medical Measures to the Decline of Mortality in the United States in the Twentieth Century. *Milbank Memorial Fund Quarterly*. 55: 405-428.

McKinney JB. 1995a. The PPBS: A Rational Framework. In *Effective Financial Management in Public and Nonprofit Agencies*. Westport and London: Quorum Books.

McKinney JB. 1995b. *Effective Financial Management in Public and Nonprofit Agencies: A Practical and Integrative Approach*. Westport, CT: Quorum Books.

McLaughlin P and J Donaldson. 1991. Education of Continuing Medical Education Programs: Selected Literature, 1984-1988. *Journal of Continuing Education Health Professions*. 11:65-84.

McMillan A. 1993. Trends in Medicare Health Maintenance Organization Enrollment: 1986-93. *Health Care Financing Review*. 15(1): 135-146.

McPake B. 1993. User Charges for Health Services in Developing Countries: A Review of the Economic Literature. *Social Science and Medicine*. 36(11): 1397-1405.

McPake B and E Banda. 1994. Address: London School of Hygiene and Tropical Medicine, UK. Contracting out of Health Services in Developing Countries. *Health Policy and Planning*. 9(1): 25-30.

McPake B, K Hanson and A Mills. 1993. Community Financing of Health Care in Africa—An Evaluation of the Bamako Initiative. *Social Science and Medicine.* 36(11): 1383-1395.

McPake B and C Hongoro. 1995. Contracting Out of Clinical Services in Zimbabwe. *Social Science and Medicine.* 41(1): 13-24.

Meade T, S Dyer, W Browne, et al. 1990. Low Back Pain of Mechanical Origin: Randomized Comparison of Chiropractic and Hospital Outpatient Treatment. *British Medical Journal.* 300: 1431.

Meerman JP. 1979. *Public Expenditure in Malaysia: Who Benefits and Why.* New York: Oxford University Press.

Meheus A, KF Schulz and W Cates. 1990. Development of Prevention and Control Programs for Sexually Transmitted Diseases in Developing Countries. In K Holmes, P Mardh, et al., eds. *Sexually Transmitted Diseases, 2nd Edition.* New York: McGraw-Hill.

Melamid E and J Luck. 1994. Reinventing Government or Reinventing Wheels? Using New Management Practices in Public Organizations. Presented at the Association for Public Policy and Management Annual Conference. Chicago, IL.

Mendell M. 1989. Market Reforms and Market Failures—Karl Polanyi and the Paradox of Convergence. *Journal of Economic Issues.* 23(2): 473-481.

Mesa-Lago C. 1991. *Social Security and Prospects for Equity in Latin America.* World Bank Discussion Paper. 140. World Bank. Washington, DC.

Michaud C and C Murray. 1994. External Assistance to the Health Sector in Developing Countries, a Detailed Analysis, 1972-1990. *Bulletin of the World Health Organization.* 72(4): 639-651.

Miller RH and HS Luft. 1994a. Managed Care Plans: Characteristics, Growth, and Premium Performance. *Annual Review of Public Health.* 15: 437-459.

Miller RH and HS Luft. 1994b. Managed Care Plan Performance Since 1980: A Literature Analysis. *Journal of the American Medical Association.* 271(19): 1512-1519.

Mills A. 1990. *Health System Decentralization: Concepts, Issues, and Country Experience.* Geneva: World Health Organization.

Mills A. 1994. Decentralization and Accountability in the Health Sector. *Public Administration and Development.* 14: 281-292.

Mills ES and EM Pernia. 1994. Introduction and Overview, Chapter 1. In EM Pernia, ed. *Urban Poverty in Asia: A Survey of Critical Issues.* Hong Kong: Oxford University Press.

Miranda E, JL Scarpaci and I Izarrazaval. 1995. A Decade of HMOs in Chile: Market Behavior, Consumer Choice and the State. *Health and Place.* 1(1): 51-59.

Mitchell M, J Thomason, D Donaldson and P Garner. 1991. The Cost of Rural Health Services in Papua New Guinea. *Papua New Guinea Medical Journal.* 34:276-84.

Mitra SN, N Ali, S Islam, et al. 1994. *Bangladesh Demographic and Health Survey, 1993-1994.* National Institute of Population Research and Training; Mitra and Associates; and Macro International, Inc. Calverton, MD.

Mittman B and L Hilborne. 1995. Applying Practice Guidelines, Outcomes Research, and Research Recommendations. *Laboratory Practice and Management.* 1(4): 39-59.

Mittman B, L Hilborne and R Brook. 1994. Unpublished research on Developing Quality and Utilization Review Criteria from Clinical Practice Guidelines: Overview of the RAND Method. RAND. Santa Monica, CA.

Mittman B, D Kanouse, L Rubenstein, et al. 1995. Effecting Change in Physician Practice as Health Care Systems Consolidate. *Journal on Quality Improvement.* 21(10): 508-511.

Mittman B, X Tonesk and PD Jacobson. 1992. Implementing Clinical Practice Guidelines: Social Influence Strategies and Practitioner Behavior Change. *Quality Review Bulletin.* 18(12):413-421.

Mittman BS. 1994. Disseminating Clinical and Health-Related Information in Small Groups: a Social Influence Perspective. *Effective Dissemination of Clinical and Health Information.* Rockville, MD: Agency for Health Care Policy and Research.

Moens F. 1990. Implementation, and Evaluation of a Community Financing Scheme for Hospital Care in Developing Countries—A Pre-Paid Health Plan in the Bwamanda Health Zone, Zaire. *Social Science and Medicine.* 30(12): 1319-1327.

Mohan D and M Varghese. 1990. Fireworks Cast a Shadow on India's Festival of Lights. *World Health Forum.* 11:323-26.

Moidu K, O Wigertz and E Trell. 1991. A Multicenter Study of Data Collection and Communication at Primary Health Care Centers. *Journal of Medical Systems.* 15(3): 205-220.

Moidu K, O Wigertz and E Trell. 1992. Multi Centre Systems Analysis Study of Primary Health Care: A Study of Socio-Organizational and Human Factors. *International Journal of Bio-Medical Computing.* 30(1): 27-42.

Monny-Lobe M, D Nichols, L Zekeng, et al. 1989. Prostitutes as Health Educators for Their Peers in Yaounde: Changes in Knowledge, Attitudes and Practices. Paper presented at the 5th International Conference on AIDS. Montreal.

Mooney G and A Creese. 1993. Priority Setting for Health Service Efficiency: The Role of Measurement of Burden of Illness. In DT Jamison, WH Mosley, et al., eds. *Disease Control Priorities in Developing Countries.* New York: Oxford University Press.

Morgenstern H, G Gellert, S Walter, et al. 1984. The Impact of a Psychosocial Support Program on Survival with Breast Cancer: The Importance of Selection Bias in Program Evaluation. *Journal of Chronic Disability.* 37(4): 273-282.

Morrow RH and JH Bryant. 1995. Health Policy Approaches to Measuring and Valuing Human Life: Conceptual and Ethical Issues. *American Journal of Public Health.* 85(10):1356-1360.

Moses LE. 1992. Statistical Concepts Fundamental to Investigations. In JC Bailar and F Mosteller, eds. *Medical Uses of Statistics.* Boston, MA: NEJM Books.

Moses S. 1992. Impacts of User Fees on Attendance at a Referral Center for Sexually Transmitted Disease in Kenya. *Lancet.* 340: 463-466.

Mosley H and C Lincoln. 1984. *Child Survival: Strategies for Research.* New York: Population Council.

Muecke M. 1992. Mother Sold Food, Daughter Sells Her Body: The Cultural Continuity of Poverty. *Social Science and Medicine.* 35(7): 891-901.

Muller M and M Young. 1986. *Health Care in China: The Availability, Utilization, and Cost of County Hospitals.* Technical Note. 86-16. World Bank, Department of Population, Health, and Nutrition. Washington, DC.

Mulrow CD. 1987. The Medical Review Article: State of the Science. *Annals of Internal Medicine.* 106(3): 485-488.

Murray CJL. 1990. Rational Approaches to Priority Setting in International Health. *Journal of Tropical Medicine and Hygiene.* 93(5): 303-311.

_____. 1994. Quantifying the Burden of Disease: The Technical Basis for Disability-Adjusted Life Years. *Bulletin of the World Health Organization.* 72(3): 495-509.

_____. 1996. *Global Health Statistics: A Compendium of Incidence, Prevalence and Mortality Estimates for Over 200 Conditions.* Global Burden of Diseas and Injury Series. Cambridge, MA: Harvard University Press.

Murray CJL and R Feachem. 1990a. Adult Mortality In Developing Countries. *Transactions of the Royal Society of Tropical Medicine and Hygiene.* 84(1): 1-2.

Murray CJL, RG Feachem, MA Phillips, et al. 1992. Adult Morbidity: Limited Data and Methodological Uncertainty. In RG Feachem, T Kjellstrom, et al., eds. *The Health of Adults in the Developing World.* Oxford: Oxford University Press.

Murray CJL, R Govindaraj and P Musgrove. 1994. National Health Expenditures—A Global Analysis. *Bulletin of the World Health Organization.* 72(4): 623-637.

Murray CJL and AD Lopez. 1994. *Global Comparative Assessments in the Health Sector: Disease Burden, Expenditures and Intervention Packages.* Geneva: World Health Organization.

Murray CJL, AD Lopez and DT Jamison. 1994. The Global Burden of Disease in 1990. Summary Results, Sensitivity Analysis and Future Directions. *Bulletin of the World Health Organization*. 72(3): 495-509.

Murray CJL, K Styblo and A Rouillon. 1993. Tuberculosis. In DT Jamison, WH Mosley, et al., eds. *Disease Control Priorities in Developing Countries*. New York: Oxford University Press.

Murray CJL, G Yang and X Qiao. 1992b. Adult Mortality: Levels, Patterns, and Causes. In RG Feachem, T Kjellstrom, et al., eds. *The Health of Adults in the Developing World*. Oxford: Oxford University Press.

Murthy TG and S Laxminarayan. 1986. Health Care Technology and Third World Nations. *Proceedings of the Institute of Electrical and Electronic Engineers (IEEE) 8th Annual Conference of Engineering in Medicine and Biology*.

Musgrave RA and P Musgrave. 1989. *Public Finance in Theory and Practice*. New York: McGraw-Hill.

Musgrove P. 1986a. What Should Consumers in Poor Countries Pay for Publicly Provided Health Services? *Social Science and Medicine*. 22(3): 329-334.

_____. 1986b. Measurement of Equity in Health. *World Health Statistics Quarterly*. 39: 325-335.

_____. 1988. Is the Eradication of Polio in the Americas Economically Justified? *Bulletin of the Pan-American Health Organization*. 22(1): 1-16

_____. 1995a. Cost-Effectiveness and the Socialization of Health Care. *Health Policy*. 32(1-3): 111-123.

_____. 1995b. Cost-Effectiveness and the Health Sector Reform. *Salud Publica De Mexico*. 37(4): 363-374.

_____. 1996. *Public and Private Roles in Health: Theory and Financing Patterns*. Discussion Paper No. 339. Washington, D.C: World Bank.

Mwabu G, J Mwanzia and W Liambila. 1995. Use Charges in Government Health Facilities in Kenya: Effect on Attendance and Revenue. *Health Policy*. 10(2): 164-170.

Myers S and N Gleicher. 1988. A Successful Program to Lower Cesarean-Section Rates. *New England Journal of Medicine*. 319: 1511-1515.

Nagendra H and R Nagarathna. 1986. An Integrated Approach of Yoga Therapy for Bronchial Asthma. *Journal Asthma*. 23: 123-137.

Najera JA, BH Liese and J Hammer. 1993. Malaria. In DT Jamison, WH Mosley, et al., eds. *Disease Control Priorities in Developing Countries*. New York: Oxford University Press.

Nath L. 1996. Data Driven Priority Setting Through Health and Population Research. *ADB Conference on Health Policy Priorities in Asia, July, 1996*. Manila, Philippines: Asian Development Bank.

National Federation of Medical Insurance (1990-1994). 1994. *Yearbook of Health Insurance Statistics*. Seoul, Korea.

National Institute of Population Studies (NIPS) and IRD/Macro International (IRD). 1992. *Pakistan Demographic and Health Survey 1990/1991*. NIPS and IRD. Calverton, MD.

National Research Council. 1991. The Epidemiological Transition: Policy and Planning Implications for Developing Countries. *Workshop on the Policy and Planning Implications of the Epidemiological Transition in Developing Countries*. Washington, DC: National Academy Press.

National Statistics Office (NSO) [Philippines] and Macro International (MI). 1994. *National Demographic Survey 1993*. NSO and MI. Calverton, MD.

Nayeri K. 1996. Book Review: Murray and Lopez, *Global Comparative Assessments in the Health Sector: Disease Burden, Expenditures and Intervention Packages. Journal of Community Health*. 21(2): 153-154.

Neff JM and G Anderson. 1995. Protecting Children with Chronic Illness in a Competitive Marketplace. *Journal of the American Medical Association*. 274(23): 1866-1869.

Nelsen KE, DD Celentano and S Eiumtrakol. 1996. Changes in Sexual Behavior and a Decline in HIV Infection Among Young Men in Thailand. *New England Journal of Medicine*. 335(5): 297-303.

Nelson RH. 1987. The Economics Profession and the Making of Public Policy. *Journal of Economic Literature*. 25(March): 49-91.

Nerem R, M Levesque and J Cornhill. 1980. Social Environment as a Factor in Diet-Induced Atherosclerosis. *Science*. 208: 1475-1476.

Newbrander W, W Barnum and H Kutzin. 1992. *Hospital Economics and Financing in Developing Countries*. Geneva: World Health Organization.

Newbrander W, G Carrin and DL Touze. 1994. Developing Countries' Health Expenditure Information: What Exists and What is Needed? *Health Policy and Planning*. 9(4): 396-408.

Newbrander W (ed.). 1997. *Private Health Sector Growth in Asia: Issues and Implications*. England: John Wiley and Sons.

Newbrander WC and JA Thomason. 1988. Computerizing a National Health System in Papua New Guinea. *Health Policy and Planning*. 3(3): 255-259.

Newhouse JP. 1992. Medical Care Costs: How Much Welfare Loss? *The Journal of Economic Perspectives*. 6(3): 179-183.

_____. 1993a. *Free for All? Lessons from the RAND Health Insurance Experiment*. Cambridge, MA: Harvard University Press.

_____. 1993b. An Iconoclastic View of Health Care Cost Containment. *Health Affairs*. 152-171.

Newhouse JP, A Williams and B McGlynn. 1988. *Taiwan Health Study*. Project Description. RAND. Santa Monica, CA.

Newman TB, WS Browner, SR Cummings, et al. 1988. Designing a New Study: II. Cross-Sectional and Case-Control Studies. In SB Hulley and SR Cummings, eds. *Designing Clinical Research: An Epidemiologic Approach*. Baltimore: Williams and Wilkins.

Nguyen TH, L Ha, S Rifken, et al. 1995. The Pursuit of Equity: A Health Sector Case Study from Vietnam. *Health Policy*. 33: 191-204.

Nguyen TH and TT Tran. 1995. Vietnam: Appropriate Management of a Pediatric Hospital in the Context of Limited Resources. *Medecine Tropicale*. 55(3): 275-280.

Nhachi C and O Kasilo. 1993. Perception of Hospital Pharmacists/Dispensing Personnel of the Essential Drugs Concepts (EDC) in Zimbabwe. *East African Medical Journal*. 70(2): 94-7.

Nichter M. 1995. Vaccinations in the Third World: A Consideration of Community Demand. *Social Science and Medicine*. 41(5): 617-632.

Nielsen CC, MA Islam, SH Thilsted, et al. 1992. Why Do Some Families Become Defaulters in a Hospital Based Nutrition Rehabilitation Follow-Up Programme. *Tropical and Geographical Medicine*. 44: 346-351.

NIH Technology Assessment Panel. 1996. Integration of Behavioral and Relaxation Approaches into the Treatment of Chronic Pain and Insomnia. *Journal of the American Medical Association*. 276: 313-318.

Nittayaramphong S and V Tangcharoensathien. 1994. Thailand: Private Health Care Out of Control? *Health Policy and Planning*. 9(1): 31-40.

Njah M, J Helali and A Tabka. 1995. Determinant Factors in the Choice of Site of Delivery and the Role of Peripheral Maternity Units in a Semi-Urban Environment in Tunisia. *Revue Francaise de Gynecologie et d'Obstetrique*. 90(3): 148, 151-154.

Nur E and H Mahran. 1988. The Effect of Health on Agricultural Labor Supply: A Theoretical and Empirical Investigation. In A Herrin, ed. *Economics, Health and Tropical Diseases*. Manila: Manila School of Economics, University of the Philippines.

O'Brien J, T Wierzba and J Pikacha. 1994. Measuring Maternal Mortality in Developing Pacific Island Countries—Experience with the Sisterhood Method in the Solomon Islands. *New Zealand Medical Journal*. 107(981): 268-269.

Okun AM. 1975. *Equality and Efficiency: The Big Tradeoff*. Washington, DC: The Brookings Institution.

Okun DA. 1988. The Value of Water Supply and Sanitation in Development: An Assessment. *American Journal of Public Health*. 78(2): 1463-1467.

Olakowski T. 1973. *Assignment Report on a Tuberculosis Longitudinal Survey, National Tuberculosis Institute, Bangalore*. SEA/TB/129. World Health Organization. Geneva.

Oranga H and E Nordberg. 1993. The Delphi Panel Method for Generating Health Information. *Health Policy and Planning*. 8: 405-412.

Organization for Economic Cooperation and Development (OECD). 1980. *La Mortalite Dans Les Pays en Developement = Mortality in Developing Countries*. OECD Publications and Information Center. Washington, DC.

_____. 1978. *The Mortality Project in Developing Countries: Report of the Fourth Expert Group Meeting*. Paris: OECD Development Center.

Ornish D, S Brown, L Sherwitz, et al. 1990. Can Lifestyle Changes Reverse Coronary Heart Disease? The Lifestyle Heart Trial. *Lancet*. 336: 129-133.

Osteria T. 1991. *The Poor in ASEAN Cities: Perspectives in Health Care Management*. Social and Cultural Studies.

Over M, RP Ellis, JH Huber, et al. 1992. The Consequences of Adult Ill Health. In RG Feachem, T Kjellstrom, et al., eds. *The Health of Adults in the Developing World*. Oxford: Oxford University Press.

Over M and P Piot. 1993. HIV Infection and Sexually Transmitted Diseases. In DT Jamison, WH Mosley, et al., eds. *Disease Control Priorities in Developing Countries*. New York: Oxford University Press.

Oyoo A, B Burstrom, B Forsberg, et al. 1991. Rapid Feedback from Household Surveys in PHC Planning: An Example from Kenya. *Health Policy and Planning*. 6(4): 380-383.

Pakistan Federal Bureau of Statistics (FBS) and UNDP. 1992. *Pakistan Integrated Household Survey: Final Results, 1991*. Islamabad, Pakistan: FBS and UNDP.

Pannarounathai S. 1995. The Bed Census Survey: A Tool for Studying Hospital Inpatient Services. *Health Policy and Planning*. 10(4): 438-440.

Paphassarang C, G Tomson, C Choprapawon, et al. 1995. The Lao National Drug Policy: Lessons Along the Journey. *Lancet*. 345(Feb 18, 1995): 433-435.

Paredes P, MDL Pena, E Flores-Guerra, et al. 1996. Factors Influencing Physicians' Prescribing Behaviour in the Treatment of Childhood Diarrhoea: Knowledge May Not Be the Clue. *Social Science and Medicine*. 42(8): 1141-1153.

Paterson MA, Ponce N, and Peabody JW. 1997. *Integrated Information Systems: Managing Decisions, Informing Policy and Measuring Quality of Health Care Reform in Macedonia*. DRU-1615-1-WB. RAND. Santa Monica, CA.

Paul BK. 1992. Health Search Behavior of Parents in Rural Bangladesh: An Empirical Study. *Environment and Planning*. 24: 963-973.

Pauley M. 1986. Taxation, Health Insurance and Market Failure in the Medical Economy. *Journal of Economics Literature*. 24(June): 629-675.

Pauly M. 1968. The Economics of Moral Hazard. *American Economic Review*. 58(1): 531-537.

Peabody JW. 1994. *The Effects of Structure and Process of Medical Care on Birth Outcomes in Jamaica*. RGSD-112. RAND. Santa Monica, CA.

_____. 1995. An Organizational Analysis of the World Health Organization: Narrowing the Gap Between Promise and Performance. *Social Science and Medicine*. 40(6): 731-742.

_____. 1996a. Economic Reform and Health Sector Policy: Lessons From Structural Adjustment Programs. *Social Science and Medicine*. 43(5): 823-835.

_____. 1996b. *Quality of Care: Key Policy Issues*. Viet Nam National Health Survey Background Paper. RAND. Santa Monica, CA.

Peabody JW, V Agadjanian, G Carter, et al. 1995a. *Advancing Health Care Reform in Ecuador: Analysis of Current Options*. DRU-963-IADB. RAND. Santa Monica, CA.

Peabody JW and P Gertler. 1996. Are Clinical Criteria Just Proxies for Socioeconomic Status? A Study of Low Birthweight in Jamaica. *Journal of Epidemiology and Community Health*. 51(1): 90-95.

Peabody JW, K Edwards, S Maerki, et al. 1996a. *Papua New Guinea National Health Plan. Technical Report: The Epidemiological and Organizational Analysis*. DRU-1223-1-ADB. RAND. Santa Monica, CA.

Peabody J, P Gertler and A Leibowitz. 1998a. The Policy Implications of Better Structure and Process on Birth Outcomes in Jamaica. *Health Policy*. 43:1-13.

Peabody JW, T Hesketh and J Kattwinkel. 1992. Creation of a Neonatology Facility in a Developing Country: Experience from a Five Year Project in China. *American Journal of Perinatology*. 5(6): 401-408.

Peabody JW, T Hesketh and P Steinberg. 1996b. Translating Clinical Practice into Health Policy: An Example From China. *Health Policy*. 35(2): 107-122.

Peabody JW, J Lawson and S Bickel. 1996c. The Health Care System in Australia: Is Down Under Right Side Up? *Journal of the American Medical Association*. 276(24): 1944-1950.

Peabody JW, J Luck, P Glassman, T Dresselhaus, and M. Lee. 1998b. Measuring the Quality of Care: A Prospective Trial Using Vignettes. [Abstract.] Presented at the Association of Health Services Research/Foundation for Health Services Research Annual Meeting, 1998.

Peabody JW, DH Lee, BM Yang, et al. 1997. Financing Health Care for the Elderly: Will an Aging Population End "Health for All" in South Korea? *Abstracts of the Society of General Internal Medicine, 1996.*

Peabody JW, SW Lee and S Bickel. 1994. Health for All in the Republic of Korea: One Country's Experience with Implementing Universal Health Care. *Health Policy.* 30(2): 29-42.

Peabody JW and S Maerki. 1995. *Papua New Guinea National Health Plan: Inception Report.* DRU-1097-ADB. RAND. Santa Monica, CA.

Peabody JW, S Maerki and JW Molyneaux. 1996d. *Papua New Guinea. The 1996-2000 National Health Plan: Budget Contingencies, Implementation Plans and Final Recommendation.* DRU-1377-1-ADB. RAND. Santa Monica, CA.

Peabody, Nordyke and Ponce. Macedonia 1998c. *Facility and Household Survey: Evaluating the Impact of Policy on Health and Provider Behavior.* DRU-1111-WB. RAND. Santa Monica, CA.

Peabody JW, O Rahman, K Fox, et al. 1994. Public and Primary Delivery of Health Care Services in Jamaica: A Comparison of Quality in Different Types of Facilities. *Bulletin of the Pan American Health Organization.* 28(2): 122-141.

Peabody JW, A Ruby and P Cannon. 1995b. An Economic Model and Policy Analysis of the Orphan Drug Act: Can the Current Legislation be Improved? *PharmoEconomics.* 8(5): 374-384.

Peabody JW and JM Schmitt. 1992. Medical Equipment in the People's Republic of China: A Survey of Medical Equipment Procurement, Utilization, and Maintenance in University Affiliated Hospitals Between 1976 and 1987. *International Journal of Technology Assessment in Health Care.* 8: 138-149.

Peabody JW, J Yu, Y Wang, et al. 1995c. Health System Reform in the Republic of China: Formulating Policy in a Market-Based Health System. *Journal of the American Medical Association.* 273(10): 777-781.

Pearson TA, DT Jamison and JT Gutierrez. 1993. Cardiovascular Disease. In DT Jamison, WH Mosley, et al., eds. *Disease Control Priorities in Developing Countries.* New York: Oxford University Press.

Pebley AR. 1992. Book Review: Child Mortality Since the 1960s—A Database for Developing Countries. *Population and Development Review.* 18(4): 760-762.

Pelc A. 1994. Presenting Economic Information for Decision Making. *Pharmoeconomics.* 6(4):346-351.

Pelletier DL. 1994. The Relationship Between Child Anthropometry and Mortality in Developing Countries—Implications for Policy, Programs and Future Research. *Journal of Nutrition*. 124(10): S2047-S2081.

Pelletier DL, EA Frongillo, DG Schroeder, et al. 1994. A Methodogy for Estimating the Contribution of Malnutrition to Child Mortality in Developing Countries. *Journal of Nutrition*. 124(October 10): S2106-S2122.

Pelletier DL, EA Frongillo, DG Schroeder, et al. 1995. The Effects of Malnutrition on Child Mortality in Developing Countries. *Bulletin of the World Health Organization*. 73(4): 443-448.

Pelto GH. 1996. Using Ethnography in the WHO Programme for the Control of Acute Respiratory Infection. *Practicing Anthropology*. 18(3): 28-31.

Peltzman S. 1976. Toward a More General Theory of Regulation. *Journal of Law and Economics*. August(19): 2.

Peto R, Z Chen and J Boreham. 1996. Tobacco—The Growing Epidemic in China. *Journal of the American Medical Association*. 275(21): 1683-1684.

Phelps C. 1991. On the New Equivalence of Cost-Effectiveness and Cost-Benefit Analysis. *International Journal of Technology Assessment in Health Care*. 7: 12-21.

Philippines National Statistics Office and Macro International. 1994. *National Demographic Survey 1993*. Calverton, MD: NSO and MI.

Phillips JD, G Carrin and M Vereecke. 1994. Strategies for Health Care Finance in Developing Countries with a Focus on Community Financing in Sub-Saharan Africa. *Journal of Developing Areas*. 29(1):146-147.

Phillips JF and JA Ross. 1992. *Family Planning Programmes and Fertility*. New York: Oxford University Press.

Phillips JF, R Simmons, MA Koenig, et al. 1988. Determinants of Reproductive Change in a Traditional Society: Evidence from Matlab, Bangladesh. *Studies in Family Planning*. 19(6): 313-334.

Phillips JF, WS Stinson, S Bhatia, et al. 1982. The Demographic Impact of the Family Planning—Health Services Project in Matlab, Bangladesh. *Studies in Family Planning*. 13(5): 131-140.

Phillips R. 1975. Role of Life-Style and Dietary Habits in Risk of Cancer Among Seventh-Day Adventists. *Cancer Research*. 35: 3513-3522.

Philpott S, M Milimo and M Mufwaya. 1993. *Mid-Term Evaluation Report, South Samfya Community Health and Development Project, Zambia, For the People and Government of Zambia, Implemented by World Vision Zambia and World Vision Australia*. Unpublished report. AIDAB. Canberra, Australia.

Physician Payment Review Commission (PPRC). 1996. *Annual Report to Congress*. Physician Payment Review Commission. Washington, DC.

Pinstrup-Anderson P, S Burger, J-P Habicht, et al. 1993. Protein-Energy Malnutrition. In DT Jamison, WH Mosley, et al., eds. *Disease Control Priorities in Developing Countries*. New York: Oxford University Press.

Piot P and KK Holmes. 1989. Sexually Transmitted Diseases. In *Tropical and Geographical Medicine*. New York: McGraw-Hill.

Pitt M, MR Rosenzweig and DM Gibbons. 1994. The Determinants and Consequences of the Placement of Government Programs in Indonesia. *World Bank Economic Review*. 7: 319-348.

Pitt MM and MR Rosenzweig. 1990. Estimating the Intrahousehold Incidence of Illness—Child Health and Gender—Inequality in the Allocation of Time. *International Economic Review*. 31(4): 969-989.

Pitt MM, MR Rosenzweig and MN Hassan. 1990. Productivity, Health, and Inequality in the Intrahousehold Distribution of Food in Low-Income Countries. *American Economic Review*. 80(5): 1139-1156.

Pohlmeier W and V Ulrich. 1994. An Econometric Model of the Two-Part Decisionmaking Process in the Demand for Health Care. *Journal of Human Resources*. 30(2): 339-361.

Poore P. 1992. Availability of Quality Vaccines: Policies of a Non-Government Organization. *Vaccine*. 10(13): 958-960.

Popkin B and E Bisgrove. 1988. Urbanization and Nutrition in Low-Income Countries. *Food and Nutrition Bulletin*. 10(1): 3-23.

Population Reports. 1980. *Radio—Spreading the Word on Family Planning*. 32. Population Information Programs, Johns Hopkins University.

Population Reports. 1985. *Radio—Spreading the Word on Family Planning*. 32. Population Information Programs, Johns Hopkins University.

Population Reports. 1986. *Radio—Spreading the Word on Family Planning*. Series J. 32. Population Information Programs, Johns Hopkins University.

Posnett J and A Street. 1996. Programme Budgeting and Marginal Analysis: An Approach to Priority Setting in Need of Refinement. *Journal of Health Services Research and Policy*. 1(3): 147-153.

Prasad B and AM De L Costello. 1995. Impact and Sustainability of a "Baby Friendly" Health Education Intervention at a District Hospital in Bihar, India. *British Medical Journal*. 310(6980): 621-623.

Preker A and R Feacham. 1995. Market Mechanisms and the Health Sector in Central and Eastern Europe. *World Bank Technical Paper*. 293(December).

Preston SH, N Keyfitz and R Schoen. 1972. *Causes of Death: List Tables for National Populations*. New York: Seminar Press.

Price M. 1992. Health Maintenance Organizations. *Nursing RSA Verpleging.* 7(6): 21-23.

Pritchett L and L Summers. 1993. *Wealthier is Healthier.* Policy Research Working Papers World Development Report. WPS 1150. World Bank. Washington, DC.

Pritchett L and L Summers. 1996. Wealthier Is Healthier. *The Journal of Human Resources.* 31(4): 841-868.

Prochaska JO and CC DiClemente. 1983. Stages and Processes of Self-Change of Smoking: Toward and Integrative Model of Change. *Journal of Consulting and Clinical Psychology.* 51: 390-395.

Prochaska JO and CC DiClemente. 1984. *The Transtheoretical Approach: Crossing the Traditional Boundaries of Therapy.* Homewood, IL: Dorsey Press.

Prochaska JO, CC DiClemente and JC Norcross. 1992. In Search of How People Change, Applications to Addictive Behaviors. *American Psychologist.* 47(9): 1102-1114.

Prochaska JO, WF Velicer, JS Rossi, et al. 1994. Stages of Change and Decisional Balance for 12 Problem Behaviors. *Health Psychology.* 13(1): 39-46.

Program for Appropriate Technology in Health (PATH). 1993. *Development and Introduction of Technologies for Health in the Developing World.* PATH. Seattle.

Propper C. 1995. Agency and Incentives in the NHS Internal Market. *Social Science and Medicine.* 40(12): 1683-1690.

Prospective Payment Assessment Commission (ProPac). 1996. *Report and Recommendations to the Congress.* Prospective Payment Assessment Commission. Washington, DC.

Prost A and M Jancloes. 1993. Rationales for Choices in Public Health: The Role of Epidemiology. In DT Jamison, WH Mosley, et al., eds. *Disease Control Priorities in Developing Countries.* New York: Oxford University Press.

Prud'homme R. 1995. The Dangers of Decentralization. *World Bank Research Observer.* 10(2):201-220.

Puska P. 1995. Health Promotion Challenges for Countries of the Former Soviet Union—Results from Collaboration Between Estonia, Russian Karelia and Finland. *Health Promotion International.* 10(3): 219-228.

Qiu RZ. 1989. Equity and Public Health Care in China. *Journal of Medicine and Philosophy.* 14(3): 283-287.

Quade ES. 1989. *Analysis for Public Decisions.* New York: North-Holland.

Quibria MG. 1994. *Rural Poverty in Developing Asia. Volume I: Bangladesh, India, and Sri Lanka.* Manila, Philippines: Asian Development Bank.

Racelis R and A Herrin. 1994. *NHA of the Philippines: Partial Estimates*. World Bank. Washington, DC.

Raghupathy S. 1996. Education and the Use of Maternal Health Care in Thailand. *Social Science and Medicine*. 43(4): 459-471.

Rahman MC, LC Chen, J Chakrabory, et al. 1982. Use of Tetanus Toxoid for the Prevention of Neonatal Tetanus. I. Reduction of Neonatal Mortality by Immunization of Non-Pregnant and Pregnant Women in Rural Bangladesh. *Bulletin of the World Health Organization*. 60: 261-267.

Rahman MM, MA Islam and D Mahalanabis. 1994. Impact of Health Education on the Feeding of Green Leafy Vegetables at Home to Children of the Urban Poor Mothers of Bangladesh. *Public Health*. 108: 211-218.

Rahman O, A Foster and J Menken. 1992. Older Widow Mortality in Rural Bangladesh. *Social Science and Medicine*. 34(1): 89-96.

Rahman O, J Strauss, P Gertler, et al. 1994. Gender Differences in Adult Health. An International Comparison. *Gerontologist*. 34(4): 131-149.

Ramachandruda G and G Kamalamma. 1991. Health Planning in India—A Critical Evaluation. *Journal of Rural Development*. 10(3): 299-310.

Rannan-Eliya R and N de Mel. 1996. *Resource Mobilization in Sri Lanka*. Draft Report. Sri Lanka, Colombo.

Ravallion M. 1992. *Poverty Comparisions: A Guide to Concepts and Methods*. Living Standards Measurement Study Working Paper. 88. World Bank. Washington, DC.

Rawls J. 1971. *A Theory of Justice*. Cambridge: Harvard University Press.

Razali MS. 1995. Psychiatrists and Folk Healers in Malaysia. *World Health Forum*. 16: 56.

Regan W. 1982. Hospital Liable for Physician Negligence Under Principal-Agent Relationship. *Hospital Progress*. 63(8): 64-66.

Registrar General of India. 1993. Estimated Infant Mortality Rates. Sample Registration System. Government of India: Delhi.

Reich J. 1987. The International Conference on Better Health for Women and Children Through Family Planning. *International Family Planning Perspectives*. 13: 86-89.

Reich MR. 1995. The Politics of Health Sector Reform in Developing Countries—3 Cases of Pharmaceutical Policy. *Health Policy*. 32(1): 47-77.

Reid AJ. 1990. Maternal Mortality—Preventing the Tragedy in Developing Countries. *Canadian Family Physician*. 36(January): 87-91.

Reports P. 1980. *Oral Rehydration Therapy (ORT) for Childhood Diarrhea*. Series L. 2. Population Information Programs, Johns Hopkins University.

Reports P. 1985. Contraceptive Social Marketing: Lessons from Experience. *Population Information Programs, Johns Hopkins University*. Series J(30).

Revisions to the National Health Accounts and Methodology. 1990. Conference Proceedings. *HCF Review*. 11(4): 42-120.

Richards DN. 1975. Methods and Effectiveness of Health Education: The Past, Present and Future of Social Scientific Involvement. *Social Science and Medicine*. 9: 141-156.

Richards FO, RE Klein, C Gonzales-Peralta, et al. 1995. Knowledge, Attitudes and Practices During a Community-Level Ivermectin Distribution Campaign in Guatemala. *Health Policy and Planning*. 10(4): 404-414.

Riegel B, D Simon, SR Bickel, et al. 1998. Teaching Ayurveda and Western Health Promotion Strategies to Healthy Adults. *American Journal of Health Promotion*. 12(4):258-61.

Riehman K. 1996. *Drug Use and AIDS in Developing Countries: Issues for Policy Consideration*. Report on AIDS and Development. World Bank. Washington, DC.

Rifkin S. 1990. *Community Participation in Maternal and Child Health/Family Planning Programmes*. World Health Organization.

Rifkin SB. 1973. Public Health in China—Is the Experience Relevant to Other Less Developed Nations? *Social Science and Medicine*. 7: 249-257.

Robertson RL. 1979. *Guidelines for Analysis of Health Sector Financing in Developing Countries*. Rockville, Maryland: Department of Health and Welfare, Public Health Service, Office of the Assistant Secretary for Health, Office of International Health.

Robey JM and SH Lee. 1990. Information System Development in Support of National Health Programme Monitoring and Evaluation: The Case of the Philippines. *World Health Statistics Quarterly*. 43: 37-46.

Robinson J. 1993. Payment Mechanisms, Nonprice Incentives, and Organizational Innovations in Health Care. *Inquiry*. 30(3): 328-333.

Rodgers GB. 1979. Income and Inequality as Determinants of Mortality: An International Cross-Section Analysis. *Population Studies*. 33(2): 343-351.

Roemer M. 1991. *National Health Systems of the World, the Countries*. Oxford University Press.

Roemer R. 1987. *Legislative Strategies for a Smoke-Free Europe*. Copenhagen: World Health Organization;

Rogers J. 1982. Medical Information Systems: Assessing Impact in Areas of Hypertension, Obesity and Renal Disease. *Medical Care*. 20:63-74.

Ron A. 1993. *Planning and Implementing Health Insurance in Developing Countries: Guidelines and Case Studies*. Macroeconomics, Health and Development Series. 7. World Health Organization. Geneva.

Roodenbeke Ed. 1994. A Future Path Toward Cooperation: Hospital Partnership. *Sante*. 4(1): 105-109.

Rosen M and L Lindholm. 1992. The Neglected Effects of Lifestyle Interventions in Cost-Effectiveness Analysis. *Health Promotion International*. 7(3): 163-170.

Rosenblatt RA. 1997. Cost of Health Care for State's Big Firms Falls 2.5% in 1996. *Los Angeles Times*. 21 January 1997. D1.

Rosenfeld A. 1981. Factors Affecting Home Health Agency Behavior: An Interactionist View. *Home Health Care Services Quarterly*. 2(2): 59-100.

Rosenfield A. 1989. Maternal Mortality in Developing Countries—An Ongoing but Neglected Epidemic. *Journal of the American Medical Association*. 262(3): 376-379.

Rosenzweig MR and KI Wolpin. 1982. Governmental Interventions and Household Behavior in a Developing Country. *Journal of Development Economics*. 10: 209-225.

Rosenzweig MR and KI Wolpin. 1986. Evaluating the Effects of Optimally Distributed Public Programs: Child Health and Family Planning Interventions. *American Economic Review*. 76: 470-482.

Ross D, B Kirkwood, F Binka, P Arthur, N Dollimore, S Morris, et al. 1995. Child Morbidity and Mortality Following Vitamin A Supplementation in Ghana. *American Journal of Public Health* . 85:1246-51.

Ross-Degnan D, R Laing, J Quick, et al. 1992. A Strategy for Promoting Improved Pharmaceutical Use: The International Network for Rational Use of Drugs. *Social Science and Medicine*. 35(11): 1329-1341.

Ross-Degnan D, SB Soumerai, PK Goel, et al. 1996. The Impact of Face-to-Face Educational Outreach on Diarrhoea Treatment in Pharmacies. *Health Policy and Planning*. 11(3): 308-318.

Rubenstein L. 1992. *Proposal, Center for the Study of Clinical Decision Making and Provider Behavior*. Sepulveda Veterans Affairs Medical Center. Los Angeles, CA.

Rutenberg N, M Ayad, L Ochoa, et al. 1991. *Knowledge and Use of Contraception*. Demographic and Health Surveys Comparative Studies. 6. Institute for Resource Development/ Macro Systems, Inc.

Rutten F. 1996a. Economic Evaluation and Health Care Decision Making. *Health Policy*. 36:215-229.

Rutten F. 1996b. The Impact of Health Economics on Health Policy and Practice. *Journal of Health Services and Resource Policy*. 1(2): 62-63.

Sachs J. 1996. Economic Growth: The Poor and the Rich. *The Economist*. 339(7967):23-35.

Sacks H. 1962. Randomized Versus Historical Controls for Clinical Trials. *American Journal of Medicine*. 72: 233-240.

Sahn D and H Alderman. 1996. The Effect of Food Subsidies on Labor Supply in Sri Lanka. *Economic Development and Cultural Change*. 45(1): 125-145.

Samuel P. 1995. *Capacity Building for Health Sector Reform*. WHO document. WHO/SHS/NHP/95.8. World Health Organization. Geneva.

Sandiford P, H Annett and R Cibulskis. 1992. What Can Information Systems Do for Primary Health Care? An International Perspective. *Social Science and Medicine*. 34(10): 1077-1087.

Satia JK, DV Mavalankar and B Sharma. 1994. Micro-Level Planning Using Rapid Assessment for Primary Health Care Services. *Health Policy and Planning*. 9(3): 318-330.

Schecter K. 1992. Soviet Socialized Medicine and the Right to Health Care in a Changing Soviet-Union. *Human Rights Quarterly*. 14(2): 206-215.

Schell F, B Allolio and O Schonecke. 1994. Physiological and Psychological Effects of Hatha-Yoga Exercise in Healthy Women. *International Journal Psychosomatics*. 41: 46-52.

Scheyer S. 1995. *Phillipines' Women's Health and Safe Motherhood Project*. Staff Appraisal Report. World Bank. Washington, DC.

Schmidt S. 1995. Social Security in Developing Countries—Basic Tenets and Fields of State Intervention. *International Social Work*. 38(1):7-26.

Schmitt J. 1996. Unpublished paper on program for optimally utilizing medical technology over its entire life cycle.

Schmitt J and D Qing. 1987. Requirements for Clinical Engineering Development. *Proceedings Zhejiang University Biomedical Society Meeting*. Hangzhou, China.

Schmitt JM. 1990. *Planned Maintenance and Repair of Medical Equipment in the Kosrae and Truk States, Micronesia*. Short-Term Consultant Report. World Health Organization (Pacific Region).

Schmitt JM. 1993. *Five-Year Follow-Up Report on Project HOPE's Biomedical Engineering Programs in Shanghai and Hangzhou, China*. Short-Term Consultant Report, Project HOPE.

Schmitt JM and H Al-Fadel. 1989. Design of Medical Instrumentation for Application in Developing Countries. *Journal of Clinical Engineering*. 14(4): 298-306.

Schmitt JM and D-R Qing. 1987a. Design of Medical Instrumentation for Application in Developing Countries. *Proceedings of the Zhejiang University, Biomedical Engineering Society Meeting*. Hangzhou, China.

Schroeder D, R Martorell, J Rivera, and MT Ruel. 1995. Age Differences on the Impact of Nutritional Supplementation on Growth. *Journal of Nutrition*. 125:1051S-1059S.

Schwartz D. 1985. Caribbean Folk Beliefs and Western Psychiatry. *Journal of Psychosocial Nursing and Mental Health Services*. 26: 26.

Schwartz WB. 1987. The Inevitable Failure of Current Cost-Containment Strategies. *Journal of the American Medical Association*. 1987(2): 220-223.

Schwiebert R and PN Fultz. 1994. Immune Activation and Viral Burden in Acute Disease Induced by Simian Immunodeficiency Virus Sivsmmpbj 14—Correlation in Vitro and in Vivo Events. *Journal of Virology*. 68(9): 5538-5547.

Schwuebel V. 1994. The DALY—An Indicator to Measure Disease Burden. *Revue D Epidemiologie Et De Sante Publique*. 42(2): 183-184.

Scrimshaw N and G Gleason. 1992. *Rapid Assessment Procedures: Qualitative Methodologies for Planning and Evaluation of Health Related Programs*. International Nutrition Foundation for Developing Countries.

Seer P and J Raeburn. 1980. Meditation Training and Essential Hypertension. *Journal of Behavioral Medicine*. 3: 59-71.

Sen A. 1985. *Commodities and Capabilities*. Amsterdam: North-Holland.

Sepehri A and J Pettigrew. 1996. Primary Health Care, Community Participation and Community-Financing—Experiences of Two Middle Hill Villages in Nepal. *Health Policy and Planning*. 11(1): 93-100.

Sewell D. 1996. The Dangers of Decentralization According to Prud'homme: Some Further Aspects. *World Bank Research Observer*. 11(1): 143-150.

Shackley P and A Healey. 1995. Creating a Market: An Economic Analysis of the Purchaser-provider Model. *Health Policy*. 25: 153-168.

Shah P, K Wagh, P Kulkarni, et al. 1975. The Impact of Hospital and Domiciliary Nutrition Rehabilitation on Diet of the Child and Other Young Children in the Family and in Neighborhood. *Indian Pediatrics*. 12(1): 95-98.

Sharma RC, HM Thaker, AS Gautam, et al. 1992. Gujarat Model of Health Management Information System with Reference to Malaria. *Indian Journal of Malariology*. 29: 11-22.

Sheldon T and I Chalmers. 1994. The UK Cochrane Centre and the NHS Centre for Reviews and Dissemination: Respective Roles Within the Information Systems

Strategy of the NHS R&D Programme, Coordination and Principles Underlying Collaboration. *Health Economics.* 3:201-203.

Shepard DS, LE Brenzel and KT Nemeth. 1986. *Cost Effectiveness of Oral Rehydration Therapy for Diarrhoeal Diseases.* PHN Technical Note. 86-26. World Bank, Population, Health and Nutrition Department. Washington, DC.

Shepard DS and SB Halstead. 1993. Dengue (with notes on yellow fever) and Japanese Encephalitis. In DT Jamison, WH Mosley, et al., eds. *Disease Control Priorities in Developing Countries.* New York: Oxford University Press.

Shi LY. 1993. Health Care in China—A Rural-Urban Comparison After the Socioeconomic Reforms. *Bulletin of the World Health Organization.* 71(6): 723-736.

Shortell S and U Reinhardt. eds. 1992. *Improving Health Policy and Management, Nine Critical Research Issues for the 1990s.* Ann Arbor: Health Administration Press.

Shucheng W. 1996. *The Reform of the Rural Cooperative Medical System in the People's Republic of China Initial Design and Interim Experience.* WHO Document. WHO/ICO/MESD.20. World Health Organization. Geneva.

Shultz T and A Tansel. 1993. *Measurement of Returns to Adult Health, Morbidity Effects on Wage Rates in Cote d'Ivoire and Ghana.* LSMS Working Paper. 95. World Bank. Washington, DC.

Sidel VW. 1993. New Lessons From China—Equity and Economics in Rural Health Care. *American Journal of Public Health.* 83(12): 1665-1666.

Simmons J. 1978. Program Planning in Health Education. *Public Health Reviews.* 7(3-4): 271-311.

Singh AK, K Moidu, E Trell, et al. 1992. Impact on Management and Delivery of Primary Health Care by a Computer-Based Information System. *Computer Methods and Programs and Programs in Biomedicine.* 37: 55-64.

Singh VA, A Wisniewski, J Britton, et al. 1990. Effect of Yoga Breathing Exercise (Pranayama) on Airway Reactivity in Subjects with Asthma. *Lancet.* 335(8702): 1381-1383.

Smego RA and PV Barrett. 1990. Health Care and the Private Sector in the Third-World. *Academic Medicine.* 65(2): 100.

Smillie JG. 1991. *Can Physicians Manage the Quality and Costs of Health Care?: The Story of the Permanente Medical Group.* New York: McGraw-Hill.

Smith CJ. 1993. (Over) Eating Success—The Health Consequences of the Restoration of Capitalism in Rural China. *Social Science and Medicine.* 37(6): 761-770.

Smith HE. 1982. Doctors and Society: A Northern Thailand Study. *Social Science and Medicine.* 16(5):515-26.

Smithson P. 1995. Quarts Into Pint Jugs? The Financial Viability of Health Sector Investment in Low Income Countries. *Health Policy and Planning*. 10(Supplement): 6-16.

Snow RW, N Peshu, D Forster, H Mwenesi, and K March. 1992. The Role of Shops in the Treatment and Prevention of Childhood Malaria on the Coast of Kenya. *Transactions of the Royal Society of Tropical Medicine and Hygiene*. 86(3):237-9.

Solon O. 1995. Addressing Possible Adverse Responses to National Health Insurance. Department of Economics working paper. University of the Philippines, Quezon City.

Solon O, S. Alalbastro, J Capuno, R Sumulong, F Quising, and C Tan. 1997. The Challenge of Health Care Financing Reforms in the Philippines. Integrative Report of the DOH-PIDS Project "Baseline Research in Health Care Financing Reform." Philippine Institute of Development Studies, Manila.

Solon O, R Gamboa, JB Schwartz, et al. 1992. *Health Sector Financing in the Philippines*. Department of Health, Republic of the Philippines. Manila.

Solon O, S Sumulong, C Tan, J Capunoi, P Quising and S. Alabastro. 1995. The Challenge of Health Care Financing Reform in the Philippines. Final Report of the DOH-PIDS, "Baseline Research on Health Care Financing Reform." Philippine Institute of Development Studies, Manila.

Sommer A, E Djunaedi, A Loeden, I Tarwotjo, K West, R Tilden, et al. 1986. Impact of Vitamin A Supplementation on Childhood Mortality. *Lancet*. 1:1169-73.

Sommerfelt A and M Stewart. 1994. *Children's Nutritional Status*. Demographic and Health Surveys Comparative Studies. 12. Institute for Resource Development/ Macro Systems, Inc.

Song Y and A Luo. 1995. Hospital Information Systems in China. *MEDINFO 95*.

Spiegel D, JR Bloom and HC Kraemer. 1989. Effect of Psychosocial Treatment on Survival of Patients with Metastatic Breast Cancer. *Lancet*. 2(8668): 888-891.

Spika JS, MH Munshi, B Wojtyniak, et al. 1989. Acute Lower Respiratory Infections: A Major Cause of Death in Children in Bangladesh. *Annals of Tropical Paediatrics*. 9: 33-39.

Srilatha V and IW Aitken. 1991. A Health Risk Index for Assessing PHC Coverage in Urban India. *Health Policy and Planning*. 6(3): 234-243.

Stanley K. 1993. Control of Tobacco Production and Use. In DT Jamison, WH Mosley, et al., eds. *Disease Control Priorities in Developing Countries*. New York: Oxford University Press.

Stansfield S. (ed). 1990. *Potential Savings Through Reduction of Inappropriate Use of Pharmaceuticals in the Treatment of ARI*. Balitmore, Maryland: Johns Hopkins University School of Hygiene and Public Health, Institute of International Programs.

Stansfield S and D Shepard. 1993. Acute Respiratory Infection. In Jamison D, Mosley W, Measham A, Bobadilla J, eds. *Disease Control Priorities in Developing Countries.* New York: Oxford University Press. 67-90.

Stanton B and A Wouters. 1992. Guidelines for Pragmatic Assessment for Health Planning in Developing Countries. *Health Policy.* 21: 187-209.

Stanton BF, JD Clemens, T Khair, et al. 1987. An Educational Intervention for Altering Water-Sanitation Behaviours to Reduce Childhood Diarrhoea in Urban Bangladesh: Formulation, Preparation and Delivery of Educational Intervention. *Social Science and Medicine.* 24(3): 275-283.

Steinglass R, L Brenzel and A Percy. 1993. Tetanus. In DT Jamison, WH Mosley, et al., eds. *Disease Control Priorities in Developing Countries.* New York: Oxford University Press.

Steiss AW. 1989. *Financial Management in Public Organizations.* Pacific Grove, CA: Brooks/Cole Pub. Co.

Stephens C, M Akerman and PB Maia. 1995. Health and Environment in Sao Paulo, Brazil: Methods of Data Linkage and Questions of Policy. *World Health Statistics Quarterly.* 48(2): 95-107.

Stiglitz J. 1998. Road to Recovery: Restoring Growth in the Region Could be a Long and Difficult Process. *Asiaweek.* 24(28):66.

Stjernsward J. 1988. WHO Cancer Pain Relief Programme. *Cancer Surveys.* 7(1): 195-208.

Strauss J, PJ Gertler, O Rahman, et al. 1993. Gender Life-Cycle Differentials in the Patterns and Determinants of Adult Health. *Journal of Human Resources.* 28(4): 791-837.

Strauss J and D Thomas. 1995. *Health, Nutrition and Economic Development.* Labor and Population Program Working Paper Series. RAND/DRU-1238-NICHD/NIA. RAND. Santa Monica, CA.

Sullivan J, S Rutstein and G Bicego. 1994. *Infant and Child Mortality.* Demographic and Health Surveys Comparative Studies. 15. Institute for Resource Development/ Macro Systems, Inc.

Sumartojo E. 1993. When Tuberculosis Treatment Fails. A Social Behavioral Account of Patient Adherence. *American Review of Respiratory Disease.* 147(5): 1311-1320.

Summers L. 1989. What Can Economics Contribute to Social Policy? Some Simple Economics of Mandated Benefits. *American Economics Association.* 79(2): 177-183.

Summers L. 1994. *Investing in All the People, Educating Women in Developing Countries.* Conference Report. 45. World Bank. Washington, DC.

Summers LH. 1992. *Investing in All the People*. Policy Research Working Paper WPS-905. World Bank. Washington, DC.

Summers L and L Pritchett. 1993. The Structual Adjustment Debate. *American Economic Review Conference Proceedings*. American Economic Association Meeting, Anaheim Calif.

Sundari TK. 1992. The Untold Story—How the Health Care Systems in Developing Countries Contribute to Maternal Mortality. *International Journal of Health Services*. 22(3): 513-528.

Suryani L and G Jensen. 1992. Psychiatrist, Traditional Healer and Culture Integrated in Clinical Practice. *Medical Anthropology*. 13(4): 301-14.

Swaddiwudhipong W, Chareewan Chaovakiratipong, P Nguntra, et al. 1995. Effect of a Mobile Unit on Changes in Knowledge and Use of Cervical Cancer Screening Among Rural Thai Women. *International Journal of Epidemiology*. 24(3): 493-498.

Swales J. 1996. Science and Medical Practice: The Turning Tide. *Journal of Health Services and Resource Policy*. 1(2): 61-62.

Swinscow T. 1978. *Statistics at Square One*. From articles published in the *British Medical Journal*. London: British Medical Association.

Taguiwalo M. 1996. Lessons Learned in Trying to Improve Public Sector Management in the Developing Countries of Asia. *Health Sector Priorities Strategic Planning Workshop*. Manila: Asian Development Bank.

Tan C, O Solon and P Gertler. 1996. Estimating the Welfare Effects of Insurance Coverage. Paper presented at Inaugural Conference of the International Health Economics Association. Vancouver, Canada.

Tan J-P and A Mingat. 1992. *Education in Asia: A Comparative Study of Cost Financing*. World Bank Regional and Sectoral Studies. Washington, DC: World Bank.

Tarimo E. 1991. *Towards a Healthy District: Organizing and Managing District Health Systems Based on Primary Health Care*. Geneva: World Health Organization.

Taylor C. 1993. Editorial: Learning From Health Care Experiences in Developing Countries. *American Journal of Public Health*. 83(11): 1531-1532.

Taylor C and R Jolly. 1988. The Straw Men of Primary Health. *Social Science and Medicine*. 26(9): 971-977.

Taylor CE. 1992. Surveillance for Equity in Primary Health Care: Policy Implications from International Experience. *International Journal of Epidemiology*. 21(6): 1043-1049.

Tekce B. 1982. Oral Rehydration Therapy: An Assessment of Mortality Effects in Rural Egypt. *Studies in Family Planning*. 13: 315-327.

Telyukov AV. 1991. A Concept of Health-Financing Reform in the Soviet Union. *International Journal of Health Services*. 21(3): 493-504.

Thailand, Bureau of Health Policy and Plan. 1997. *Health in Thailand: 1995-1996.* Ministry of Public Health, Thailand.

Thomas D. 1994. Like Father Like Son, Like Mother Like Daughter: Parental Resources and Child Height. *The Journal of Human Resources*. 29(4):950-988.

Thomas D, V Lavy and J Strauss. 1996. Public Policy and Anthropometric Outcomes in the Cote d'Ivoire. *Journal of Public Economics*. 61(2): 155-192.

Thomason J. 1994. A Cautious Approch to Privatization in Papua New Guinea. *Health Policy and Planning*. 9(1): 41-49.

Tielsch JM and A Somner. 1984. The Epidemiology of Vitamin A Deficiency and Xerophthalmia. *Annual Review of Nutrition*. 4: 183-205.

Timaus I and W Graham. 1989. *Measuring Adult Mortality in Developing Countries: A Review and Assessment of Methods*. WPS 155. World Bank. Washington, DC.

Tipping G and M Segall. 1995. *Health Care Seeking Behaviour in Developing Countries: An Annotated Bibliography and Literature Review*. Development Bibliography. 12. Institute of Development Studies.

Tipping G and M Segall. 1996. Using a Longitudinal Illness Record to Study Household Health Care Decision-Making in Rural Communes in Viet Nam. *Health Policy and Planning*. 11(2): 206-211.

Tokyo Metropolitan Government. 1989. *Basic Study of Tokyo's National Health Insurance*. Tokyo Metropolitan Governement. Tokyo.

Tollman S, D Schopper and A Torres. 1990. Health Maintenance Organizations in Developing Countries: What Can We Expect? *Health Policy and Planning*. 5(2): 149-160.

Tomkins A. 1981. Nutritional Status and Severity of Diarrhoea Among Pre-School Children in Rural Nigeria. *Lancet*. 1: 860-862.

Trussell J. 1988. Does Family Planning Reduce Infant Mortality? *Population and Development Review*. 14: 171-178.

Trussell J and AR Pebley. 1984. The Potential Impact of Changes in Fertility on Infant, Child, and Maternal Mortality. *Studies in Family Planning*. 15(6): 267-280.

Tulchinsky TH and EA Varavikova. 1996. Addressing the Epidemiologic Transition in the Former Soviet Union—Strategies for Health System and Public Health Reform in Russia. *American Journal of Public Health*. 86(3): 313-320.

Uemura K. 1989. Excess Mortality Ratio with Reference to the Lowest Age-Sex-Specific Death Rates Among Countries. *World Health Statistics Quarterly*. 42(1): 26-48.

United Nations International Children's Emergency Fund (UNICEF). 1992. *The State of the World's Children*. Oxford: Oxford University Press.

_____. 1993. *The State of the World's Children*. Oxford: Oxford University Press.

_____. 1996. *The State of the World's Children*. Geneva: Oxford University Press.

United Nations (UN). 1985a. *Modern Management Information Systems for Public Administration in Developing Countries*. United Nations Department of Technical Cooperation for Development.

_____. 1985b. *Socio-Economic Differentials in Child Mortality in Developing Countries*. New York: Department of International Economic and Social Affairs.

_____. 1986a. *Age Structure of Mortality in Developing Countries: A Data Base for Cross-Sectional and Time Series Research*. New York: United Nations, Department of International Economic and Social Affairs.

_____. 1986b. *Determinants of Mortality Change and Differentials in Developing Countries: The Five-Country Case Study Project*. Population Studies. New York: United Nations: Departments of International Economic and Social Affairs.

_____. 1990. *Application of Government Auditing Standards in Developing Counries*. United Nations Department of Technical Cooperation for Development.

_____. 1991a. *Child Mortality in Developing Countries: Socioeconomic Differentials, Trends, and Implications*. New York: United Nations Department of International Economic and Social Affairs.

_____. 1991b. *Government Financial Management in Least Developed Countries*. New York: United Nations Department of Technical Co-operation for Development.

_____. 1992. *Child Mortality Since the 1960s: A Database for Developing Countries*. New York: United Nations Department of Economic and Social Development.

_____. 1994. *World Contraceptive Use*. ST/ESA/SER.A/143. Department for Economic and Social Information and Policy Analysis, Population Division, New York, NY.

_____. 1995. *Economic and Social Survey of Asia and the Pacific, 1995*. New York.

Uplekar M and D Shepard. 1991. Treatment of Tuberculosis by Private General Practitioners in India. *Tubercle*. 72: 284-290.

U.S. Bureau of the Census. 1996. *Statistical Abstract of the United States: 1996*. Washington, DC.

U.S. Department of Health and Human Services (USDHHS). 1989a. *Reducing the Health Consequences of Smoking: 25 years of Progress*. Report of the Surgeon General. CDC-89-8411. DHHS Office on Smoking and Health.

_____. 1989b. *Smoking, Tobacco, and Health: A Fact Book*. Washington, D C: Office on Smoking and Health.

_____. 1992. *Smoking and Health in the Americas*. A 1992 report of the Surgeon General, in collaboration with the Pan American Health Organization. (CDC)92-8419. DHHS.

University of New Mexico/WHO Collaborating Center for the Dissemination of Community-Oriented Problem-Based Medicine. 1991. *Community Medical Education in China: An Experiment in Community-Oriented Problem-Based Learning at Xian Medical University's Hanzhong and Ankang Branch Colleges*.

Vallin J. 1992. Causes of Adult Mortality in Countries with Low Mortality Rates—A Comparison Between Several Industrialized and Developing Countries. *Population*. 47(3): 555-582.

Van de Walle D. 1992. *The Distribution of the Benefits from Social Services in Indonesia, 1978-1987*. Washington, DC: World Bank.

_____. 1995. *Public Spending and the Poor: What We Know, What We Need to Know*. Policy Research Working Paper. 1476. World Bank. Washington, DC.

Van de Walle D, M Ravallion and M Gautam. 1994. *How Well Does the Social Safety Net Work?* Washington, DC: The World Bank.

van der Gaag J. 1995. *Private and Public Initiatives, Working Together for Health and Education*. Directions in Development. Washington, DC: World Bank.

Van Der Walt H and L Gilson. 1994. Reforming the Health Sector in Developing Countries. *Health Policy and Planning*. 9(4): 353-370.

Van Der Walt H and C Matthews. 1995. How Do Health Service Managers Respond to Qualitative Research? *Social Science and Medicine*. 41(12): 1725-1729.

Van Doorslaer E and A Wagstaff. 1993. Equity in the Finance of Health Care: Methods and Findings. in E Van Doorslaer, A Wagstaff, et al., eds. *Equity in the Finance and Delivery of Health Care: An International Perspective*. New York: Oxford University Press.

Van Doorslaer E, A Wagstaff and F Rutten. 1993. *Equity in the Finance and Delivery of Health Care: An International Perspective*. New York: Oxford University Press.

Vandeven W and R Vanvliet. 1995. Consumer Information Surplus and Adverse Selection in Competitive Health Insurance Markets—An Empirical Study. *Journal of Health Economics*. 14(2): 149-169.

Vaughan JP, L Gilson and A Mills. 1993. Diabetes. In DT Jamison, WH Mosley, et al., eds. *Disease Control Priorities in Developing Countries*. New York: Oxford University Press.

Venkataswamy G. 1993. Can Cataract Surgery be Marked like Hamburgers in Developing Countries? *Archives of Ophthalmology*. 115:580.

Verhasselt Y and GF Pyle. 1993. Geographical Inequalities of Mortality in Developing Countries—Introduction. *Social Science and Medicine*. 36(10): 1239-1241.

Victora CG, PG Smith, JP Vaughan, et al. 1988. Water Supply, Sanitation and Housing in Relation to the Risk of Infant Mortality from Diarrhoea. *International Journal of Epidemiology*. 17: 651-654.

Vinicor P, S Cohen, S Mazzuca, et al. 1987. DIABEDS: A Randomized Trial of the Effects of Physician and/or Patient Education on Diabetes Patient Outcomes. *Journal of Chronic Disease*. 40:345-356.

Virgilio GD. 1993. Problem-Based Learning for Training Primary Health Care Managers in Developing Countries. *Medical Education*. 27(3):266-273.

Visschedijk JH, IM Liywalii and J Van Oosterhout. 1995. Pilot Project for Financial Decentralization in Senanga, Zambia. *Geographical Medicine*. 47(1):39-42.

Vlassoff C and M Tanner. 1992. The Relevance of Rapid Assessment to Health Research and Interventions. *Health Policy and Planning*. 7(1): 1-9.

Waddington CJ and KA Enyimayew. 1989. A Price to Pay: The Impact of User Charges in Ashanti-Akim District, Ghana. *International Journal of Heath Planning and Management*. 4(1): 17-47.

Wagner EH, BT Austin and M Von Korff. 1996. Organizing Care for Patients with Chrionic Illness. *Milbank Quarterly*. 74(4): 511-44.

Wagstaff A and E Van Doorslaer. 1993. Equity in the Finance and Delivery of Health Care: Concepts and Definitions. in E Van Doorslaer, A Wagstaff, et al., eds. *Equity in the Finance and Delivery of Health Care: An International Perspective*. New York: Oxford University Press.

Wallack S, K Skwara and J Cai. 1996. Redefining Rate Regulation in a Competitive Environment. *Journal of Health Politics, Policy, and Law*. 21(3): 489-510.

Wallis M. 1989. *Bureaucracy: Its Role in Third World Development*. London: Macmillan.

Wallman S and M Baker. 1996. Which Resources Pay for Treatment? A Model for Estimating the Informal Economy of Health. *Social Science and Medicine*. 42(5): 671-680.

Walsh J and M Simonet. 1995a. Data Analysis Needs for Health Sector Reform. *Health Policy*. 32(1-3): 295-306.

Walsh J and M Simonet. 1995b. Data Needs for Policy Reform. In P Berman, ed. *Health Sector Reform in Developing Countries: Making Health Development Sustainable*. Boston: Harvard School of Public Health.

Walsh J and K Warren. 1979. Selective Primary Health Care—An Interim Strategy for Disease Control in Developing Countries. *New England Journal of Medicine*. 301(November): 967-974.

Walsh JA, CM Feifer, AR Measham, et al. 1993. Maternal and Perinatal Health. In DT Jamison, WH Mosley, et al., eds. *Disease Control Priorities in Developing Countries.* New York: Oxford University Press.

Walt G. 1994. *Health Policy—An Introduction to Process and Power.* Johannesburg: Witwatersrand University Press.

Wang C. 1993. Developing Countries: A Report from China. *Medical Informatics.* 18(1): 1-10.

Walt G and L Gilson. 1994. Reforming the Health Sector in Developing Countries: The Central Role of Policy Analysis. *Health Policy and Planning.* 9(4):353-70.

Wang J, DT Jamison, E Bos, A Preker and J Peabody. 1998. *Measuring Country Performance on Health: Selected Indicators for 115 Countries.* Appendix A—East Asia and the Pacific: Regional and Country-Specific Indicators of Performance on Health, Appendix B—Europe and Central Asia: Regional and Country-Specific Indicators of Performance on Health, and Appendix E—South Asia: Regional and Country-Specific Indicators of Performance on Health. World Bank Sector Strategy Paper. Washington, DC.

Wang J, DT Jamison, E Bos and MT Vu. 1997. Poverty and Mortality Among the Elderly: Measurement of Performance in 33 Countries, 1969-92. *Tropical Medicine and International Health.* 2:1001-1010.

Wang D, Z Zhang and S Zheng. 1993. Computers Against Disease. *World Health Forum.* 14: 298-300.

Wang Y-Y and S-H Yang. 1985. Occult Impaired Hearing Among "Normal" School Children in Endemic Goiter and Cretinism Areas Due to Iodine Deficiency in Guizhou. *Chinese Medical Journal.* 98(2): 89-94.

Wang'ombe JK. 1995. Public Health Crises of Cities in Developing Countries. *Social Science and Medicine.* 41(6): 857.

Ward VM, D Maine, J MacCarthy, et al. 1994. A Strategy for the Evaluation of Activities to Reduce Maternal Mortality in Developing Countries. *Evaluation Review.* 18(4): 438-457.

Warren KS, D Bundy, RM Anderson, et al. 1993. Helminth Infection. In DT Jamison, WH Mosley, et al., eds. *Disease Control Priorities in Developing Countries.* New York: Oxford University Press.

Wasserheit JN. 1989. The Significance and Scope of Reproductive Tract Infections Among Third World Women. *International Journal of Gynecology and Obstetrics.* 3 (Supplement): 145-168.

Wassermann J, W Manning, J Newhouse, et al. 1991. The Effects of Excise Taxes and Regulations on Cigarette Smoking. *Journal of Health Economics.* 10(1): 43-64.

Weaver M, H Wong, AS Sako, et al. 1994. Prospects for Reform of Hospital Fees in Sub-Saharan Africa: A Case Study of Niamey National Hospital in Niger. *Social Science and Medicine*. 38(4): 565-574.

Weinberger M, E Oddone and W Henderson. 1996. Does Increased Access to Primary Care Reduce Hospital Readmissions? *New England Journal of Medicine*. 334(22): 1441-1447.

Weiner J, A Dobson, S Maxwell, et al. 1996. Risk-Adjusted Medicare Capitation Rates Using Ambulatory and Inpatient Diagnoses. *Health Care Financing Review*. 17(3): 77-100.

Weiner JP and GD Lissovoy. 1993. Razing a Tower of Babel: A Taxonomy for Managed Care and Health Insurance Plans. *Journal of Health Politics, Policy and Law*. 18(1): 75-103.

Weisbrod BA. 1991. The Health Care Quadrilemma: An Essay on Technological Change, Insurance, Quality of Care, and Cost Containment. *Journal of Economic Literature*. 21: 523-552.

Weiss W. 1988. Cultural Models of Diarrheal Illness: Conceptual Framework and Review. *Social Science and Medicine*. 27: 5-16.

Weissman MM, RC Bland, GJ Canino, et al. 1996. Cross-National Epidemiology of Major Depression and Bipolar Disorder. *Journal of the American Medical Association*. 276(4): 293-298.

Weniger B and T Brown. 1996. The March of AIDS Through Asia. *New England Journal of Medicine*. 335(5): 343-4.

Wennberg J and A Gittleson. 1982. Variations in Medical Care Among Small Areas. *Scientific American* 246: 120-135.

Wessels W. 1985. The Traditional Healer and Psychiatry. *Australian and New Zealand Journal of Psychiatry*. 19: 283.

West-Bengal. 1992. Privatisation of Health Care. *Economic and Political Weekly*. 27(19): 977-978.

White C and J Bailar. 1956. Retrospective and Prospective Methods of Studying Association in Medicine. *American Journal of Public Health*. 46: 35-44.

White K. 1985. Health Surveys. *World Health Statistics Quartely*. 38(1): 2-14.

White R and E Frank. 1994. Health Effects and Prevalence of Vegetarianism. *Western Journal of Medicine*. 160: 465-471.

Whorewell P, A Prior and S Colgan. 1987. Hypnotherapy in Severe Irritable Bowel Syndrome: Further Experience. *Gut*. 28: 423-425.

Wig N. 1982. Methodology of Data Collection in Field Surveys. *Acta Psychiatria Scandanavia*. 296(Supplement): 77-86.

Wilbulpolprasert S. 1991. Community Financing: Thailand's Experience. *Health Policy and Planning*. 6(4): 354-360.

Wildavsky A. 1977. Doing Better and Feeling Worse. The Political Pathology of Health Policy. In *Doing Better and Feeling Worse. Health in the United States*. Boston: Proceedings of the American Academy of Arts and Sciences.

_____. 1984. *The Politics of the Budgetary Process*. Boston: Little, Brown.

_____. 1992. *The New Politics of the Budgetary Process, Second Edition*. New York: Harpers Collins.

Wilkinson M, W Njogu and N Abderrahim. 1993. *The Availability of Family Planning and Maternal and Child Health Services*. Demographic and Health Surveys Comparative Studies. 7. Institute for Resource Development/ Macro Systems, Inc.

Williamson OE. 1987. *The Economic Institutions of Capitalism: Firms, Markets, Relational Contracting*. New York: Collier Macmillan Publishers.

Wilson RG and DL Smith. 1991. Microcomputer Applications for Primary Health Care in Developing Countries. *Infectious Disease Clinics of North America*. 5(2): 247-264.

Winslow R. 1997. Health-Care Costs May Be Heading up Again. *Wall Street Journal*. 21 January 1997. B1.

Wolf C. 1986. *Markets or Governments: Choosing Between Imperfect Alternatives*. N-2505-SF. RAND. Santa Monica, CA.

Wolfe JH, PL Harris and CV Ruckley. 1994. Trust Hospitals and Vascular Services. *British Medical Journal*. 309(6951):414.

Wolinsky A. 1996. The Illusion of Certainty. *New England Journal of Medicine*. 335(1): 46-49.

Wong GC, VC Li, MA Burris and Y Xiang. 1995. Seeking Women's Voices: Setting the Context for Women's Health Interventions in Two Rural Countries in Yunnan, China. *Social Science and Medicine*. 41(8):1147-57.

Wong H. 1996. *Health Financing In Tuvalu*. HFS Technical Report. Bethesda, MD: Abt Associates, Inc.

Wong H and S Govind. 1992. *Health Financing In Fiji: The Role of And Potential For Cost Recovery*. HFS Technical Report. Bethesda, MD: Abt Associates, Inc.

Wonnacott T and R Wonnacott. 1990. *Introductory Statistics for Business and Economics*. New York: John Wiley & Sons.

Woodall JP. 1988. Epidemiological Approaches to Health Planning, Management and Evaluation. *World Health Statistics Quarterly*. 41: 2-10.

Woodward D. 1992. *Debt, Adjustment and Poverty in Developing Countries. Volume II: The Impact of Debt and Adjustment at the Household Level in Developing Countries.* London: Printer Publishers in association with Save the Children.

Woolley F, R Kane, C Hughes, et al. 1978. The Effects of Doctor-Patient Communication on Satisfaction and Outcome of Care. *Social Science and Medicine.* 12: 121-128.

World Bank. 1984. *China: The Health Sector.* World Bank Country Study. World Bank. Washington, DC.

_____. 1987. *Financing Health Services in Developing Countries: An Agenda for Reform.* Washington, DC: The World Bank.

_____. 1988a. *World Development Report 1988.* New York: Oxford University Press.

_____. 1988b. *Staff Appraisal Report, India: Fifth.* 7077-IN. World Bank. Washington, DC.

_____. 1988c. *Pakistan, Population and Health Sector Report.* Draft. 7349-PAK. World Bank. Washington, DC.

_____. 1988d. *Staff Appraisal Report, Sri Lanka: Health and Family Planning Project.* 7050-CE. World Bank. Washington, DC.

_____. 1989a. *Sri Lanka Nutrition Review.* World Bank. Washington, DC.

_____. 1989b. *Staff Appraisal Report, Phillipines Health Development Project.* 7665-PH. World Bank. Washington, DC.

_____. 1989c. *Indonesia: Health Planning and Budgeting.* World Bank Country Study. World Bank. Washington, DC.

_____. 1989d. *Staff Appraisal Report, China: Integrated Regional Health Development Project.* 7632-CHA. World Bank. Washington, DC.

_____. 1989e. *Staff Appraisal Report, India: Sixth (National Family Welfare Training and Systems Development) Population Project.* 7731-IN. World Bank. Washington, DC.

_____. 1989f. *Staff Appraisal Report, Indonesia: Third Health Project.* 7542-IND. World Bank. Washington, DC.

_____. 1990a. *Poverty.* World Development Report 1990. New York: Oxford University Press.

_____. 1990b. *Lao People's Democratic Republic, Population, Health and Nutrition Sector Review.* 8181-LAO. World Bank. Washington, DC.

_____. 1990c. *Fiji, Performance and Prospects of Education, Training and Health Services.* 8119-FIJ. World Bank. Washington, DC.

_____. 1990d. *India: Strengthening the Role of Non-Governmental Organizations in the Health and Family Welfare Program in India, Volume 1.* 8521-IN. World Bank. Washington, DC.

_____. 1990e. *India-Tamil Nadu Integrated Nutrition Project Completion Report.* World Bank. Washington, DC.

_____. 1990f. *China, Long Term Issues and Options in the Health Transition.* World Bank Country Study. Washington, DC: World Bank.

_____. 1990g. *Indonesia: Strategy for a Sustained Reduction in Poverty.* Washington, DC: The World Bank.

_____. 1991a. *Indonesia: Health Planning and Budgeting.* World Bank Country Study. 7291-IND. World Bank. Washington, DC.

_____. 1991b. *New Directions in the Philippines Family Planning Program.* World Bank. Washington, DC.

_____. 1991c. *Papua New Guinea, Management, Manpower, Money: A Select Review of Health and Population in Papua New Guinea.* 8959-PNG. World Bank. Washington, DC.

_____. 1991d. *Staff Appraisal Report, China: Infectious and Endemic Disease Control Project.* 9894-CHA. World Bank. Washington, DC.

_____. 1991e. *Staff Appraisal Report, Bangladesh: Fourth Population and Health Project.* 9400-BD. World Bank. Washington, DC.

_____. 1991f. *Staff Appraisal Report, Republic of Korea: Health Technology Project.* 9280-KO. World Bank. Washington, DC.

_____. 1991g. *The Challenge of Development.* World Development Report 1991. New York: Oxford University Press.

_____. 1992a. *Vietnam: Population, Health and Nutrition Sector Review.* World Bank. Washington, DC.

_____. 1992b. *Staff Appraisal Report, Republic of Korea Public Hospital Modernization Project.* 10283-KO. World Bank. Washington, DC.

_____. 1992c. *India: Health Sector Financing.* 10859-IN. World Bank. Washington, DC.

_____. 1993a. *Investing in Health.* World Development Report 1993. New York: Oxford University Press.

_____. 1993b. *Indonesia: Public Expenditures, Prices, and the Poor.* Washington, DC: The World Bank.

_____. 1993c. *The East Asian Miracle: Economic Growth and Public Policy.* World Bank Policy Research Reports. Washington, DC: Oxford University Press.

_____. 1993d. *Staff Appraisal Report, Indonesia: Third Community Health and Nutrition Project.* 11255-IND. World Bank. Washington, DC.

_____. 1993e. *Staff Appraisal Report, India: Uttar Pradesh Basic Education Project.* 11746-IN. World Bank. Washington, DC.

_____. 1993f. *Staff Appraisal Report, Republic of the Philippines: Urban Health and Nutrition Project.* 11702-PH. World Bank. Washington, DC.

_____. 1993g. *Staff Appraisal Report, Papua New Guinea: Population and Family Planning Project.* 11264-PNG. World Bank. Washington, DC.

_____. 1993h. *Staff Appraisal Report, China: Rural Health Workers Development Project.* 11404-CHA. World Bank. Washington, DC.

_____. 1993i. *Elderly Family Planning Programs.* Washington, DC.

_____. 1993j. *Indonesia: Public Expenditures, Prices, and the Poor.* Washington, DC: World Bank.

_____. 1993k. *Implementing the World Bank's Strategy to Reduce Poverty: Progress and Challenges.* Washington, DC: World Bank.

_____. 1993l. *Staff Appraisal Report, Islamic Republic of Pakistan: Health Sector Study, Key Issues and Concerns.* 10391-PAK. World Bank. Washington, DC.

_____. 1993m. *Staff Appraisal Report, Malaysia: Health Development Project.* 10995-MA. World Bank. Washington, DC.

_____. 1994a. *Health Priorities and Options in the World Bank's Pacific Member Countries.* 11620-EAP. World Bank. Washington, DC.

_____. 1994b. *World Population Projections, 1994-95.* Washington, DC: World Bank.

_____. 1994c. *Staff Appraisal Report, India: District Primary Education Project.* 13072-IN. World Bank. Washington, DC.

_____. 1994d. *Staff Appraisal Report, Lao People's Democratic Republic: Health System Reform and Malaria Control Project.* 13107-LA. World Bank. Washington, DC.

_____. 1994e. *Infrastructure for Development.* World Development Report. New York: Oxford University Press.

_____. 1994f. *Staff Appraisal Report, Nepal: Population and Family Health Project.* 10812-NEP. World Bank. Washington, DC.

_____. 1994g. *Staff Appraisal Report, Kyrgyz Republic: Social Safety Net Project.* 12986-KG. World Bank. Washington, DC.

_____. 1994h. *Philippines Devolution and Health Services: Managing Risks and Opportunities.* Report. 12343-ph. World Bank. Washington, DC.

_____. 1994i. *Indonesia's Health Work Force: Issues and Options.* 12835-IND. World Bank. Washington, DC.

_____. 1994j. *Staff Appraisal Report, China: Comprehensive Maternal and Child Health Project.* 13025-CHA. World Bank. Washington, DC.

_____. 1994k. *Staff Appraisal Report, India: Andhra Pradesh First Referral Health System Project.* 13402-IN. World Bank. Washington, DC.

_____. 1995a. *Workers in an Integrating World.* World Development Report 1995. New York: Oxford University Press.

_____. 1995b. *World Tables.* Washington, DC: World Bank.

_____. 1995c. *Viet Nam Poverty Assessment and Strategy.* 13442-VN. The World Bank. Washington, DC.

_____. 1995d. *Staff Appraisal Report, Phillipines Women's Health and Safe Motherhood Project.* 13566-PH. World Bank. Washington, DC.

_____. 1995e. *Staff Appraisal Report, Indonesia: Fourth Health Project, Improving Equity and Quality of Care.* Washington, DC: The World Bank.

_____. 1995f. *An International Assessment of Health Care Financing: Lessons for Developing Countries.* Washington, DC: World Bank.

_____. 1995g. *China NHA Assessment.* World Bank. Washington, DC.

_____. 1996a. *From Plan to Market.* World Development Report 1996. New York: Oxford University Press.

_____. 1996b. *World Tables.* Washington, DC: World Bank.

_____. 1996c. *Socio-Economic Time Series Access and Retrieval System (STARS).* Washington, DC: World Bank.

_____. 1997c. Financing Health Care: Issues and Options for China. Washington, DC: World Bank. China 2020 Series, 1-92.

World Bank_____. 1997a. Sector Strategy Paper R97-168. *Health, Nutrition & Population.* World Bank. Washington, DC.

World Bank_____. 1997b. *World Development Report.* World Bank. Washington, DC.

World Health Organization (WHO). 1946. *The Constitution of World Health Organization.* International Health Conference. New York, NY: United Nations Economic and Social Council.

_____. 1978. Primary Health Care. *International Conference on Primary Health Care.* Alma Ata, USSR: World Health Organization.

_____. 1979. *Formulating Strategies for Health for All by the Year 2000*. Health for All. Geneva: World Health Organization.

_____. 1981a. *Global Strategy for Health for All by the Year 2000*. Health for All. Geneva: World Health Organization.

_____. 1981b. *Development of Indicators for Monitoring Progress Towards Health for All by the Year 2000*. Geneva: World Health Organization.

_____. 1983. *Smoking Control Strategies in Developing Countries*. Technical Report. 695.

_____. 1984. A Programme for Controlling Acute Respiratory Infections in Children: Memorandum from a WHO Meeting. *Bulletin of the World Health Organization*. 62: 47-58.

_____. 1985. *Control of Sexually Transmitted Diseases*. World Health Organization. Geneva.

_____. 1986a. *Cancer Pain Relief*. World Health Organization. Geneva.

_____. 1986b. *Maternal Mortality Rates: A Tabulation of Available Information*. Family Health Division.

_____. 1987. Available Data on Blindness. *Bulletin of the World Health Organizations*. 87(14): 1-23, 34.

_____. 1988. *Strengthening Ministries of Health for Primary Care*. Technical Report. 766. World Health Organization.

_____. 1990a. *Acute Respiratory Infections in Children: Case Management in Small Hospitals in Developing Countries: A Manual for Doctors and Senior Health Workers*. Monograph. WHO/ARI/90.5. World Health Organization. Geneva.

_____. 1990b. *Priority for the Poorest*. Geneva: World Health Organization.

_____. 1991. *Organization and Financing of Health Care Reform in Countries of Central and Eastern Europe*. Report by WHO Task Force on Health Development in Countries of Central and Eastern Europe for a Meeting at the World Health Organization, April 22-26. Geneva: World Health Organization.

_____. 1992. *The Use of Essential Drugs, Model List of Essential Drugs (Seventh List)*. WHO Technical Report Series. World Health Organization. Geneva.

_____. 1993a. *Evaluation of Recent Changes in the Financing of Health Services*. HFS technical report series. Geneva: World Health Organization.

_____. 1993b. *Guidelines for the Development of Health Management Information Systems*. Manila: World Health Organization.

_____. 1994a. *Progress Towards Health for All*. Statistics of Member States, 1994. Geneva: World Health Organization.

_____. 1994b. *Global Comparative Assessments in the Health Sector: Disease Burden, Expenditures, and Intervention Packages—Collected Reprints from the Bulletin of the World Health Organization*. Geneva: World Health Organization.

_____. 1994c. *Health Sector Reform Report on a Consultation*. WHO document. WHO/SHS/NHP/94.5 Unpublished. World Health Organization.

_____. 1995a. *Health Situation in the South-East Asia Region, 1991-1993*. New Delhi: Regional Office for South East Asia.

_____. 1995b. *Bridging the Gap*. The World Health Report. Geneva: World Health Organization.

_____. 1995c. *Western Pacific Region Data Bank on Socioeconomic and Health Indicators*. Manila: World Health Organization.

_____. 1995d. *Interregional Consultation on Health Insurance Reform*. Conference. WHO/SHS/NHP/95.9. World Health Organization. Seoul, Korea.

_____. 1996a. *Fighting Disease Fostering Development*. The World Health Report. Geneva: World Health Organization.

_____. 1996b. *EMRO-Memorandum on Afghanistan and Pakistan*. Data tables. World Health Organization. Geneva.

_____. 1996c. *Western Pacific Region Data Bank on Socioeconomic and Health Indicators*. World Health Organization. Geneva.

_____. 1996d. *State of the World's Vaccines and Immunization*. Geneva: WHO/UNICEF.

_____. 1996e. *The Tobacco Epidemic: A Global Public Health Emergency*. Tobacco Alert. Special Issue, World No-Tobacco Day. World Health Organization. Geneva.

_____. 1996f. *Demographic Data for Health Situation Assessment and Projections*. Geneva: World Health Organization.

_____. 1996g. *District Hospitals: Guidelines for Development, Second Edition*. World Health Organization Regional Office for the Western Pacific (WPRO).

_____. 1996h. *EPI Information System, Summary for the WHO European Region*. CEPI Series. WHO/EPI/CEIS/96.04. World Health Organization. Geneva.

_____. 1996i. *EPI Information System, Summary for the WHO Western Pacific Region*. CEPI Series. WHO/EPI/CEIS/96.06. World Health Organization. Geneva.

_____. 1996j. *Expanded Program on Immunization. Summary for the WHO Southeast Asia Region*. World Health Organization. Geneva.

_____. 1996k. *WHO Reform and Response to Global Change Role of WHO Country Offices Revised Report of the Development Team.* WHO Document. EB97/5. World Health Organization. Geneva.

_____. 1997a. Frances McCaul, WHO. Personal communication. February 17, 1997.

_____. 1997b. Report of the Third Evaluation of the Implementation of HFS Strategies—South-East Asia Region. World Health Organization. Geneva.

_____. 1998. *Health Implications of the Economic Crisis in the South-East Asia Region.* Report of a Regional Consultation, Bangkok, Thailand, 23-25 March 1998. New Delhi: Regional Office for South East Asia.

WHO Ad Hoc Committee. 1996. *Investing in Health Research and Development.* Ad Hoc Committee on Health Research Relating to Future Intervention Options. TDR/GEN96.1, Annex 5. World Health Organization.

WHO/ARI. 1988. *Case Management of Acute Respiratory Infection in Children: Intervention Studies.* 88-2. World Health Organization. Geneva.

_____. 1991. *Programme for Control of Acute Respiratory Infections: Interim Programme Report.* 91-19. World Health Organization. Geneva.

WHO/SEARO. 1995a. *Interim Programme Report.* CDD Unit. World Health Organization. Geneva.

_____. 1995b. *Interim Programme Report.* GPA Unit. World Health Organization. Geneva.

WHO/TDR. 1995. *Tropical Disease Research Progress 1975-94. Highlights 1993-94 Twelfth Programme Report of the UNDP/World Bank/WHO.* Conference Report. WC-680-95TR. WHO/Special Programme for Research and Training in Tropical Diseases (TDR). Geneva.

WHO/UNICEF. 1978. *ALMA-ATA Primary Health Care.* Health for All. Geneva: World Health Organization.

Wouters A. 1992. Health Care Utilization Patterns in Developing Countries—Role of the Technology Environment in Deriving the Demand for Health Care. *Bulletin of the World Health Organization.* 70(3): 381-389.

Yang BM. 1991. Health Insurance in Korea: Opportunities and Challenges. *Health Policy Planning.* 6(2): 119.

Yang BM. 1995. Health Financing Korea. Presented at ADB Workshop on Financing Human Resource Development in Asia. Seoul National University.

Yank PL and J Lawson. 1991. Health Policy Reform in the People's Republic of China. *International Journal of Health Services.* 21(3): 481-491.

Yazbeck A and E Gemmen. 1995. *Data Collection as a Policy Tool: A Description of HFS Collection Methods and Data Sets*. HFS Theme Paper. Abt Associates, Inc. Bethesda, MD.

Yesudian C. 1994. Behaviour of the Private Sector in the Health Market in Bombay. *Health Policy and Planning*. 9(1): 72-80.

Yin RK. 1994. Case Study Research, Design and Methods. In *Applied Social Research Methods Series, 2nd Edition*. Thousand Oaks, CA: Sage Publications. 5:1-125.

You CM. 1994. Privatization in China—A Case Study of Health-Care Management (Reconciliation Between Human and Ideals and Economic Limitations). *International Review of Administrative Sciences*. 60(4): 595-607.

Young M. 1990. Maternal Health in China—Challenges of the Next Decade. *Health Policy*. 14(2): 87-125.

Yucun S, A Weixi, S Liang, et al. 1981. Investigation of Mental Disorders in Beijing Suburban District. *Chinese Medical Journal*. 94(3): 153-156.

Zang J. 1990. Immediate Antiasthmatic Effect of Acupuncture in 192 Cases of Bronchial Asthma. *Journal of Traditional Chinese Medicine*. 10(2): 89-93.

Zeckhauser R. 1975. Procedures for Valuing Lives. *Public Policy*. 23:419-64.

Zivkovic M, J Marinkovic, B Legetic, et al. 1994. Evaluation Techniques for the Healthy School Project in Yugoslavia. *Health Promotion International*. 9(2): 73-79.

John W. Peabody is Attending Physician at the West Los Angeles Veterans Affairs Medical Center, Senior Scientist at RAND headquarters in Santa Monica, and Assistant Professor of Medicine at the University of California, Los Angeles (UCLA). The holder of advanced degrees in medicine, public health, and policy, he is an international health specialist who has conducted medical, economic and policy evaluations in over 30 Asian and Pacific countries, Latin America and Eastern Europe. Prior to joining RAND, Dr. Peabody held staff positions with WHO in Geneva and Manila and with Project HOPE in China. The author of over 40 scientific publications, he currently leads projects investigating the impact of health care reforms on access, quality of care, and health outcomes.

M. Omar Rahman is Assistant Professor of Demography and Epidemiology at Harvard University's School of Public Health. He has served as a Visiting Professor at UCLA and Behavioral Scientist in RAND's Labor and Population Department. Holding advanced degrees in medicine, epidemiology, and health policy and management, Dr. Rahman is the author of over 25 publications in medical and policy journals. His research, which focuses on socio-economic determinants of adult and elderly health among other areas, has been sponsored by the National Institute on Aging and the Asian Development Bank.

Paul J. Gertler is Professor of Economic Analysis and Policy at the Haas School of Business and Professor of Health Care Finance and Management, School of Public Health, University of California, Berkeley. He has also taught at Harvard University and SUNY, Stony Brook and served as Senior Researcher at RAND. The coauthor of *The Willingness to Pay for Medical Care* (1990) as well as numerous book chapters and refereed papers, Professor Gertler has been a Faculty Research Associate of NBER since 1985 and is a former editor of the *Journal of Human Resources*. He has conducted economic and health research in over 20 Asian nations for several international agencies.

Joyce Mann has been a Resident Consultant at RAND since 1989 and has also served as a lecturer at UCLA's School of Public Health. A specialist in public health and policy analysis, she has conducted research on health sector reform in Asia for the Asian Development Bank, the five-year national health plan in Indonesia for that country's government, rural health insurance in China for the World Bank, and alternative health payment systems in Taiwan. Dr. Mann has also undertaken numerous projects on health care provision in the United States, Africa, and Ecuador, and has coauthored many articles on health care financing and research.

Donna O. Farley is Senior Health Policy Analyst at RAND. She served as Senior Analyst at the Physician Payment Review Commission in Washington in 1993-96, and as president, director, or senior officer in a number of private and non-profit firms in health care management, financing, and planning. Dr. Farley is the author of numerous articles, book chapters, and RAND publications on health policy in the United States and overseas. Her current research interests include managed care, insurance for vulnerable populations, and evaluation of payment designs.

Jeff Luck is Assistant Professor in the Department of Health Services in the School of Public Health, UCLA, Program Manager at the VA Medical Center, West Los Angeles, and Consultant to RAND. He has also served as a consultant to the Asian Development Bank on Papua New Guinea and as a technical advisor to the California Public Health Improvement Project. Dr. Luck has coauthored a number of publications on managed care, management development, and public health programs.

David Robalino is a Doctoral Fellow at the RAND Graduate School. He has also served as a consultant on the implementation of information systems to Ecuador's Ministry of Foreign Affairs and on the economic impacts of reform to Ecuador's National Commission on Modernization. He has written or coauthored a number of professional publications, including RAND Working Papers on diffusion of competing technologies and modeling health choices.

Grace M. Carter serves as a Consultant in RAND's health program following a 30-year career on RAND's staff. She most recently directed the Center for Health Care Financing Policy Research cosponsored by RAND, UCLA and Harvard, investigating risk and retrospective payment adjustments systems and prospective payment systems among other topics, and has consulted on health services research projects in Taiwan, Ecuador, Canadian provinces, and the Kyrgyz Republic. Dr. Carter is the author and coauthor of numerous refereed articles on health care financing, organization, and management.

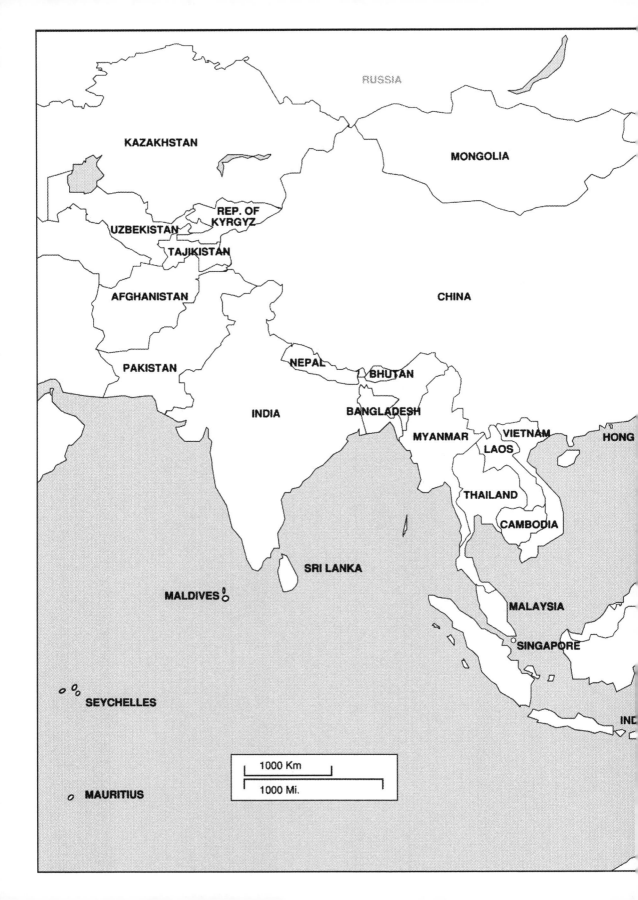

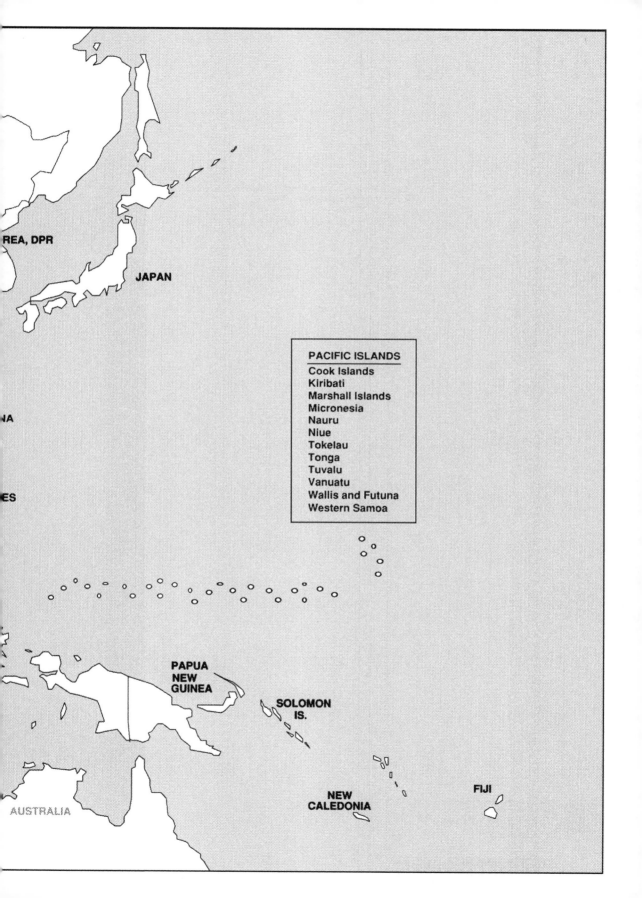

KOREA, DPR

JAPAN

PACIFIC ISLANDS
Cook Islands
Kiribati
Marshall Islands
Micronesia
Nauru
Niue
Tokelau
Tonga
Tuvalu
Vanuatu
Wallis and Futuna
Western Samoa

PAPUA
NEW
GUINEA

SOLOMON
IS.

NEW
CALEDONIA

FIJI

AUSTRALIA

For EU product safety concerns, contact us at Calle de José Abascal, 56–1°,
28003 Madrid, Spain or eugpsr@cambridge.org.

www.ingramcontent.com/pod-product-compliance
Ingram Content Group UK Ltd.
Pitfield, Milton Keynes, MK11 3LW, UK
UKHW030856150625
459647UK00021B/2778